TUMOR MARKERS

Cancer Research Monographs, Vol. 4

Other volumes in Series

TUMOR MARKERS

Biology
and
Clinical Applications

edited by

Nasser Javadpour, M.D.

PRAEGER

New York
Westport, Connecticut
London

Library of Congress Cataloging-in-Publication Data
Main entry under title:

Tumor markers.

(Cancer research monographs ; v. 4)
Includes index.
1. Tumor markers—Diagnostic use.   2. Tumor
antigens—Diagnostic use.   3. Tumors—Diagnosis.
4. Immunodiagnosis.   I. Javadpour, Nasser, 1937–
II. Series. [DNLM: 1. Histocytochemistry—methods.
2. Immunologic Technics.   3. Neoplasms—diagnosis.
W1 CA692C v.4 / QZ 241 T9254]
RC270.3.T84T85   1986   616.99'407583   85–30014
ISBN 0-275-92145-X (alk. paper)

Library of Congress Catalog Card Number: 85–30014
ISBN: 0-275-92145-X
First published in 1987

Praeger Publishers, 521 Fifth Avenue, New York, NY 10175
A division of Greenwood Press, Inc.

Printed in the United States of America

The paper used in this book complies with the Permanent
Paper Standard issued by the National Information Standards
Organization (Z39.48-1984).

10   9   8   7   6   5   4   3   2   1

List of Contributors

N. Bashirelahi
Associate Professor of Biochemistry
University of Maryland
Dental and Medical Schools
Baltimore, Maryland

Magdalena Blaszczyk
The Wistar Institute of Anatomy and
    Biology
36th & Spruce Streets
Philadelphia, Pennsylvania

Harris Busch
Baylor College of Medicine
Department of Pharmacology
Houston, Texas

T. Ming Chu
Diagnostic Immunology Research
    and Biochemistry Department
Roswell Park Memorial Institute
Buffalo, New York

Frank H. DeLand, M.D.
University of Kentucky and Veterans
    Administration Medical Centers
Lexington, Kentucky

D. B. Ekiko
University of Maryland
Dental and Medical Schools
Baltimore, Maryland

E. G. Elias
Professor of surgery, and Director of
    Surgical Oncology

University of Maryland
Baltimore, Maryland

S. Ganesan
University of Maryland
Dental and Medical Schools
Baltimore, Maryland

David M. Goldenberg, D.Sc., M.D.
Center for Molecular Medicine and
    Immunology
University of Medicine and Dentistry
    of New Jersey
Newark, New Jersey

Ariel C. Hollinshead, Ph.D.
Professor of Medicine
Division of Hematology and Oncology
Department of Medicine
The George Washington University
    Medical Center
Washington, D.C.

Nasser Javadpour, M.D.
Director
Section of Urologic Oncology
Department of Surgery
University of Maryland
School of Medicine
Baltimore, Maryland

H. Kohail
University of Maryland
Dental and Medical Schools
Baltimore, Maryland

Hilary Koprowski
Staff Scientist
The Wistar Institute of Anatomy and
    Biology
36th & Spruce Streets
Philadelphia, Pennsylvania

Cornelius G. McWright, Ph.D.
Adjunct Professor of Biological
    Sciences and Forensic Sciences
The George Washington University
Washington, D.C.

Jose V. Ordonez
Department of Microbiology and
    Program of Oncology
University of Maryland
655 W. Baltimore Street
Baltimore, Maryland

N. M. Papadopoulos, Ph.D.
Clinical Chemistry, Clinical
    Pathology
Clinical Center
National Institutes of Health
Bethesda, Maryland

Avery A. Sandberg
Chief of Cytogenetics
Roswell Park Memorial Institute
Buffalo, New York

Zenon Steplewski
The Wistar Institute of Anatomy and
    Biology
36th & Spruce Streets
Philadelphia, Pennsylvania

J. D. Young, Jr.
University of Maryland
Dental and Medical Schools
Baltimore, Maryland

Contents

Preface

The quest for finding biologic markers associated with cancer has attracted the attention of physicians who manage cancer. These biologic markers may be classified into groups, the first of which consists of onco-fetoproteins such as alpha-fetoprotein (AFP), carcino-embryonic antigen (CEA), certain placental proteins, and prostatic-specific antigens (PSA). These markers are generally present in the embryonic stage, disappear during adult life, but appear again during malignant cellular transformation.

The second group of biologic markers consists of enzymes. These enzymes include prostatic acid phosphatase and creatine kinases.

The third group consists of hormones. These include human chorionic gonadotropin, calcitonin, adrenocortical-stimulating hormone (ACTH), and parathyroid hormones.

The fourth group includes spermine, putrescine, spermitidine, and other tumor-associated proteins.

During the past several years, the development of sensitive and specific radioimmunoassays and immunocytochemical techniques has helped physicians to detect minute amounts of these markers in sera and cells of patients with cancer. These markers may help to detect, stage, characterize, and monitor certain cancers. An enormous amount of basic and clinical information is available concerning these biologic markers, and it is hoped that this simple yet comprehensive book will assist physicians who are dealing with cancer.

The early portion of the book presents discussions of the principles of various techniques in the detection of tumor markers. Subsequent chapters have been designed to cover steroid receptors, monoclonal antibodies, flow cytometry, chromosomal abnormalities, radio-immunodetection, ectopic hormones, cell markers in leukemia, nucleo-lar antigens, and certain other nonspecific markers. A chapter has also been allocated to the discussion of clinically useful markers.

Attempts have been made to select only key references to avoid an encyclopedic review of the literature. The contributors of the chapters have been chosen on the basis of their recognized authority on the various topics.

We are grateful to these authors, as well as to Mrs. Suzanne Mosteller and Peter Klamkin for their valuable contributions and skillful assistance in compiling this book.

Nasser Javadpour, M.D.

1

Introduction

Nasser Javadpour, M.D.

Although recent advances in radiologic, endoscopic, and pathologic techniques have led to the earlier diagnosis of cancers and improvements in the care of cancer patients, the limits of sensitivity of these methods preclude the detection of cancers smaller than 10^9 cells (1 Gm). This corresponds to 30 doubling times (Fig. 1–1). The period of time between diagnosis of cancer and the death of a patient is relatively short, although it does depend on the natural history of the cancer. We therefore need means to detect tumors earlier, to stage them more accurately, and to monitor and determine the length of therapy (Fig. 1–2).

During the past several years, the development of specific and sensitive immunocytochemical techniques—such as radioimmunoassay (RIA), immunoperoxidase (IP), peroxidase antiperoxidase (PAP), and radioimmunodetection (RID)—has made a remarkable contribution to the diagnosis and management of cancer patients. These modalities have provided the means for early diagnosis and treatment and a potential for radioimmunotherapy (RIT) of cancer. The current progress has been made even more promising through the development of specific and sensitive antisera-utilizing monoclonal antibodies by fusing sensitized spleen cells with myeloma cells of the mouse.[1,5]

CRITERIA FOR RELIABLE TUMOR MARKERS

A number of critera are essential for a marker to be useful in the diagnosis and management of cancer patients. Among these criteria

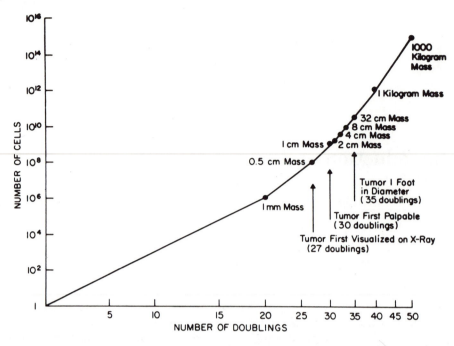

Figure 1–1. Doubling time of a tumor plotted against the number of cancer cells. Note that for a tumor to be first palpable requires 30 doubling times, or one billion cells.

are specificity for malignant disease, detectability in body fluids and tissue extracts, a relatively short biologic half-life, and correlation of a positive marker assay result with the presence of a tumor. The assay result should reflect the tumor-bearing status and prognosis of the patient. It should also reflect the amount of tumor burden and correlate this with the effectiveness of anti-cancer therapeutic modalities.

PROBLEM OF FALSE-POSITIVE AND FALSE-NEGATIVE

Clinical evaluation of the efficacy of diagnostic tests has often produced misleading results, so that tests that were initially regarded as valuable were later rejected as worthless. The initial optimism and subsequent disillusionment with carcinoembryonic antigens as a

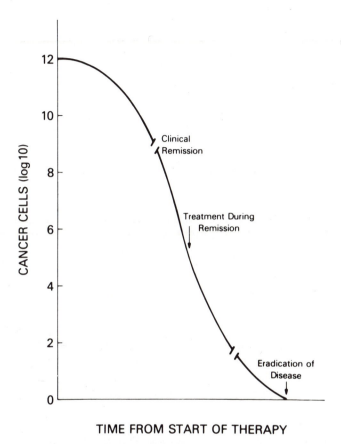

TIME FROM START OF THERAPY

Figure 1–2. Remission.

marker for different cancers serves as a classic example of such disappointment.

The sensitivity and specificity of a diagnostic test may be detected by simple algebraic formulas (Table 1–1). Sensitivity [a/(a + b)] refers to the question: is this test sensitive enough to detect the minimal amount of disease? If it is not, then the test would produce false-negative results. Specificity [d/(b + d)] refers to the question: if the test is negative, what is the likelihood of the patient being free of disease? Failure of the test to predict this correctly would produce a false-positive result.

To have a low false-negative initially, one should examine a large number of patients with minimal disease. To avoid false-positive results requires examination of a large number of patients with an inflammatory disease and a number of normal controls without disease

Table 1–1   Efficacy of Tumor Markers

Test Results	Cancer		Total (patients)
	Present	Absent	
Positive	a	b	a + b
Negative	c	d	c + d
Total	a + c	b + d	a + b + c + d

of the organ under investigation. These comparative studies should be performed in a blind fashion to avoid any bias.

CURRENT CLINICALLY USEFUL MARKERS

A number of tumor markers are available to detect cancer. Although a few of them fulfill the criteria for a near-perfect marker of a given cancer like hCG for choriocarcinoma, nevertheless, when utilized in the context of clinical problems, they may be useful at least in monitoring the therapy. The various cancer markers are tabulated in Tables 1–2 to 1–4.

The discovery and characterization of specific tumor markers will help to expand the utilization of these techniques. The development of monoclonal antibody technology will make it possible to raise large amounts of potentially specific and sensitive antibodies. Furthermore, with the advent of γ-emission tomography, the imaging of small lesions may be possible, and the ultimate objective of achieving a high tumor:nontumor ratio will be brought closer. This will, perhaps, enable clinicians to detect small metastatic tumors for staging and make possible the specific delivery of anti-cancer therapy to a tumor (Figs. 1–3, 1–4).

It appears attractive to attempt to label, with a γ-emitting radioactive material, the T-antigen or some other tumor-associated antigen for the purpose of localization of metastatic bladder cancer by chemo- or radioimmunotherapy. These approaches are attractive because of the current lack of sensitive and reliable techniques to localize and deliver specific cytotoxic agents to tumor-sparing normal cells.

Table 1–2   Onco-Fetoproteins and Ectopic Hormones

Marker	Malignant	Nonmalignant
1. hCG	Testicular and ovarian cancers	Placenta
2. AFP	Liver, ovarian, testicular, gastric, and pancreatic cancers	Yolk sac and fetal liver
3. Calcitonin	Thyroid, breast, and lung cancers	Renal insufficiency
4. Placental alkaline phosphatase	Testicular, ovarian, breast and lung cancers	Placenta
5. Placental lactogen	Testicular and ovarian cancers	Placenta
6. Gammaglutamyl transpeptidase	Testicular cancer and metastases to the liver	Liver diseases
7. Placental protein 5, 10, and 15	Testicular cancer, ? other cancers	Placenta
8. Pregnancy-specific B_1 glycoprotein	Testicular, ovarian, and breast cancers	Placenta

LIMITATIONS OF MARKERS

Understanding the biologic half-life and other characteristics of tumor markers is important in their clinical application. The problems of false-positive, false-negative, sensitivity, and specificity of the given tumor marker should be considered.

FUTURE PROSPECTS

Perhaps the most outstanding progress in cancer immunology has occurred in the field of immunodiagnosis, in particular the development of specific and sensitive immunocytochemical techniques to measure and localize cell markers in the sera and cancer cells of cancer patients. In this chapter, the development and utilization of cell markers in urologic cancer with newer techniques such as IP, PAP, RID, RIT, and monoclonal antibodies have been presented.

Table 1–3 Enzymes and Antigens

Marker	Malignant	Nonmalignant
1. Acid phosphatase	Prostatic and breast cancers	Prostate
2. Alkaline phosphatase	Sarcoma, bony metastatic tumors	Liver, bone
3. Galactosyl transferase	Carcinoma of the pancrease liver, colon, and gallbladder	Polycytemia vera
4. Ribonuclease	Pancreatic cancer	Pancreatitis, renal insufficiency
5. Sialyal transferase	Cancer of the colon, breast, and prostate, melanoma	
6. Hydroxyproline	Metastases to the bone	Inflammatory disease, hepatitis
7. Cell surface antigen and T antigen	Breast and bladder cancers	Red blood cells and certain normal cells

Table 1–4 Metabolic and Other Products

Marker	Malignant	Nonmalignant
1. Polyamines, spermine, putrescine, cadaverine	Breast, prostatic, bladder, and colon cancers	Rheumatoid arthritis, liver disease
2. Complement components	Liver, prostate, breast, lung, and stomach cancers	Peritonitis, hemochromatons
3. Fibrin degradation products	Ovarian and prostatic cancers	Renal diseases, genitourinary infection
4. Lactic dehydrogenase	Testicular and ovarian cancers, leukemia	Liver and heart diseases

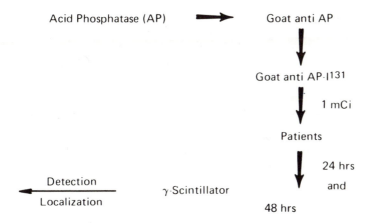

Figure 1–3. Staging of prostatic cancer.

The findings from these techniques have exceeded even the wildest dreams of immunologists and are revolutionizing serology. Utilization of immunochemical techniques has made the localization of these cellular markers a new dimension in the histopathologic diagnosis of certain tumors. Radioimmunoimaging and the potential for radiochemotherapy or radioimmunotherapy is encouraging.[2–4]

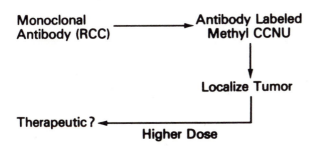

Figure 1–4. Affinity therapy of RCC by chemotherapeutic agent-labeled antibody.

REFERENCES

1. Diamond, B. A., Dale, E., Yelton, B. A., and Scharff, M. D. Monoclonal antibodies—a new technology for producing serologic reagents. N. Engl. J. Med. 304: 1344, 1981.

2. Javadpour, N., McIntire, R. K., and Waldmann, T. A. Immunochemical determination of human chorionic gonadotropin and alpha-fetoprotein in sera and tumors of patients with testicular cancer. JNCI 49: 209–213, 1978.

3. Javadpour, N. Recent advances in the detection of metastatic testicular cancer. Int. J. Andrology 4: 222, 1981.

4. Kurman, R. J., Scardino, P. T., McIntire, R. K., and Javadpour, N. Cellular localization of alpha-fetoprotein and human chorionic gonadotropin in germ cell tumors of the testis using an indirect immunoperoxidase technique: A new approach to classification utilizing tumor markers. Cancer 40: 2136, 1977.

5. Milstein, C., Adetugbo, K., and Cowan, N. J. Somatic cell genetics of antibody-secreting cells: Studies of clonal diversification and analysis by cell fusion. Cold Spring Harbor Symp. Quant. Biol. 41: 793, 1977.

2

Principles and Application: Radioimmunoassay and Enzyme-Linked Immunoassays

Ariel C. Hollinshead, Ph.D.,
& Cornelius G. McWright, Ph.D.

INTRODUCTION

Reliable immunochemistry must be tempered with basic immunobiology. There are very few reliable assays that are sensitive enough for the important task of sorting out and cross-comparing the hundreds of candidate substances for eventual designation as biologic markers in human cancer.

Two assays have been useful in microdetermination and microdistinction between well-defined, appropriately prepared candidate biologic markers—namely, radioimmunoassay (RIA), and enzyme-linked immunoassay (EIA) or one form of EIA, enzyme-linked immunosorbent assay (ELISA).

In the current era of rapidly developing technology—in both the hybridoma and monoclonal antibody and the genetic engineering fields—the use of automated, highly sensitive RIA and EIA methods will be applied, along with further modifications and a battery of additional methods, for detection of relevant reactive molecules in millions of different cells, cell fluids, and intracellular materials.

In this chapter, we outline the relatively simple principles behind these assays, the remarkable ability of these assays to detect picogram amounts of any molecule, and the high specificity of a properly applied assay methodology for detection and measurement of biologic markers in human cancer. Selected examples of the usefulness of the assays will serve to illustrate the way in which such tests sharpen our scientific observations.

RADIOIMMUNOASSAY

Numerous substances such as steroids, peptide hormones, drugs, and biologic markers can be quantitatively determined, at the picogram level, from a patient's serum by radioimmunoassay. RIA was introduced by Berson and Yalow in 1960 as a method to measure serum insulin concentrations. Since then it has achieved widespread use as a sensitive and discriminating method that is used in both the clinical and the research laboratory.

The general principles of RIA are relatively simple. They are based upon competition for an antibody between a radiolabeled indicator substance and its unlabeled counterpart at unknown concentration in a test sample. For example, a purified candidate biologic marker (CBM) is radioactively labeled. Antibodies to the CBM which have been generated in heterologous species are added in sufficient amounts to the labeled CBM to produce from 50 to 80% binding. Known amounts of unlabeled CBM are added to a mixture of labeled CBM and anti-CBM and compete for the antibody binding sites. Labeled CBM bound to antibody is then separated from unbound labeled CBM (Fig. 2–1). Based upon the amount of labeled CBM bound at various known concentrations of unlabeled CBM, a standard curve can be constructed that will permit the determination of an unknown concentration of CBM (Fig. 2–2).

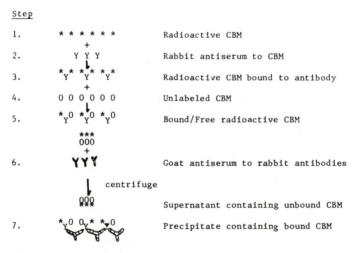

Figure 2–1. Radioimmunoassay. The radioactive candidate biologic marker (CBM) antibody complexes formed in step 3 are precipitated by goat antiserum prepared against rabbit antibodies. The radioactivity of either the supernatant or the precipitate can be counted (step 7).

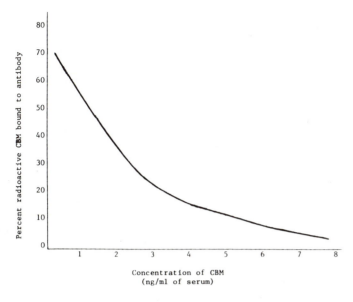

Figure 2–2. Theoretical standard curve for determining the concentration of CBM in serum. As the amount of CBM increases, the percentage of radioactive CBM bound to antibody decreases. At approximately equal amounts of radioactive CBM to unlabeled CBM, there is equal binding to antibody.

Various techniques have been used for the separation of bound antibody from unbound CBM. The double-antibody method is the more widely used approach. The complexes are precipitated with an antiserum whose specificity is directed at the Fc region of anti-CBM, thus leaving unbound CBM in the supernatant (Fig. 2–1). However, a number of other procedures, such as electrophoresis and chromatography, may be used that eliminate the need for a second antiserum for this separation.

Solid-phase RIA also eliminates the need for a second antiserum. With this method, specific antibody is either adsorbed to the walls of plastic tubes or covalently linked to a solid matrix. When tubes are used, the free antibody is removed by washing. The tube surface is then coated with an unrelated protein to prevent nonspecific binding to the plastic surface of subsequently added CBM. Unlabeled CBM is then added, followed by radiolabeled CBM. Both the labeled and unlabeled CBM compete for the specific antibody-binding sites. After equilibration, the radioactivity is counted. The difference between the amount of labeled CBM added and the amount remaining in solution is the amount bound by adsorbed antibody.

ENZYME-LINKED IMMUNOASSAYS

Enzyme-linked immunoassays (EIA) avoid the hazards and expense of RIA and are equally as sensitive. They depend upon the use of covalently linked enzyme–antibody complexes whereby the complexes are both immunologically and enzymatically active. Detection is by enzymatic activity rather than radioactivity. Horseradish peroxidase and alkaline phosphatase are examples of enzymes that are commonly used for coupling to antibody. They can convert colorless substrates to colored products, which, under defined conditions, can be measured.

Many variations of EIA exist, but the most appropriate for measuring CBM in human serum is the enzyme-linked immunosorbent assay (ELISA) as shown in Fig. 2–3. Two different antibodies bind to CBM. The first antibody of the system, which is specific for CBM, is adsorbed to a solid matrix. The second antibody, which has been generated in a different species, also binds CBM. The antibody of the enzyme–antibody complex binds to the second antibody in the system, and the enzyme converts substrate to products. A variation on this scheme is the sandwich-type ELISA (Fig. 2–4).

APPLICATIONS

Currently biologic markers in human cancer are most useful in monitoring the disease during and after treatment. None is clearly tumor-specific; such a designation can never be applicable for random-bred humans. Rather, the term tumor-associated antigen (TAA) has been used for purified, separated polypeptides that may share common chemical or immunologically cross-reactive sites of identity when each is compared with TAA from individual primary tumors of a given type or group. The alterations and modulations of TAA in metastatic sites have been shown, for example, in melanoma.[6] The value of each biologic marker is determined in each clinical situation by its concentration in biologic fluids and the sensitivity limits of the analytical procedures used.[20] Many substances have been investigated that have present and potential value as biologic markers in human cancer. One of the best characterized of these that has wide clinical application is the carcinoembryonic antigen.

Carcinoembryonic Antigen

The carcinoembryonic antigen (CEA) is a complex glycoprotein with a molecular weight of approximately 200 kd, with many antigenic sites.

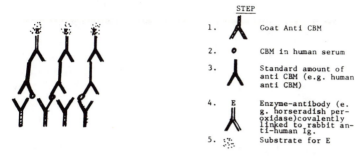

STEP

1. Goat Anti CBM

2. CBM in human serum

3. Standard amount of anti CBM (e.g. human anti CBM)

4. Enzyme-antibody (e. g. horseradish per- oxidase)covalently linked to rabbit an- ti-human Ig.

5. Substrate for E

Figure 2–3. Enzyme-linked immunosorbent assay. This is one of several variations of enzyme-linked immunoassays for measuring CBM in human serum. To measure CBM, add in order 1–2–3–4–5.

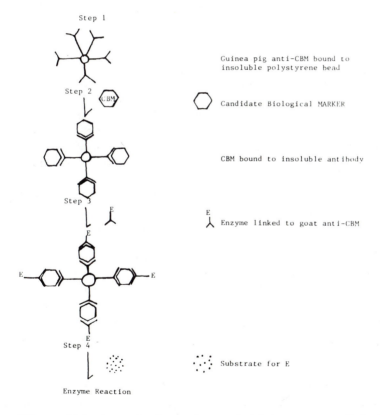

Step 1

Guinea pig anti-CBM bound to insoluble polystyrene bead

Step 2

Candidate Biological MARKER

CBM bound to insoluble antibody

Step 3

Enzyme linked to goat anti-CBM

Step 4

Substrate for E

Enzyme Reaction

Figure 2–4. General scheme for sandwich-type enzyme-linked immunosorbent assay.

It is produced by early embryonic tissue and in various carcinomas. Small amounts are also produced by normal cells of the gastrointestinal tract. Although CEA was first described as a specific marker for adenocarcinoma of the gastrointestinal tract, elevated levels have been found in some apparently normal individuals who are heavy smokers as well as in some patients with nonmalignant inflammatory diseases and infections. In more recent years, improved analytical techniques have also led to CEA testing in several malignancies, including breast cancer.[14]

The two most widely used assays for detection of CEA are RIA and EIA. Since the broad acceptance of the significance of CEA, many variations of RIA and EIA have been reported upon, and a number of commercial kits are available for CEA detection. However, in any immunoassay system, specificity and sensitivity are the factors that govern its usefulness.

Abbott Laboratories have produced a CEA–EIA solid-phase system based on a noncompetitive sandwich-type principle. The assay is carried out by first treating a plasma sample with an acid buffer. The supernatant is then incubated with polystyrene beads that have been coated with anti-CEA antibodies produced in guinea pigs. Unbound material is then washed away. The solid phase is then incubated with an excess of goat anti-CEA–peroxidase complex, and the excess labeled antibody is washed away. Enzyme activity is assayed by the addition of substrate, which is converted to a colored product. The CEA concentration is proportional to the absorbance of the colored product. The general scheme for this procedure is shown in Fig. 2–4.

Maiolini et al. have evaluated the Abbott CEA–EIA system and have found that the characteristics of the assay are good sensitivity (about 0.25 u/liter) and satisfactory reproducibility.[12] They found little cross-reactivity between CEA and molecules such as nonspecific cross-reacting antigens that are known for their high potential of cross-reactivity.

Kuroki et al. investigated and compared the antigenic reactivities of different CEA preparations from tumor tissues or of various CEA-related antigens from normal tissues using three commercially available RIA kits and their own RIA system.[11] In general, all CEA preparations including CEA standards gave similar reactions with the RIA systems. Differences in reaction intensity were, however, observed among the CEA preparations, and the order of reaction intensity among the preparations varied, based upon the assay system employed. That is, a given CEA preparation that reacted most strongly with one assay system reacted very weakly with another, and vice versa. Also, nonspecific cross-reacting antigen-2(NCA-Z) from meconium and normal fecal antigen-2(NCA-Z), which possessed physicochemical properties similar to those of CEA, revealed reactivities indistinguishable from those of the CEA preparations in all systems.

Although it appears that the RIA systems that are currently available for CEA carry some limitations in specificity and in radioimmunological heterogeneity, monoclonal antibodies have the potential to greatly improve this situation. In practice this potential has not been realized, because in using monoclonal antibodies it has been difficult to obtain quantitative binding of antigen, quantitative precipitation of antigen–antibody complexes, or determination of optimum working conditions for immunoassays. Wagener et al. reported on a general precipitation method that can easily be applied to any homogeneous phase in which monoclonal antibodies are employed, and they characterized five monoclonal antibodies, each recognizing a different epitope on CEA.[18] The method employs biotin-labeled antibody, radiolabeled antigen, and avidin as a precipitating agent in a homogeneous-phase competitive radioimmunoassay. This method eliminates incomplete or variable precipitation of antigen–antibody complexes often encountered in immunoassays in which monoclonal antibodies are employed.

A two-site monoclonal antibody-enzyme immunoassay (MEIA) for CEA was developed by Hedin et al.[5] This assay uses two monoclonal anti-CEA antibodies that recognize two different epitopes in the peptide moiety of CEA. The assay was sensitive to 0.5 μg/liter and had a measuring range of 0.5–200 μg of CEA per liter. It was highly specific inasmuch as none of three known CEA-related substances—nonspecific cross-reacting antigen-1(NCA-1) and NCA-2 and biliary glycoprotein I(BGP-I)—reacted in the assay. Sera tested in MEIA were also assayed in parallel with a conventional sandwich RIA, Phadebas CEA PRIST (Pharmacia, Uppsala, Sweden). This assay uses specific sheep and rabbit antisera and has a lower limit of sensitivity of approximately 1 μg of CEA per liter. The following additional commercial assays were also investigated in this study: CEA Roche Test Kit (Z-gel assay) and CEA EIA-Test (sandwich test using one monoclonal antibody), both from Hoffman-LaRoche (Basel, Switzerland); Abbott CEA RIA Diagnostic Kit (sandwich assay—Abbott Laboratories); and Serono Diagnostic CEA Kit (double-antibody assay—Serono, Rome).

None of the commercially available CEA assays was able to differentiate between CEA and NCA-2. With the exception of colon, normal tissue extracts did not react in MEIA even when tested at very high concentrations.

A comparative analysis of CEA levels in sera from healthy individuals and patients with malignant and nonmalignant diseases by using MEIA in parallel with a conventional RIA demonstrated that the MEIA was more specific for carcinomas than the RIA. This was essentially due to the MEIA giving lower CEA values than the RIA in sera from patients with nonmalignant diseases. Carcinoma patients, on the other hand, gave almost identical values in the two assays.

Prostate Antigen

The incidence of prostate cancer is second highest among all cancers in males and is the third highest cause of cancer deaths for men. Wang et al. described a new prostate-specific antigen (PA) distinct from prostatic acid phosphatase which is of potential value as a diagnostic and prognostic marker in prostate cancer.[19] Human PA was identified in the prostate (normal, benign hypertrophic, and cancerous) and seminal plasma as well as in human prostate carcinoma cells in culture and in nude mice. The antigen was not found in other human tissues. In crude extract of human prostate it appears to exist in several isomeric forms, one of which was purified and found to have a molecular weight of 33–34 kd and contains a single polypeptide.

Kuriyama et al. developed a sensitive sandwich-type EIA for the detection of PA. With this method, PA concentrations as low as 0.10 ng/ml could be detected.[10] The assay was reproducible. PA was not detectable in sera from normal females or female cancer patients. Sera from male patients with nonprostatic cancer contained a PA range similar to that of normal males. Patients with prostate cancer and benign prostatic hypertrophy were shown to have elevated levels of circulating PA. Although no quantitative difference in PA levels was found between the benign prostatic hypertrophy group and stage A of prostatic cancer, patients with stages C and D prostatic cancer showed significantly elevated levels of PA qualitatively and quantitatively. The results indicate that PA may be used as an adjunct in the diagnosis of prostate cancer.

Prostatic Acid Phosphatase

Prostatic acid phosphatase (PAP) has been used as a biologic marker in the diagnosis of metastatic prostatic cancer for over 40 years. PAP is immunologically distinct from acid phosphatase from other tissues but antigenically indistinguishable from preparations from prostatic fluid, prostatic tissue, and seminal plasma. Additionally, we have found no immunologic difference between PAP and acid phosphatase present in vaginal fluid, although electrophoretic differences can be seen. Choe and Rose combined the immunological precipitation step with the conventional enzyme assay procedure and called it immunoenzyme assay (IEA).[3] The RIA measures free and bound antigen in equilibrium. The IEA measures the concentration of antigen by its catalytic activity after the precipitation of antigen–antibody complexes. The sensitivity for both methods was reported as 1.95 ng/ml. However, the sensitivity of RIA is highly affected by antibody affinity because it measures free and bound antigen in equilibrium, whereas IEA is less affected by the affinity of antibodies. Although IEA is as sensitive as, or superior to, RIA, the clinical application of this technique has not been extensive.

Lung Tumor-Associated Antigen

Several reports have appeared concerning human lung tumor-associated antigens (LTA). In most cases the antigens are shared by the various histological types. Braatz et al. reported on the purification and partial characterization of a protein isolated from a human lung tumor which appeared to be an LTA.[2] In order to better define the distribution and occurrence of the LTA, a competitive protein-binding RIA was developed capable of detecting less than 10 ng of LTA. They examined a panel of 215 sera for LTA from normal individuals and pretreatment patients with lung cancer, benign lung disease, and nonlung cancers. Positive rates in lung cancers of the following histological types were found: adenocarcinoma, 60% (9/15); squamous cell, 42% (13/31); large cell, 17% (3/18); and small cell, 19% (3/16). In addition, 13% (3/23) of other cancers, 0% (0/24) of benign lung disease, and 2% (2/88) of normals were positive. Approximately one-third of stage I patients in the squamous cell and adenocarcinoma groups were positive, while two-thirds of patients with more advanced stage III disease in these categories showed elevations.

Using a method based upon the same principles as RIA and EIA, a sensitive thin-layer immunoassay employing an adaptation of the visualization of condensation on plastic surface method (VCS-TLI), Hollinshead et al. tested both the purified polypeptide TAAs from squamous cell and adenocarcinomas and the selected, monoclonal-antibody-derived TAA fragments (epitopes) against a series of coded sera in 684 assays.[7] Both TAA and TAA epitopes reacted similarly with the lung cancer test sera at a given dilution, with 89 out of 95 test sera positive with one or both antigens. When both epitopes were positive, results showed a comparison with pathological evaluations in which there had been noted characteristics of shared adeno-epidermoid features. Further serum titrations of positive reactions indicated greater sensitivity in tests with monoclonal antigens. Of 6 sera that were negative in the test, 3 of these were taken during the first two weeks after operation, at a time when many patients are immunosuppressed, but there is no explanation for the other 3 negative tests. The TAA chosen are not shared by other types of lung cancer, and tests with 18 other lung cancer types and 12 normal sera were negative. Although the TAA had not shown a high degree of cross-reactivity using the less sensitive double-immunodiffusion–immunoelectrophoresis tests, it was of interest that a high degree of cross-reaction was seen with other cancer types of the squamous cell and adenocarcinoma categories (28/40), although this was reduced when the same sera were tested against the TAA epitopes (5%). Not all the TAA epitopes derived using several monoclonal TAA antibodies were as specific, indicating that the TAA polypeptide chains contain sections that are more cross-reactive and sections that are more specific. Precancerous conditions were detected in patients with asbestosis using retrospective sera from those known to develop lung cancer later, indicating possible usefulness in high-risk groups.

The most encouraging aspect of these studies by Braatz et al. and by Hollinshead et al. was the ability of the RIA to discriminate patients with benign lung or nonlung malignant disease using partially purified antigen, and of the VCS-TLI to detect differences between monoclonal-antibody-derived antigen fragments, with both tests discriminating lung cancer patients from normal individuals. It is highly possible that further studies, such as those by Hedin et al. in the MEIA test using anti-CEA monoclonal antibodies[5] and by Hollinshead et al. in the VCS-TLI test using monoclonal antibody-derived lung TAA epitopes,[7] will provide an opportunity to establish further the role of antigens and antibodies in the evolution of disease patterns, both at the primary developmental, malignant, and metastatic phases. It would be useful to automate such tests, to computerize the data, and to test thousands of test materials to provide a more complete understanding of such patterns.

Fibronectin

Fibronectin (FN) is a high molecular weight extracellular adhesive glycoprotein of a variety of adherent cells. It is distributed in loose connective tissue and basement membranes and interacts with collagen, fibrin, actin, heparin, hyaluronic acid, DNA, and *Staphylococcus aureus*. It is also found in plasma and other body fluids and mediates macrophage clearance of nonbacterial particulates. Reports have indicated that FN is consistently reduced or absent in transformed cell lines and is therefore of potential value as a biologic marker in malignant disease. Pearlstein and Baez developed a solid-phase RIA for the determination of FN levels in plasma which is sensitive in the range of 0.5–5 μg/ml and utilizes antiserum at a 1:1,000 dilution.[13] In addition, the iodination procedure employed to label FN results in a biologically intact protein.

Kawamura et al. developed a competitive EIA using polystyrene beads as a solid phase and glucose oxidase as a marker enzyme.[9] This method gave a reproducible standard curve for plasma FN in the range of 0.5–50 μg/ml. The plasma FN levels in patients with malignant, collagen, and liver diseases were also measured. The mean plasma FN level in patients with collagen disease was significantly higher than that in normal persons, whereas the mean plasma FN levels in patients with malignant and liver diseases were not significantly different.

Neuron-Specific Enolase

Neuron-specific enolase (NSE) is a glycolytic enzyme widely distributed in mammalian tissues. In the brain, three forms of enolase ($\alpha\alpha$, $\alpha\gamma$ and $\gamma\gamma$) exist. The γ subunit is identical with the nervous system-specific and species-nonspecific protein, and thus $\alpha\gamma$ and $\gamma\gamma$ types of enolase are referred to as NSE. Subsequent studies have revealed that NSE is present in endocrine cells of the central and peripheral divisions of the diffuse neuroendocrine system. Additionally, NSE has been identified in the gut, lung, pancreas, pituitary thyroid, and adrenal glands.

Tapia et al. demonstrated that NSE is present in large amounts in tissue extracts from all classes of peripheral neuroendocrine tumors, including islet cell tumors, phaeochromocytomas, medullary thyroid carcinomas, oat-cell carcinoms, and carcinomas of the gut, pancreas, and lung.[16] Using a double-antibody solid-phase RIA with ^{125}I-labeled NSE purified from human brain to determine NSE concentration, they found that NSE could be detected in plasma samples and that significantly raised levels are seen in patients with neuroendocrine tumors.

Ishiguro et al. used a sensitive solid-phase sandwich EIA to determine serum levels of NSE in patients with neuroblastoma and in control subjects.[8] Serum levels of NSE in healthy adults ranged from 1.4 to 5.7 ng/ml (2.87 ± 1.18 ng/ml, $n = 20$), and in control children (1–7 years old) from 2.6 to 10.8 ng/ml (5.76 ± 2.42 ng/ml, $n = 20$). Serum samples ($n = 13$) from patients with neuroblastoma contained high levels of NSE ranging from 13.6 to 330 ng/ml (mean, 96 ng/ml). However, those ($n = 7$) from ganglioneuroblastoma patients were within a normal range (3.0–25.0 ng/ml; mean, 8.3 ng/ml). Their results suggest that NSE in serum may be a valuable biologic marker for the screening and therapeutic monitoring of neuroblastoma.

A study was also undertaken by Ariyoshi et al. using the same solid-phase sandwich EIA to evaluate NSE as a biologic marker for carcinoma of the lung.[1] They measured serum NSE in 80 normal individuals, 20 patients with small cell carcinoma of the lung (SCCL). and 54 patients with non–small cell carcinoma (non-SCCL). The mean value of the control group was 2.1 ± 0.4 ng/ml (range, 1.3–3.0 ng/ml). Serum levels exceeding 7.5 ng/ml were considered to be positive. Thirteen of 20 patients (65%) with SCCL had positive serum NSE levels, whereas 6 of 54 patients (11%) with non-SCCL had positive levels. Positive NSE in sera of patients was observed only in patients with an advanced clinical stage of SCCL or non-SCCL. No correlation between serum NSE levels and metastatic sites could be found. The serum NSE levels in subtypes of SCCL were positive in 9 of 10 patients with oat cell carcinoma and in 4 of 10 patients with intermediate cell carcinoma. Serum NSE levels changed in parallel with the clinical course during the treatments. Their data suggest that serum NSE may be a useful marker for monitoring the clinical course of lung carcinoma, especially of SCCL. Additionally, the detection of NSE in non-SCCL is of interest in relation to the histogenesis of lung carcinomas that exhibit the properties of neuroendocrine tumors.

Sarcoma

Studies have demonstrated tumor-associated antigens (TAA) present on metastases that were not detected on the primary tumor. The combination of a highly sensitive ELISA technique with soluble sarcoma-associated antigen (SAA) has enabled Roth and Wesley to investigate autologous humoral immune responses to primary and metastatic human sarcomas.[15] They observed the binding of antibodies in autologous sera to extracts of both primary tumor and its metastases.

It has been known for some time that TAA elicits the formation of antibodies in sera from patients with the disease. These circulating antibodies react *in vivo* with the antigens on the tumor cell and may also complex with TAA that is shed from the cells. However, several problems have limited their usefulness as diagnostic and prognostic indicators. Most assays are dependent on tissue culture cell lines as the source of TAA. Accordingly, they are susceptible to a variety of artifacts, including contamination. Recently, Gupta et al. reported on a procedure for the separation and isolation of antibody and TAA fractions from the plasma of melanoma patients by immunoadsorption with protein A-bearing *Staphylococcus aureus*.[4] The activity and specificity of the TAA were determined by RIA. Although this method is sensitive, it has the major disadvantage of requiring isotopes.

The ELISA technique developed by Roth and Wesley for the detection of TAA overcomes many of the problems that have been mentioned.[15] Soluble extracts from fresh tumors are used as the antigen source, thereby eliminating the need for cultured cell lines. Butanol extracts of fresh sarcoma tissue contain antigens that are recognized by antibodies in autologous sera from sarcoma patients. The use of these soluble extracts provides a continuous and consistent source of antigen that undoubtedly contributes to the reproducibility of the ELISA. The importance of these antigens to the host tumor response remains to be determined, but clearly there are determinants present that can at least quantitatively be distinguished from normal adult tissues. Additionally, it is a sensitive assay capable of detecting nanogram levels of TAA. Thistlethwaite et al. have also used the methodology for this assay to study syngeneic humoral immune response to a primary tumor and its metastases in an UV-light-induced murine melanoma system.[17]

Alpha-Fetoprotein

As with CEA, alpha-fetoprotein (AFP) has been extensively studied and characterized. It is a glycoprotein with a molecular weight of 69 kd and is produced in early fetal life by the yolk sac, parts of the gut, and the liver. Malignancies developing in these organs in later life may produce AFP and release it into circulation.

In the nonpregnant individual, raised serum AFP levels are found in most cases of primary hepatoma and in nonseminomatous germ cell tumors. AFP is measured by RIA with antisera of minimal cross-reactivity with albumin. Because of organ specificity, AFP has proven useful in the screening for certain tumors in clinical situations.

Generally, only values above 100 ng/ml should be considered suspect, whereas those showing values between 25 and 100 ng/ml should be checked again within a few months.[14]

CONCLUSION

We have presented the principles of radioimmunoassay and enzyme-linked assay, the various indirect, direct, competitive, noncompetitive, and additional modifications of these assays, and the advantages and disadvantages of each form of assay. We have given major examples of the uses of these assays in the study of biologic markers: two-site monoclonal antibody–enzyme immunoassay (MEIA) for CEA; sandwich-type EIA for prostate antigen; an immunoenzyme assay combining a precipitation step for prostate acid phosphatase; a radioimmunoassay using antisera to alpha-fetoprotein; a competitive protein-binding RIA to detect lung TAA; a variation of EIA, called VCS-TLI, which detects nanogram quantities of lung TAA epitopes; a competitive solid-phase EIA with marker enzyme, which tests for fibronectin; a solid-phase sandwich EIA which tests neuron-specific enolase; an ELISA using sarcoma TAA which detects at nanogram levels; and others.

These assays are the workhorses in the current studies of biologic markers, and the agents being tested must be further evaluated in studies employing immunoperoxidase or radiolabeled-imaging studies. In addition, there is the great advantage of multitests, in which several markers for a particular disease are tested on the same material and plotted together for better categorization and identification. Not all materials are ideal for these tests, and the ease with which enzymes or normal tissue components are tested by seeking antigen levels may not apply to the problems involved in the testing of tumor-associated antigens. In some cases, normal sera and cancer sera may not detect a low level of antigen, and hyperimmune sera may be necessary. In many cases, it may be necessary to remove nonspecific antigen–antibody complexes by use of drugs or other chemicals for cellular complexes or by use of blood-clearance procedures or other precipitation methods for circulating interfering competing substances or complexes. The assays are only as good as the materials used for testing and depend a great deal on an in-depth understanding of the biological changes and immunologic aspects of the disease under study. Use of highly purified materials, use of monoclonal antibodies and secondary monoclonal antibodies, use of a variety of carefully defined epitopes, and fresh, well-selected sera or tissue specimens or cloned cells and cell-sorted populations from a given tumor and many other variables may result in a highly efficient use of RIA and EIA to provide candidate biologic markers worth pursuing for further evaluation by other forms of testing. With most solid tumors, the levels of antibody are more reliable for monitoring the disease state, and tests with nanogram amounts of standard epitopes for tests of patient sera are best. In tests developed for aid in diagnosis, levels of antigen in the bloodstream may be more helpful. In any case, it is now possible to devise tests that detect both antigen and antibody, and more will be learned about the individual forms of cancer. Rapid automation and the testing of large numbers of well-defined sera and tissues will permit a greater understanding of the way in which these biologic markers interact at different stages of the premalignant and malignant processes.

REFERENCES

1. Ariyoshi, Y., Kato, K., Ishiguro, Y., Ota, L., Sato, T., and Suchi, T. Evaluation of serum neuron-specific enolase as a tumor marker for carcinoma of the lung. Gann *74*: 219–225 (1983).

2. Braatz, J.A., Hua, D. T., and Princier, G. L. Serum levels of a human lung tumor-associated antigen using an improved radioimmunoassay. Cancer Res. *43*: 110–113 (1983).

3. Choe, B. K., and Rose, N. R. Prostatic acid phosphatase: A marker for human prostatic adenocarcinoma. In: *Methods in Cancer Research* Vol. 19 (H. Busch and L. C. Yeoman, eds.), 199–232 (1982).

4. Gupta, R. K., Leitch, A. M., and Morton, D. L. Detection of tumour associated antigen in eluates from protein A columns used for *ex vivo* immunoadsorption of plasma from melanoma patients by radioimmunoassay. Clin. Exp. Immunol. *53*: 589–599 (1983).

5. Hedin, A., Carlsson, L., Berglund, A., and Hammarstrom, S. A monoclonal antibody–enzyme immunoassay for serum carcinoembryonic antigen with increased specificity for carcinomas. Proc. Natl. Acad. Sci. *80*: 3470–3474 (1983).

6. Hollinshead, A., Arlen, M., Yonemoto, R., Cohen, M., Tanner, K., Kundin, W., and Scherrer, J. Pilot studies using melanoma tumor-associated antigens (TAA) in specific active immunochemotherapy of malignant melanoma. Cancer *49*: 1387–1404 (1982).

7. Hollinshead, A. Stewart, T. H. M., Hamilton, R. L., and DiAngelo, C. R. Lung tumor-associated antigens: Thin layer immunoassay. Cancer Detec. Prev. *6*: 185–191 (1983).

8. Ishiguro, Y., Kato, K., Shimizu, A., Ito, T., and Nagaya, M. High levels of immunoreactive nervous system-specific enolase in sera of patients with neuroblastoma. Clin. Chim. Acta *121*: 173–180 (1982).

9. Kawamura, K., Tanaka, M., Kamiyama, F., Higashino, K., and Kishimoto, S. Enzyme immunoassay of human plasma fibronectin in malignant, collagen and liver diseases. Clin. Chim. Acta *131*: 101–108 (1983).

10. Kuriyama, M., Wang, M. C., Papsidero, L. D., Killian, C.S., Skimano, T., Valenzuela, L. A., Nishimura, T., Murphy, G. P., and Chu, T. M. Quantitation of prostate-specific antigen in serum by a sensitive enzyme immunoassay. Cancer Res. *40*: 4658–4662 (1980).

11. Kuroki, M., Yamaguchi, A., Koga, Y., and Matsuoka, Y. Antigenic reactivities of purified preparations of carcinoembryonic antigen (CEA) and related normal antigens using four different radioimmunoassay systems for CEA. J. Immunol. Methods *60*: 221–233 (1982).

12. Maiolini, R., Bagrel, A., Chavance, C., Krebs, B., Herbeth, B., and Masseyeff, R. Study of an enzyme immunoassay kit for carcinoembryonic antigen. Clin. Chem. *26*: 1718 (1980).

13. Pearlstein, E., and Baez, L. A solid-phase radioimmunoassay for the determination of fibronectin levels in plasma. Anal. Biochem. *116*: 292–297 (1981).

14. Pohl, A. L., Francesconi, M., Ganzinger, V. C., Graninger, W., Lenzhofer, R. S. and Moser, K. V. Present value of tumor markers in the clinic. Cancer Detec. Prev. *6*: 17–20 (1983).

15. Roth, J. A. and Wesley, R. A. Human tumor-associated antigens detected by serologic techniques: Analysis of autologous humoral immune responses to primary and metastatic human sarcomas by an enzyme-linked immunoabsorbant solid-phase assay (ELISA). Cancer Res. *42*: 3978–3985 (1982).

16. Tapia, F. J., Polak, J. M., Barbosa, A. J. A., Bloom, S. R., Marangos, P. J., Dermody, C., and Pearse, A. G. E. Neuron specific enolase is produced by neuroendocrine tumours. Lancet *1*: 808–811 (1981).

17. Thistlethwaithe, P., Davidson, D. D., Fidler, I. J., and Roth, J. A. Syngeneic humoral immune responses to tumor-associated antigens expressed by K-1735 UV-induced melanoma and its metastases. Cancer Immunol. Immunother. *15*: 11–16 (1983).

18. Wagener, C., Clark, B. R., Rickard, K. J., and Shively, J. E. Monoclonal antibodies for carcinoembryonic antigen and related antigens as a model system: The determination of affinities and specificities of monoclonal antibodies by using biotin-labeled antibodies and avidin as precipitating agent in a solution phase immunoassay. J. Immunol. *130*: 5, 2302–2307 (1983).

19. Wang, M. C., Kuriyama, M., Papsidero, L. D., Loor, R. M., Valenzuela, L. A., Murphy, G. P., and Chu, T. M. Prostate antigen of human cancer patients. In: *Methods in Cancer Research* Vol. 19 (H. Busch and L. Yeoman, eds.), 179–197 (1982).

20. Winters, W. D. New techniques for detecting tumor markers: A prospective. Cancer Detec. Prev. *6*: 21–31 (1983).

3

Immunocytochemistry: Principles and Clinical Applications

Nasser Javadpour, M.D.

During the past several years, the development of specific and sensitive immunocytochemical techniques has made remarkable contributions to the diagnosis and management of cancer. Among these techniques are specific and sensitive radioimmunoassay (RIA), immunoperoxidase (IP), peroxidase antiperoxidase (PAP), and radioimmunodetection (RID). These modalities have provided the means for early diagnosis and treatment and a potential for radioimmunotherapy (RIT) of cancer. The current progress has been made even more promising through the development of specific and sensitive antisera utilizing monoclonal antibodies by fusing sensitized spleen cells with myeloma cells of the mouse. This chapter discusses the development and utilization of these techniques in the detection of cell markers in tumor and cancer cells and their potential impact on the detection, localization, and therapy of urologic cancer.[1-7]

IMMUNOCYTOCHEMICAL TECHNIQUES

There are a number of immunocytochemical techniques (ICCT) available; however, the most reproducible and convenient ones are IP and PAP (Fig. 3–1). The advantages of these techniques over fluorescent microscopy include the following: (1) No specialized equipment is necessary. (2) No fresh tissue is required; the paraffin block, formaldehyde-fixed tissues that are usually available in pathology departments are sufficient for prospective studies. (3) The storage

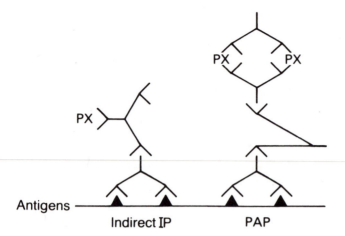

Figure 3–1. Schema of immunocytochemical techniques.

of material and slides does not pose any particular problems. (4) The slides can be filed and kept as permanent records. (5) Finally, undesirable background staining is minimized and the detail of tissue and exact locations of a given cell marker may be precisely localized in various parts of a cell by a simple counterstain.[7]

IMMUNOPEROXIDASE TECHNIQUE

Immunoperoxidase methods have much in common with established immunofluorescence procedures. Both have the potential for demonstration of specific cell and tissue antigens, with similar limitations demanding rigorous control of specificity. In any study the choice of an immunofluorescence method or an IP method can be made according to the desired objective, the degree of morphologic detail required, the material available for study, and the ease of access to specialized UV microscopy. The major advantage of IP is that it can be utilized in either a prospective or a retrospective study, since the tissue to be stained can be fixed in formaldehyde—and this is usually available—whereas immunofluorescence requires fresh or frozen tumor specimens. Thus, IP has certain features that make the immunocytochemistry more convenient and practical.

The IP technique utilizes a 4- to 6-micron-thick section of formaldehyde-fixed tumor which is deparaffinized in xylene and cleared in the usual fashion. The section is incubated in a humid chamber for 30–60 min with appropriate antisera to a given marker.

Table 3–1   Immunoperoxidase Staining Technique

1. Deparaffinize sections by immersing in xylene 5 min ×2.
2. Wash the section by immersing in absolute alcohol 5 min ×2.
3. Dehydrate the section by immersing the sections in Tris buffer 0.5 *M*, pH 7.6, 5 min ×3.
4. Neutralize the endogenous peroxidase by immersing the section in methanol–H_2O_2 mixture for 20 min (0.6% H_2O_2).
5. Wash the sections with Tris buffer 5 min ×2.
6. Incubate the sections with 3% normal goat solution in Tris buffer.
7. Incubate the sections with first antibody with appropriate controls for 1 h in humidity chamber.
8. Wash the excess antibody with Tris buffer 5 min ×3.
9. Incubate the sections with second antibody for 1 h in humid chamber.
10. Wash the sections with Tris buffer ×3 to remove all excess second antibody.
11. Develop the color by diaminobenzidine (5 mg/40 ml of buffer and 30 λ of H_2O_2 in 200 ml of diaminobenzidine solution).
12. Develop the color by examining the test section under the microscope (this usually takes 4–6 min).
13. Wash the section with tap water and counterstain with hematoxylin.
14. Dehydrate the sections and mount cover slips with permount.

The second antibody is a gamma globulin that is conjugated with horseradish peroxidase. The section is washed again and exposed for 10 min to diaminobenzidine containing 0.05% hydrogen peroxide. All the appropriate controls, including sections exposed to normal serum and absorbed antiserum, are included (Table 3–1).

We have recently utilized the peroxidase-antiperoxidase (PAP) technique with equally reliable results. Because of scarcity of information in the literature, it is discussed briefly below.

PEROXIDASE-ANTIPEROXIDASE TECHNIQUE

In principle, PAP is similar to IP, with perhaps more sensitivity and less background. As with IP, the technique requires antisera—for example, a rabbit antiserum—to a given marker, plus a second antibody, which is usually a goat anti-rabbit IgG. The PAP technique also utilizes a third antiserum—namely, peroxidase antiperoxidase—which is raised in rabbits. The remainder of the technique is similar to that of the conventional IP technique (Table 3–2).

Table 3–2   Peroxidase–Antiperoxidase Protocol

1. Take slides through xylol 3 min ×2, absolute alcohol 2 min ×2, and phosphate buffered saline 2 min ×2.
2. To block endogenous peroxide, immerse slides in freshly made 0.3% hydrogen peroxide in methanol for 25 min.
3. Wash in PBS 2 min ×3.
4. Cover sections with 3% NGS for 20 min to block nonspecific staining. Drain and blot around section, but *do not wash*.
5. Incubate with antiserum in 20% NGS for 16 h (overnight) at room temperature in humidity chamber.
6. Wash in PBS 5 min ×3.
7. Incubate with goat anti-rabbit Ig 1:20 for 30 min at room temperature.
8. Wash in PBS 5 min. ×3.
9. Incubate with freshly thawed and prepared PAP 1:50 in 1% NGS for 30 min at room temperture.
10. Wash in PBS 5 min ×3.
11. Stain with freshly prepared DAB (40 mg/100 ml PBS with 175 λ H_2O_2/100 ml) for 7 min. Filter solution before using and dispose of all contaminated materials properly.
12. Rinse in distilled water 2 min ×3.
13. Counterstain with hematoxylin for 60 sec.
14. Wash in warm tap water for 2 min.
15. Wash in distilled water for 2 min.
16. Take slides through absolute alcohol 2 min ×2, and xylol 3 min ×2.
17. Allow slides to dry, and mount cover slips with permount.

Although it was hoped that steroid receptors could be detected and localized through the use of this immunologic technique with specific and sensitive antisera to various steroids, so far it has not worked satisfactorily. Hopefully, preparation of specific antibodies to estrophilin may open the way for further progress in this area.[2]

PREPARATION OF MONOCLONAL ANTIBODIES

The prospects for IP, PAP, RID, and RIT are becoming more promising with the recent advent of hybridoma technology, which can produce massive, yet pure, desired antibodies. Due to the importance of this technology we present a brief discussion of monoclonal antibodies.

Immunologic assays have always been plagued by uncertainties and unpredictability in the heterogeneity of the immune response.

Immunization is still more of an art than a science, and serologists have had to be satisfied with whatever quality and quantity of antibodies an immunized animal will provide. However, hybridoma technology has eliminated some of these technical problems.[6] To appreciate the advances that have been made and the difficulties that remain, it is necessary to understand how antibody-producing hybridoms are generated by hybridoma.

Mice are immunized with the antigen of interest and are then usually given another injection to obtain a secondary response. Two to four days later, the spleen is removed and teased apart to form a suspension of spleen cells. The spleen cells are mixed with mouse myeloma cells that have previously been adapted to grow continuously in culture. Polyethylene glycol is added to the mixture to promote the fusion of cell membranes, and the cells are suspended in tissue culture medium. Because only one of every 2×10^5 spleen cells actually forms a viable hybrid with a myeloma cell, it is necessary to eliminate all the unfused myeloma and the spleen cells to allow recovery of that hybrid. Such hybrids can be isolated by growth in a selective medium. Variants of mouse myeloma cells that lack the enzyme hypoxanthine phosphoribosyltransferase are used; then hypoxanthine, aminopterin, and thymidine are added to the growth medium. Since the myeloma cells lack the enzyme, they cannot use exogenous hypoxanthine to synthesize purines. The aminopterin blocks their endogenous synthesis of purine and pyrimidines, and the myeloma cells die. However, a hybrid between a myeloma cell and a spleen cell contains the transferase provided by the normal spleen cell, uses the exogenous hypoxanthine and thymidine, and survives. The normal spleen cells are not killed by this selective medium, but they do not survive the culture. The hybrids, which double approximately every 24–48 hours, rapidly outgrow the few nondividing but persistent spleen cells. Clones that are producing antibodies are grown to mass culture and are recloned as soon as possible. This procedure eliminates contaminating non–antibody-producing clones and cells that have lost the ability to produce an antibody as a result of chromosomal loss. The specificity of the antibody is confirmed by more extensive testing.

AVIDIN–BIOTIN METHOD

The affinity of biotin for avidin is 1,000-fold more than that of antigen for antibody, and this property can be taken advantage of to detect the presence of T-antigen. Our technique is summarized in Table 3–3.

Table 3–3   Avidin–Biotin Technique

1. Deparaffinize in xylene, hydrate in alcohol, and wash in phosphate buffer solution.
2. Incubate with normal serum and H_2O_2.
3. Incubate with biotin-labeled antibody for 30 min.
4. Incubate with avidin-labeled peroxidase for 45 min.
5. Incubate with diaminobenzidine for 5–7 min.
6. Wash and counterstain with hemotoxylin, clean, and mount.

Briefly, four slides are selected from each specimen and deparaffinized, washed, and rehydrated, as before. Then, using the avidin–biotin method, one can test for the presence of T-antigen. Endogenous peroxidase is first blocked by incubating all slides in 3% H_2O_2 in absolute methyl alcohol for 25 min. The slides are then washed in three 5-min Tris buffer (pH 2.4) baths (Fig. 3–2). Alternatively, this technique can be modified to detect T-antigen as follows: Two slides from each specimen are treated with neuraminidase, as before. One nonneuraminidase slide and one neuraminidase slide are treated with PNA (peanut agglutinin), while the two other slides are treated with a 3% concentration of normal goat serum (control specimens) for 1 h. Each slide is then incubated with normal horse serum for 30 min. The excess antibody and serum is rinsed in three Tris buffer washes. The slides are then incubated with diaminibenzidine for 5–7 min, then washed and counterstained with hemotoxyline.

CLINICAL APPLICATION

The use of immunocytochemistry has made a substantial contribution to the localization of cell markers in lymphoid cells and their malignancies including leukemia, lymphoma, and Hodgkin's disease. It has also made a contribution to immunocytologic localization in ABO (H) antigens in normal, fetal, and cancer tissue. Detection of these cell-surface antigens in a number of cancers, including urothelial, cervical, and certain other cancers, has helped to forecast the prognosis of such tumors. The use of immunocytochemistry has proven its clinical application in detecting hCG and AFP in germ cell testicular cancer and ovarian cancer. The immunohistologic classifications of germ cell tumors has also helped in the understanding of the origin and histopathology of these tumors. This has also been essential

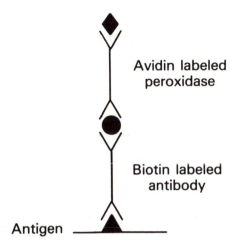

Avidin labeled
peroxidase

Biotin labeled
antibody

Antigen

Figure 3–2. Schema of avidin-biotin technique (affinity of avidin for biotin is high).

in diagnosing germ cell tumors when these occur in extragonadal sites. Also, in hepatoma one may localize AFP in hepatocellular cancer cells. Immunoenzymatic techniques have also been helpful in the localization of carcinoembryonic antigens, calcitonin, and acid phosphatase and prostatic-specific antigen. One may conclude that these techniques have brought a new dimension to histopathology in addition to morphologic diagnosis.

In summary, the investigators utilizing immunoenzymatic techniques may be able to detect the cellular origin of, distribution of, presence or absence of, and changes in any cellular products that are capable of producing an antibody.

RADIOIMMUNODETECTION OF CANCER

We have recently reported a technique for locating γ-hCG-producing tumors in the retroperitoneal area not detectable with the conventional modalities, but this approach requires multiple venous catheterizations and use of the alpha subunit of hCG. Another method developed recently for locating tumors *in vivo* is based on injecting radioactive antibodies made against a tumor-associated marker and then performing total-body scintigraphy to pinpoint foci of abnormal radioactivity, corresponding to sites of tumor. This procedure has been

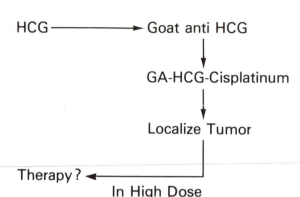

Figure 3–3. Schema of affinity therapy of cancer by chemotherapeutic agent-labeled antibody.

termed radioimmunodetection (RID) of cancer. The first extensive application of this approach was with antibodies to carcinoembryonic antigen (CEA).[1] More recent studies have included the use of antiodies to AFP and hCG[3] (Fig. 3–3).

Radioantibody Preparation

Hyperimmune goat antiserum is prepared with purified urinary hCG. The anti-hCG serum is absorbed with urinary protein using an automated chromatography system with a solid-phase (Sepharose 4B, Pharmacia, Piscataway, NJ) immunoabsorbent column. The immunoglobulin G (IgG) fraction of the absorbed antiserum is chromatographically purified, as previously discussed. Goat anti-hCG is labeled with [131]I (Amersham/Searle, Arlington Heights, IL) by the chloramine-T method. Individual preparations of ^{131}I-labeled goat anti-hCG IgG are tested for pyrogenicity in rabbits, and for sterility and acute toxicity. Once they have been proven to be nontoxic and pyrogen-free, they are utilized for patients. Goat anti-human AFP is labeled with ^{131}I utilizing the same techniques.

Scintillation Technique

The radioiodinated anti-hCG or anti-AFP IgGs are administered intravenously at a total dose of approximately 1 μCi in 20 ml of sterile normal saline over a period of 10–15 min. To subtract the free iodine in bladder and stomach and to suppress the background caused by antigen–antibody complexes, 500 μCi of ^{99m}Tc-labeled human serum albumin is injected intravenously before imaging. Images of the anterior chest and anterior and posterior abdomen are obtained by gamma scintillation 24–48 h after the intravenous injection of the radioantibody. The data obtained are stored in a computer capable of computing digital images of the ^{131}I-labeled antibody alone, ^{99m}Tc and ^{99m}Tc-albumin or ^{131}I-labeled antibody minus the technetium components.

RID and Management of Cancer

Cancer RID with antibodies to hCG and to AFP appears to be a useful procedure for the pretreatment and posttreatment evaluation of patients with testicular cancer and can reveal sites of tumor not detectable by other methods for hCG-producing tumor. This technique may be utilized in RIT by using a therapeutic dosage of antibody labeled with radioactive material. An experimental design using athymic mice with xenographic human yolk sac tumor is in progress in our laboratory.

RID has the potential for making a remarkable impact on the treatment of prostatic cancer. If this technique is proven reliable, it will play an important role in the staging of the disease and perhaps in RIT since one may attach a number of radioisotopes including ^{131}I, for the purpose of therapy. This approach appears to be promising in light of the development of massive pure monoclonal antibody techniques.

CONCLUSIONS AND FUTURE PERSPECTIVES

Perhaps the most outstanding progress in cancer immunology has been in the field of immunodiagnosis—mainly the development of specific and sensitive immunocytochemical techniques to measure and localize cell markers in the sera and cancer cells of cancer patients. In this chapter, we have discussed the development and utilization of cell markers in urologic cancer with newer techniques such as IP, PAP, RID, RIT, and monoclonal antibodies.

These findings have exceeded even the wildest dreams of immunologists, and they are revolutionizing serology. Not only is it now possible to generate a homogeneous antibody, but the production of that antibody is immortalized, and the only limitation on the amount of antibody available is the number of mice to which one is willing to give injections. In addition, impure antigens can be used, since the technique for generating antibody-forming hybrids results in the identification and propagation of cloned cell lines producing a single antibody that will react with the antigen and will not react with any contaminating material. Basic researchers in all areas of biology and clinical investigators studying a wide variety of systems have recognized the enormous potential of large amounts of monoclonal homogeneous antibodies and have begun to generate such reagents. These developments have become an important part of contemporary urologic practice.

REFERENCES

1. Goldenberg, D. M., Deland, F. H., Kim, E., Bennett, F. J., Primus, J. R., Van Nagel, G., Estes, N., De Simone, P., Rayburn, P. Use of radiolabeled antibodies to carcinoembryonic antigen for the detection and localization of diverse cancers by external photoscanning. N. Engl. J. Med. 298: 1384–1388, 1978.

2. Howard, D. R., Batsakis, J. G. Cytostructural localization of a tumor associated antigen. Science 210: 201, 1980.

3. Javadpour, N., Goldenberg, D., and Deland, F. H. Radioimmunodetection of metastatic cancer. JAMA 246: 45, 1981.

4. Javadpour, N. Serum and cellular biologic tumor markers in patients with urologic cancer. Human Pathol. 10: 557–68, 1979.

5. Kurman, R. J., Scardino, P. T., McIntire, R. K., Javadpour, N. Cellular localization of alpha-fetoprotein and human chorionic gonadotropin in germ cell tumors of the testis using an indirect immunoperoxidase technique: A new approach to classification utilizing tumor markers. Cancer 40: 2136–2151, 1977.

6. Milstein, C., Adetugbo, K., Cowan, N. J. Somatic cell genetics of antibody-secreting cells: Studies of clonal diversification and analysis by cell fusion. Cold Spring Harbor Symp Quant Biol. 41: 793–803, 1977.

7. Taylor, C. R. Immunoperoxidase techniques. Theoretical and practical aspects. Arch. Path. Lab. Med. 102: 113–121, 1978.

4

Enzymes as Markers in the Detection and Management of Cancer

T. Ming Chu

INTRODUCTION

Abnormality in enzyme activity is one of the major biochemical characteristics of tumor cells. Qualitative or quantitative difference in enzyme activity has long been used as a parameter in distinguishing a tumor cell from its normal counterpart, and as the target in developing therapeutic agents against cancer. The use of enzymes as tumor markers is based on the concept that alterations in the gene expression in malignant transformation can be detected at the level of the end products, the enzymes or isoenzymes. Although qualitative differences in enzyme expression between normal and tumor cells would be the ideal probe to indicate the presence of a tumor, at the present stage of development no such specific enzyme has been clinically utilized. Findings on the enzymatic imbalance in cancer cells have been applied to the development of diagnostic tests for cancer.

Technology has not yet advanced to the point where a single tumor cell or even a tiny tumor mass can be detected clinically by an enzymatic method alone. This is because the diagnostic enzyme assay is commonly used to measure activity in serum, urine, and other extracellular fluids, where the abnormality of enzyme activity is vastly diluted or the active enzyme is metabolized, although recent

Our work reported in this chapter was supported in part by research grants CA-15126, CA-15437, and CA-18410 awarded by NCI, DHHS.

immunochemical assay has in part solved the latter problem. Despite these inherent difficulties, enzymatic assay for cancer has yielded promising results as an aid for initial detection, for differential diagnosis, for defining the possible organ site, for providing information for additional work-up on a patient, and for evaluating the progression or regression of the disease, as well as for monitoring the efficacy of treatment.

This chapter reviews the most recent developments in the use of enzymes as markers for the diagnosis and treatment of cancer patients. Readers are also referred to other published materials for review (Schwartz, 1982).

PROSTATIC ACID PHOSPHATASE

Acid phosphatase of the prostate was the first tumor marker to be discovered, perhaps with the exception of Bence Jones protein. Serum acid phosphatase assay has been used for over 50 years as a laboratory aid for the diagnosis of metastatic prostate cancer. As far as organ and cell type specificity is concerned, prostatic acid phosphatase (PAP) is one of the few enzyme markers exhibiting such a unique characteristic. It also is the best-known and most extensively investigated marker enzyme in cancer.

Biochemically, PAP is a glycoprotein with a molecular weight of 100 kd, consisting of 2 dimers, 13% carbohydrates, and 87% peptides with multiple isoelectric points. *N*-Terminal amino acid is lysine, and partial sequence has also been reported recently. Over the past several years, PAP has been measured by three generations of techniques: spectrophotometry or biochemistry, hetero-antiserum, and monoclonal antibody immunochemistry. Several unique antigenic determinants specific to PAP have been identified by monoclonal antibodies, supporting the immunologic specificity of this enzyme (Lee et al., 1982). At least ten different biochemical and immunological methods, including several commercial kits, are readily available. Indeed, the specificity and sensitivity of the diagnostic test for this enzyme has reached a point second to none, reflecting the significant clinical interest in this "oldest" enzyme marker (Chu et al., 1982).

Clinically, the biochemical and the immunological methods commonly in use serve equally well for identifying the patients with advanced stage of prostate cancer. Although it is generally assumed that either assay is adequate as a monitor for the majority of metastatic prostate cancer patients, the major difference in clinical utilization between these two types of assay occurs where serial measurements are required for detecting early disease recurrence and for monitoring efficacy of treatment response (Killian et al., 1982).

In a group of 57 patients with pathological stages A_2 to D_1 prostate cancer who had received either a definitive surgical or radiation therapy, and who were receiving adjuvant chemotherapy, serum acid phosphatase activity as measured by a biochemical method (designated AcP) and prostatic acid phosphatase as measured by an immunochemical method (designated PAP) were compared for their relative values in monitoring these patients. Likewise, in a group of 33 patients with newly diagnosed stage D_2 disease with no prior therapy, who were receiving surgical, hormonal, or chemotherapy, AcP and PAP were similarly compared. The analysis revealed that an elevated PAP in disease recurrence and disease progression generally precedes an elevated AcP and thus represents a more sensitive parameter. Variation in serially increased PAP is more predictive than that of AcP for disease recurrence and progression. Additionally, PAP was shown to be a more sensitive monitor than AcP for change in objective treatment response. These observations can be attributed to the fact that PAP as measured by a defined sensitive immunological method is more specific than AcP for the activity of prostate cancer.

It should be noted that PAP is prostate specific, rather than prostate-tumor specific. Thus, a slight elevation of serum PAP in some patients with benign prostatic hypertrophy can be expected and has been detected. Because of this possible false-positivity in patients with benign disease and true-negativity in a significant number of patients with very early prostate cancer, PAP has not been judged as a suitable screening modality for prostate cancer.

Clinical utilization of the PAP assay can be greatly enhanced if it is combined with other prostate cancer-related markers. For example, in advanced prostate cancer, bone isoenzyme of serum alkaline phosphatase and PAP have been shown to be of increased and reliable value as quantitative markers of tumor load and of bone matastasis. When combined with human prostate-specific antigen (PA) assay, a recently reported marker of prostate cancer, an additive clinical value in the immunodiagnosis of prostate cancer was demonstrated. Although neither PAP nor PA is prostate-tumor specific, one apparent advantage of this combination test is the increase in the sensitivity of detection of an elevation of either marker. Another obvious advantage is that adjustments can be made of various cutoff points for each marker assay, allowing selection of the values that result in best sensitivity and specificity. Since both PAP and prostate antigen are specific to the prostate, false-positives occur extremely rarely, if at all.

In addition to serum assay, tissue stain of PAP with specific anti-PAP antibody by means of the immunohistochemical technique has been shown to be of great value in identifying the prostate origin of a tumor. This is used to explore the specificity of PAP in the histogenesis of tumor affecting the prostate gland and to demonstrate the prostate origin of metastasis in various sites. A conventional peroxidase–antiperoxidase procedure was performed on formalin-fixed, paraffin-embedded, routine pathology material. Using specific anti-PAP prepared in our laboratory, all cases of primary and metastatic prostate adenocarcinomas stained positively, while none of the specimens from cases of non-prostatic primary and secondary tumors stained. The results demonstrated that the immunohistochemical stain of PAP is a practical, sensitive, and specific diagnostic test for the prostate origin of an otherwise unclassifiable primary or metastatic tumor.

Although PAP is predominatly a cytoplasmic protein, not cell surface or plasma membrane associated, it has been used with some degree of success as the target for radioimmunodetection of prostate tumor.

Specific polyclonal antiserum to PAP, labeled with radioactive iodine, has been able to localize tumor, particularly bone metastasis. Equally surprising is the recent report on the *in vivo* application of PAP monoclonal antibody in antibody-directed experimental chemotherapy in human prostate tumor xenograft in animals with an antibody–drug (such as 5-fluorouracil deoxyriboside) conjugate. This experimental animal work with monoclonal anti-PAP will hopefully provide useful information toward the possible addition of new clinical modalities to prostate cancer.

Despite the extensive laboratory and clinical investigation of PAP during the past five decades, the basic biology of PAP in prostate or prostate cancer is totally unknown. In absolute quantitative values, PAP in malignant prostate is less than that in normal or benign prostate in terms of protein or DNA. Why does PAP in circulation indicate otherwise? This is just one of the most simple and intriguing questions to be faced with PAP.

NEURON-SPECIFIC ENOLASE

Neuron-specific enolase (NSE), or nervous system-specific enolase ($\gamma\gamma$-isoenzyme of enolase), is a relatively new tumor marker enzyme. Although enolase is a common, yet important, enzyme and best known for its role involving the synthesis of ATP in glycolysis, its clinical significance in oncology has only been appreciated in the past two years. NSE was first identified in brain tissue and is found only in the cells associated with amine precursor uptake and decarboxylation (APUD) and in the neurons of the diffuse neuroendocrine system. Antiserum directed against purified NSE is highly specific and possesses no cross-reactivity with enolase of non-neuron origin. This characterisitic makes NSE a suitable marker enzyme for tumors of a neuroendocrine or APUD nature. Availability of specific antiserum reagent ensures an easy immunologic assay (ELIA or RIA) for NSE. Again, it should be emphasized that NSE is not a tumor-specific enzyme.

Using serum NSE as the marker, small cell carcinoma of the lung was the first tumor shown to be associated with an elevated NSE level (Carney et al., 1982). In a group of 94 newly diagnosed untreated patients, including 38 with limited disease and 56 with extensive disease, serum NSE was raised (> 12 ng/ml) in 39% and 87% of patients, respectively (overall 69%). Quantitative NSE level was related to extent of disease, as extensive-stage patients had a significantly higher mean NSE level (59 ng/ml) than did limited-stage patients (13.8 ng/ml). In extensive-disease patients, NSE was elevated in 34/41 of patients with metastases at 1 or 2 sites and in all 15 patients who had metastases at 3 or more sites. Additionally, serum NSE was shown to be an effective monitor for treatment response, as serial measurements revealed an excellent clinical correlation in 23 patients receiving combination chemotherapy. Furthermore, the source of serum NSE was shown to originate from tumor cells, as continuous cell lines established from 10 patients of the study expressed significant levels of NSE. These results are extremely interesting from at least two points of view: first, a "new" enzyme tumor marker, NSE, has been identified; second, a simple NSE assay alone has been shown to be effective in monitoring the clinical response of small cell lung cancer, one of the few tumors that can be treated with presently available means.

Serum NSE has also been shown to be of clinical value in neuroblastoma as a prognostic biochemical marker. Serum NSE was measured in 122 patients with metastatic neuroblastoma (clinical stage IV), and 96% of these patients had an elevated NSE. Those patients exhibiting a NSE of above 100 ng/ml were generally associated with poor prognosis, particularly in infants less than 1 year old at diagnosis. All 7 patients with NSE below 100 ng/ml were alive up to 3 years after diagnosis, whereas 7 of 8 with NSE above 100 ng/ml died within 1 year of diagnosis.

Combining NSE with other markers, such as pancreatic polypeptide and HCG, could be useful in determining prognosis and in monitoring response to therapy in pancreatic islet cell tumors and carcinoid tumors of the gastrointestinal tract. NSE is commonly elevated in nonfunctioning pancreatic islet cell tumors, but infrequently in glucagonomas and intestinal islet cell tumors.

Immunohistochemical staining of NSE has been used as a diagnostic tool. Differential diagnosis of neuroblastoma, which expresses NSE, from Wilm's tumor has been reported. Additionally, in one series of 157 pancreatic endocrine tumors where α-HCG and NSE immunohistochemical stains were examined, α-HCG immunoreactive cells were present in 42/56 functioning malignant pancreatic endocrine tumors, but in only 1/67 functioning benign tumors, in only 1/17 nonfunctioning malignant, and in none of 17 nonfunctioning benign tumors; in all but 1 of these tumors NSE was detected (Kloppel et al., 1983). Thus, α-HCG represents a reliable marker for malignancy in functioning pancreatic endocrine tumors, and the presence of NSE established the neuroendocrine nature of the tumors. Further diagnostic value of immunostaining on NSE has been shown in Merkel cell tumor, in thyroid cell tumor, in thymic carcinoid tumor, and in a few melanomas. It can be expected that further clinical value of NSE will be derived from tumors of neuroendocrine origin and those of APUD cells.

In the remainder of this chapter, some "old" enzyme markers associated with cancer are briefly updated with recent information.

RIBONUCLEASE

Ribonuclease (RNAase) as an enzyme marker for cancer, in particular for pancreatic cancer, is perhaps the most controversial subject in recent biochemical oncology. The use of serum RNAase in the diagnosis of pancreatic cancer was received with great enthusiasm in 1976, when a paper in the *Proceedings of the National Academy of Sciences* (USA) reported strikingly abnormal elevation of serum RNAase activity in patients with pancreatic cancer (Reddi & Holland, 1976). RNAase was measured biochemically with poly(C) as substrate. Ninety percent of pancreatic cancer patients exhibited an elevated activity (> 250 U/ml) of serum RNAase, while 90% of patients with various cancers (breast, lung, colon, stomach, liver) were below this level. Severe renal insufficiency was the only nonmalignant clinical condition where a markedly elevated serum RNAase activity was observed. There was no elevation in the serum RNAase level of patients with pancreatitis. Serum RNAase was thus advocated— because of its unique specificity, its pancreas origin, and its high elevation in pancreas cancer as indicated in this report—as a reliable enzyme marker for pancreatic carcinoma.

This promising report was confronted three years later by a report, published in the same journal, which demonstrated that serum RNAase was not useful in the diagnosis of pancreas cancer (Peterson, 1979). Data were presented to show that, using poly(C) as substrate also, serum RNAase activity was equally elevated in patients with pancreatic cancer, with pancreatitis, and with nonpancreatic disease or malignancy. Patients with pancreas carcinoma could not be separated from those with others. Additionally, patients with total pancreatectomy still exhibited elevated serum RNAase activity after surgery. Patients with early and "curable" pancreatic cancer had normal serum RNAase activity, as did those with extensive malignancy without obstructive jaundice.

These two major papers on the role of serum RNAase in the diagnosis of pancreas cancer generated a series of reports in the following years. Although a few supported the positive report, the majority of recent publications indicated that serum RNAase measurement has limited value, if any at all, in biochemical diagnosis of pancreas cancer. In fact, pancreatic cancer is such a dismal type of cancer that there is no marker at all at present that is useful for the early detection of this malignancy, which has the poorest prognosis of all.

It should not be construed that RNAase is no longer a viable marker for cancer of the pancreas or other cancers. It suggests that further basic investigation is required to delineate the exact nature of RNAase in cancer. RNAase is well known for its presence as multiple forms with various molecular weights, isoelectric points, sources of origin, substrate affinity, and reaction kinetics, as well as possible immunologic specificity as reported recently. For example, several RNAases have been purified from the pancreas, malignant pancreatic ascites, and the prostate, as well as other tissues (Lee et al., 1983). Amino acid composition and sequence were reported for some of the RNAases of various origins. These are some important issues to be addressed by additional research before any clinical investigation is further attempted on RNAase.

TERMINAL DEOXYNUCLEOTIDYL TRANSFERASE

Very few enzyme markers have been identified to be associated with non-solid tumors. Among them, terminal deoxynucleotidyl transferase (TdT) is the most extensively investigated and promising enzyme parameter, at least for certain forms of leukemia. TdT was first identified in calf thymus over 20 years ago. Clinical importance of this enzyme was not appreciated until TdT was found about 10 years ago to be present in ALL cells and T-ALL cell lines. TdT is an enzyme that polymerizes DNA by catalyzing the addition of deoxynucleotide residue to the 3′-hydroxyl group of a primer polydeoxynucleotide, regardless of its length (at least 3), from deoxyribonucleoside triphosphates without the requirement of a template polynucleotide. Although antibody specific to TdT, without cross-reactivity with other DNA polymerases (α, β, γ), is available, the biochemical approach is also a commonly used analytical technique for TdT.

TdT activity in lymphocytes from normal peripheral blood is generally low or not detectable, although it can be slightly induced in the short term by PHA stimulation. Highly elevated TdT activity is found in almost all patients with ALL, 30% of patients with blast CML, and approximately 10% of patients with AML, as well as in a small percentage of patients with non-Hodgkin's leukemia. It should be noted that in patients with elevated TdT activity, not all cells were always positive for TdT. For example, with the use of the immunofluorescence technique, in ALL the portion of cells positive for TdT was 20–80% during relapse and less than 1% during remission. In CML, positive cells for TdT would moderately increase during "lymphoblastic" crisis.

TdT has been shown to be of prognostic significance in adult patients with leukemia and malignant lymphoma. The activity of TdT is correlated with remission frequency and duration, and with survival in patients with ALL, ANLL, and malignant non-Hodgkin's lymphoma (Mertelsmann, 1982). However, quantitative activity of TdT alone in blasts at time of diagnosis of children with typical ALL generally did not necessarily convey prognostic information.

When combined with adenosine deaminase, TdT can be used for the subclassification of ALL. In T-ALL, TdT is positive and there is a very high level of adenosine deaminase activity; in non–T-, non–B-ALL TdT is positive with an intermediate level of adenosine deaminase; and in B-ALL, TdT is negative or very low along with a low level of adenosine deaminase. Similar observations have been reported for malignant lymphoma; only those with T- or non–T-, non–B-lymphoblastic lymphoma were found to have TdT activity comparable to that of ALL cells.

LACTATE DEHYDROGENASE ISOENZYME

Lactate dehydrongenase (LDH) is a well-known enzyme that is routinely analyzed in the clinical laboratory. Serum LDH activity is a nonspecific parameter for a variety of abnormal physiologic and pathologic conditions and has not been used as a specific enzyme marker for neoplastic disease. Isoenzyme pattern (I to V) of LDH has also been commonly examined by the electrophoretic technique and had added limited value for cancer diagnosis. Although occasionally an "abnormal" peak within the traditional LDH isoenzymes is detected in some diseases, including cancer, its clinical significance is not well understood. A new LDH isoenzyme, designated LDH_k, was recently reported to be of importance in cancer (Anderson et al., 1983).

LDH_k, or asp56/LDH_k, is more basic electrophoretically than other common isoenzymes of LDH. It was originally identified as a gene product as expressed by the Kirsten murine sarcoma virus under anaerobic conditions. It is generally assumed that the molecular weight of LDH_k is 56 kd. Since it is also an anaerobic shock polypeptide, it is designated asp56/LDH_k, representing the protein as asp56 and the activity as LDH_k. In addition to the cells infected with Kirsten murine sarcoma virus, LDH_k has been purified from other sources, including human colon carcinoma. Biochemically, LDH_k is reversibly inhibited by oxygen and is noncompetitively inhibited by GTP and ATP, which exhibited no effect on the activity of other common LDH isoenzymes.

The rationale for examining LDH_k as a tumor marker comes from the observation that many human cancers have been reported recently to express a cellular oncogene related to that of the Kirstein virus, and that LDH_k represents a transforming activity of the virus. Preliminary results on LDH_k obtained from human tumor tissues and cancer patients' serum have been encouraging. The assay is generally performed on the imidazole/borate electrophoretic gel system with the LDH_k from Kirsten murine sarcoma virus-transformed cells as the reference. Gel is stained for LDH activity, which is then quantitatively scanned by a densitometer.

Examination of human tissue revealed that tumor tissue usually demonstrated an LDH_k peak, with an activity 10- to 100-fold greater than that of adjacent "normal" tissue. Specimens examined were those of colon carcinoma, mammary carcinoma, laryngeal carcinoma, stomach carcinoma, renal carcinoma, melanoma, and liposarcoma. It is noted that traditional LDH isoenzymes showed much less activity in both tumor and normal tissues and exhibited no differences in their activities when assayed in the presence or absence of oxygen. These results therefore showed that a variety of human tumors express quantitatively an elevated LDH_k activity when compared with their normal counterparts.

Serum specimens from cancer patients and normal controls also revealed a quantitative difference between these two groups. Approximately 50% of cancer patients demonstrated the presence of serum LDH_k, while normal controls seldom did.

This initial study involving a limited number of patients has clearly presented a promising role for LDH_k as a possible cancer marker. Its ultimate significance in clinical oncology awaits additional investigations, particularly on specimens from the early stages of cancer, and from those undergoing therapeutic treatment.

GLYCOSYLTRANSFERASES

Glycosyltransferases are a group of enzymes involving the transfer and addition of a specific carbohydrate from a primer donor to a specific protein and glycoprotein acceptor. They occur widely in animal tissues and have been known for some time. However, the importance of glycosyltransferases in clinical oncology was not appreciated until the late 1970s. Although their role in cancer metastasis has been largely speculative, clinical investigation on these enzymes as potential tumor markers has been extensive. Three enzymes in the group are better known—galactosyltransferase, sialyltransferase, and fucosyltransferase, which catalyze the addition of galactose, sialic acid, and fucose, respectively, to their specific acceptors. The former two enzymes have been studied the most.

Galactosyltransferase activity in serum was found to be elevated in a variety of cancer patients. As with other tumor markers, the percentage of early cancer patients exhibiting an elevated serum enzyme level was less than that of advanced cancer patients. For example, in breast cancer, only 15% of stage I patients showed an elevated serum galactosyltransferase (UDP-galactose:*N*-acetylglucosamine) activity, whereas 65% of stage II, 80% of stage III, and over 95% of stage IV patients, respectively, registered a positive reading. However, this is not necessarily the case in some tumor tissues—e.g. transitional cell carcinoma of the bladder, where an increased activity of galactosyltransferase (UDP-galactose:glycoprotein) showed no correlation with tumor stage or grade. Galactosyltransferase (UDP-galactose:glycoprotein) has been claimed to be a very useful marker, more sensitive than 5′-nucleotidase, for ovarian cancer. It also appeared to be correlated with patients' clinical status.

As in many other enzymes, serum galactosyltransferase activity is derived from a combination of isoenzymes. An isoenzyme designated galactosyltransferase II (GT-II) has been identified, by polyacrylamide gel electrophoresis fortified with ^{3}H-labeled UDP-galactose, to be primarily associated with cancer (Podolsky et al., 1981). With this more defined procedure, elevated serum GT-II was detected in 85/117 patients with colorectal cancer, 18/23 with breast cancer, 13/20 with lung cancer, 15/18 with pancreas cancer, and 12/16 with stomach cancer, along with a series of other cancers including prostate, gallbladder and bile duct, kidney, lymphoma, and hepatoma, but not in patients with melanoma or osteosarcoma. An overall positive rate of 71% (165/232) was reported.

The most interesting clinical report on GT-II was from a prospective study of 270 patients for detecting pancreas carcinoma with GT-II; the report compared this method with other serological tumor markers and with commonly practiced physical diagnostic skills for sensitivity and specificity of each test (Podolsky et al., 1981). These included carcinoembryonic antigen (CEA), α-fetoprotein, ferritin, C1q binding, and RNAase, plus ultrasound, computerized body tomography (CBT), and endoscopic retrograde cholangiopancreatography (ERCP). The final diagnosis of the 270 patients evaluated was 61 with pancreas cancer, 28 with other gastrointestinal or intraabdominal primary cancers, as well as 14 with other cancers, along with 167 patients with benign diseases including 24 with cholelithiasis or biliary-tract disease, 16 with acute pancreatitis, and 27 with chronic pancreatitis or depression. Among the serological markers determined, GT-II was shown to be the most sensitive (67%) and specific (98%) for discrimination between benign and malignant pancreatic disease (CEA was the next most useful marker). In comparison with ultrasound or CBT, GT-II showed no significant difference in sensitivity in detecting pancreas carcinoma. Only ERCP was more sensitive (98%) than GT-II. GT-II combined with radiologic or endoscopic tests resulted in a sensitivity greater than any single diagnostic test alone. However, the combination of GT-II with any of the other serologic markers did not yield a statistically significant increase in pancreas cancer detection.

In this prospective study, an elevated serum RNAase was detected in 30% of patients with pancreas cancer and in 14% of patients with benign diseases. As discussed earlier in this chapter, RNAase activity apparently is not a useful diagnostic test, and this is further documented in the above report.

Indeed, this is a very interesting study on GT-II as an enzyme marker for cancer, especially for carcinoma of the pancreas. Data for early and localized pancreatic cancer are, unfortunately, not available in this report. If GT-II were able to detect asymptomatic patients, it really would be a "break-through" marker for this malignancy. One of the current research activities involves development of a simplified

GT-II assay, such as RIA or ELISA, specific for this isoenzyme of galactosyltransferase.

An ELISA using "monospecific" rabbit antibodies against galactosyltransferase (lactose synthase) purified from human milk was recently reported (Verdon et al., 1983). The assay was able to detect 10 μg of enzyme/liter of sample. Healthy blood donors were found to contain 60–436 μg/liter. From an initial study with a limited number of patients, the serum level of the enzyme in ovarian cancer appeared to correlate with tumor burden of the patients. A highly elevated level was predominately found in ovarian cancer patients, particularly those with persistent or progressive disease (FIGO stage III and IV). In patients with cancer of the breast and lung, slightly but not significantly higher values were found. Thus, the ELISA assay for this galactosyltransferase appeared to be "specific" for ovarian cancer to some extent. Serum level may serve mainly for patient monitoring, although enzyme level in ascites was reported useful for diagnosis by this procedure.

Sialyltransferase catalyzes the transfer of sialic acid from the nucleotide cytidine monophosphate sialic acid to the galactose residue of desialylated fetuin. Serum sialyltransferase activity has been extensively studied in cancer patients (Henderson & Kessel, 1977). Abnormal activity was generally found in a significant number (> 80%) of all patients, as observed in some reports. However, elevated sialyltransferase activity was detected in patients with a variety of benign and non-neoplastic diseases, such as chronic and acute liver disorders and rheumatoid arthritis.

Serum sialyltransferase appears to be most effective in monitoring the clinical status of cancer patients. Some patients with primary breast carcinoma, without metastasis, had elevated levels. Mastectomy caused a rapid fall of abnormal enzyme activity, to within the normal range in patients with stage I breast cancer, but not in those with stage II or III diseases. In some patients with metastatic breast cancer, elevated enzyme levels decreased only after responding to treatment. The enzyme activity increased when disease recurrence developed. Thus, serum sialyltransferase may be associated with the extent of the disease and correlated with success or failure of treatment in breast carcinoma.

The fucosyltransferases are a family of enzymes that catalyze the transfer of the monosaccharide fucose from a GDP-fucose donor to specific acceptors. At least three serum fucosyltransferases have been described. Elevated levels of fucosyltransferase activity were found in some patients with cancer of the colon, breast, and other solid tumors, as well as in AML and non-Hodgkin's lymphoma. Although it has been disputed that the different acceptors used in the assay would alter enzyme mechanism and may measure a different fucosyltransferase activity, it is generally agreed that an elevated enzyme level is associated with proliferative and secretory processes of both normal and noeplastic cells (Kessel & Bauer 1979). Therefore, the most promising utilization of serum fucosyltransferase activity, like sialyltransferase, is in the monitoring of patients, perhaps with the exception of GDP-fucose:*N*-acetylglucosaminide fucosyltransferase.

OTHER ENZYME CANCER MARKERS

The enzymes described above are those that have been more extensively studied or utilized in clinical oncology in recent years. There are many other enzymes that have been reported to be associated with cancer. Some of these putative markers are briefly reviewed.

γ-Glutamyltranspeptidase (γ-GTP) was originally studied in experimental animals with liver cancer. It is present in preneoplastic liver and hepatoma, but not in the normal adult rat liver. γ-GTP has been shown in human cancer to be a useful laboratory parameter for the detection of secondary liver metastasis when combined with other assays, such as carcinoembryonic antigen or phosphohexose isomerase. Recent reports also indicated that γ-GTP level can be used as an aid in the management of human cancer (Sahm et al., 1983). In a study where plasma γ-GTP was measured in 435 cancer patients along with 120 normal healthy controls and 24 non-neoplastic immunologic disorders, the mean γ-GTP levels in cancer patients were significantly elevated, with the exception of those with malignant lymphoma. Additionally, serially increasing γ-GTP was associated with disease progression or metastasis, whereas a normal level was detected in disease-free patients. Patients responding to therapy were associated with decreasing levels.

Although creatine kinase (CK), specifically the brain-type isoenzyme CK-BB, is present in epithelial cells of various normal tissues and neoplasms (Tsung, 1983), CK-BB has been advocated by some investigators as a tumor marker, particularly for carcinoma of the prostate and breast. Total CK activity was usually very low in tumor tissues. Presumably a bulky tumor or an advanced stage of malignancy is a requisite to the release of detectable CK-BB in circulation.

Several isoenzymes of alkaline phosphatase have been identified in the circulation of cancer patients, such as the Nagao isoenzyme in ovarian cancer, liver isoenzyme in hepatic metastatis, and bone isoenzyme in bone metastasis. A variety of cancers have also been found to be associated with elevated serum alkaline phosphatase isoenzymes (Kottel & Fishman, 1982). The identification of variants on electrophoresis and characterization of these isoenzymes, as well as recent development of monoclonal antibodies specific to variant isoenzymes, should provide additional information on the role of alkaline phosphatase in cancer. At present, the most important clinical value of alkaline phosphatase is in its combination with other markers. For example, the combination of alkaline phosphatase and CEA can be used economically to screen for liver metastasis and to determine which patients should undergo a liver scan (Chu, 1982). The combination of alkaline phosphatase bone isoenzyme, prostatic acid phosphatase, and prostate antigen is an extremely effective indicator for monitoring prostate cancer.

A relatively new assay for 5'-nucleotide phosphodiesterase isoenzyme V activity has been shown by a few investigators to be very effective in detecting hepatic metastasis and primary hepatocellular carcinoma. This enzyme is different from the one commonly known as 5'-nucleotidase. It is an exonuclease hydrolyzing a phosphodiester to produce a nucleotide and an alcohol. Technical complicity in measuring this enzyme is the major factor that has limited this assay to a very selected group of investigators.

Adenosine deaminase is a fairly well known enzyme, and its clinical value, along with TdT, in ALL was discussed previously. In addition, it has been shown to be a biochemical marker for chronic myelogenous leukemias, because nearly 90% of patients in the accelerated phase had an elevation of adenosine deaminease activity. The elevation was not a direct reflection of an increased absolute blast count.

Thymidine kinase isoenzymes were shown to be of prognostic relevance in a subgroup of adult non-Hodgkin's lymphoma. Peripheral blood thymidine kinase I was used as an independent marker for identifying a subgroup of patients who responded poorly to current therapy and required new therapeutic approaches.

An elevation of enzyme activity or protein mass is usually used, as previously discussed, as the parameter for the manifestation of malignancy. In contrast to this increase in enzyme activity in cancer, a decrease was recently reported in the activity of an enzyme, α-L-fucosidase, in the serum of ovarian cancer patients (Barlow et al., 1981). The frequency of low α-fucosidase level was 3 times greater in ovarian cancer patients when compared with a control female population. Low levels appeared to have no correlation with disease stage, tumor burden, histologic type, or grade of differentiation.

However, a familial study suggested that the enzyme deficiency may be heritable and associated with an increased risk for the development of ovarian cancer. This interesting observation requires additional study for confirmation; if it is indeed so, then this enzyme may be a potential epidemiological biochemical marker for ovarian cancer.

REFERENCES

Anderson, G. R., Polonis, V. R., Petell, J. K., Saavedra, R. A., Manly, K. F., and Matovcik, L. M. Asp56/LDH$_k$ in human cancer. Isoenzymes 11: 155–172, 1983.

Barlow, J. J., DiCoccio, R. A., Dillard, P. H., Blumenson, L. E., and Matta, K. L. Frequency of an allele for low activity of focusidase in sera. J. Natl. Cancer. Inst. 67: 1005–1009, 1981.

Carney, D. N., Ihde, D. C., Cohen, M. H., Marangos, J., Bunn, P. A., Minna, J. D., and Gazdar, A. F. Serum neuron-specific enolase: A marker for disease extent and response to therapy of small cell lung cancer. Lancet I: 583–585, 1982.

Chu, T. M. The detection of liver metastasis by laboratory tests. In: Liver Metastasis (eds. L. Weiss and H. A. Gilbert), pp. 255–265, 1982. G. K. Hall Medical Publishers, Boston.

Chu, T. M., Wang, M. C., Lee, C. L., Killian, C. S., and Murphy, G. P. Prostatic acid phosphatase in human prostate cancer. In: Biochemical Markers for Cancer (ed. T. M. Chu), pp. 117–136, 1982. Marcel Dekker, Inc., New York.

Henderson, M., and Kessel, D. Alterations in plasma sialyltransferase level in patients with neoplastic disease. Cancer 39: 1129–1134, 1977.

Kessel, D., and Bauer, C. H. Human serum fucosyltransferase and tumor therapy. Science 204: 647, 1979.

Killian, C. S., Vargas, F. P., Slack, N. H., Murphy, G. P., and Chu, T. M. Prostate-specific acid phosphatase versus acid phosphatase in monitoring patients with prostatic cancer. Ann. N.Y. Acad. Sci. 390: 122–132, 1982.

Kloppel, G., Girard, J., Polak, J. M., Vaitukaitis, J. L., Kasper, M., and Heitz, P. U. Alpha-human chorionic gonadotropin and neuron-specific enolase as markers for malignancy and neuroendocrine nature of pancreatic endocrine tumors. Cancer Detect. Prev. 6: 161–166, 1983.

Kottel, R. H., and Fishman W. H. Developmental alkaline phosphatase as biochemical tumor markers. In: Biochemical Markers for Cancer (ed. T. M. Chu), pp. 93–116, 1982. Marcek Dekker, Inc., New York.

Lee, C. L., Li, S. L., and Chu, T. M. Purification and characterization of ribonucleases from human seminal plasma. Biochem. J. 215: 605–612, 1983.

Lee, C. L., Li, C. Y., Jou, Y. H., Murphy, G. P., and Chu, T. M. Immunochemical characterization of prostatic acid phosphatase with monoclonal antibodies. Ann. N.Y. Acad. Sci. 390: 52–61, 1982.

Mertelsmann, R. The prognostic significance of terminal deoxynucleotidyl transferase in patients with leukemias and malignant lymphomas. Adv. Exp. Med. Biol. 145: 259–277, 1982.

Peterson, L. M. Serum ribonuclease in the diagnosis of pancreatic carcinoma. Proc. Natl. Acad. Sci. USA. 76: 2630–2634, 1979.

Podolsky, D. K., McPhee, M. S., Alpert, E., Warshaw, A. L., and Isselbacher, K. J. Galactosyltransferase isoenzyme II in the detection of pancreatic cancer: Comparisons with radiologic, endoscopic and serologic tests. New Eng. J. Med. 304: 1313–1318, 1981.

Reddi, K. K., and Holland, J. F. Elevated serum ribonuclease in patients with pancreatic cancer. Proc. Natl. Acad. Sci. USA 73: 2308–2310, 1976.

Sahm, D. F., Murray, J. L., Munson, P. L., Nordquist, R. E., and Lerner, M. P. Gamma-glutamyltranspeptidase levels as an aid with the management of human cancer. Cancer 52: 1673–1678, 1983.

Schwartz, M. K. Enzymes as tumor markers. In: Biochemical Markers for Cancer (ed. T. M. Chu), pp. 81–92, 1982. Marcel Dekker, Inc., New York.

Tsung, S. H. Creatine kinase activity and isoenzyme pattern in various normal tissues and neoplasms. Clin. Chem. 29: 2040–2043, 1983.

Verdon, B., Berger, E. G., Salchli, S., Goldrisch, A., and Gerber, A. An enzyme-linked immunosorbent assay for lactose synthase (galactosyltransferase) in serum and its application as a tumor marker in ovarian carcinoma. Clin. Chem. 29: 1928–1933, 1983.

5

Agglutination Tests
in Detecting Cell Surface Antigens

Nasser Javadpour, M.D.

The cell surface antigens are antigens that may appear, delete, and/or undergo some changes as a result of carcinogenesis.[8,9] The presence of these cell markers is normally controlled by the genetic make-up of the cells. As the cells undergo transformation, the control and synthesis of these antigens may also undergo some changes.[6,14] ABO (H) cell surface antigens serve as an example of cell surface antigens that may undergo changes according to the severity of malignant transformation of normal tissue harboring such antigens. These changes may happen prior to and independent of morphologic changes: therefore, presence or absence of these cell surface antigens may serve as another parameter in the diagnosis and staging of and therapeutic approaches to a given cancer.

In this chapter, we discuss the methods for detecting these antigens and their clinical significance in terms of management of patients with various cell surface antigens and their changes in malignancy. The cell surface antigens that may be clinically useful and are currently under intensive investigation are: ABO (H) cell surface antigens, T antigen, and tumor-associated antigens.

ABO (H) CELL SURFACE ANTIGENS

Davidsohn and co-workers developed the specific red cell adherence test (SRCA) to determine the presence or absence of ABO (H) cell surface antigens.[3] In applying the test to cancer of the cervix, they found that as cells from the cervix undergo malignant dedifferentiation from atypia to anaplasia, there appears to occur a progressive loss of the ABO (H) cell surface antigens.

Detection of ABO (H) cell surface antigens has become increasingly important over the last several years, not only in research but also in clinical medicine. Recent work by several authors in the field of urology has shown a correlation between loss of ABO (H) cell surface antigens and potential for metastasis or recurrence of transitional cell carcinoma of the bladder.[1] Although cell surface antigens have been detected and correlated with other cancers (Table 5–1), the major studies have been in bladder cancer. Before examining the value of ABO (H) cell surface antigens, we will discuss the SRCA tests for detecting these cell surface antigens.

Techniques of SRCA

Five-micron-thick histologic sections are deparaffinized and cleared in several changes of xylene and alcohol and rinsed in three changes of 0.5 M Tris buffered saline, pH 7.4, for 5 min each (Table 5–2). The slides are then incubated with isoantibody (anti-A or anti-B blood grouping human sera) in moist petri dishes for 15 min. The slides are then washed in three changes of buffered saline for 15 min each and are then incubated with isologous indicator erythrocytes for 15 min.

Table 5–1 Normal Tissue Having ABO (H) Isoantigens

	SRCA	
Organs	Positive	Negative
Adrenal		Cortex and medulla
Blood	Erythrocytes	Leukocytes
Blood vessels	Endothelial cells	
Bronchus	Epithelium	
Nervous system		Cell and glia
Endocervis	Squamous epithelium	Basal layer
Esophagus	Squamous epithelium	
Fallopian tube	Columnar epithelium	
Gallbladder	Columnar epithelium	
Kidney	Glomeruli	Convoluted tubule
Ureter	Transitional cells	Submucosa of muscularis
Urinary bladder	Transitional cells	Submucosa of muscularis

Table 5–2 Technique for Detecting ABO (H) Antigen

1. Deparaffinize the section by immersing in xylene 5 min ×2.
2. Wash the section by immersing in absolute alcohol 5 min ×2.
3. Rehydrate the section by immersing the section in phosphate buffer, pH 7.4, 5 min ×3.
4. Incubate the section with appropriate antibody.
5. Wash the excess antibody with phosphate buffer, pH 7.4, ×3.
6. Overlay isologous blood cells (3% whole blood cell suspension on the section) and spread uniformly; incubate for 5 min.
7. Invert the slide and rest on two small pieces of applicator stick in petri dish, fill the dish with buffer in such a way that the lower portion of the slide is submerged, and let it stand for 5 min.
8. Examine the section for the presence or absence of adhered red cells under a low-powered microscope.

The erythrocytes are outdated blood bank cells washed three times in buffered saline and resuspended to give a 3–5% suspension. The slides are then carefully inverted on wood applicator sticks in petri dishes filled with just enough buffered saline to cover the inverted surface of the slide. This allows the unreacted erythrocytes to settle off the slide. The slides are then gently moved to a clear area of the petri dish and are read and photographed while inverted in saline (Fig. 5–1).

For blood group O patients, H antigen is assayed for by using a *Ulex europaeus* extract in place of an antiserum. Twenty grams of *Ulex europaeus* seeds are ground up and then homogenized in 11 ml of buffered saline at 0°C. This preparation is then centrifuged on the Beckman preparatory ultracentrifuge at 15,000 rpm for 30 min, and the supernatant is recentrifuged at 36,000 rpm for 120 min at 0°C. The supernatant is immediately frozen at −20°C until needed. This preparation is used in place of the human blood grouping antisera and is incubated with the slides for 1 h. The O erythrocytes are treated with 0.01% papain (Sigma) for 30 min at 37°C and then washed in buffered saline, to increase their reactivity. The O erythrocytes are incubated with the slides for 30 min prior to inverting the slides in saline.

ABO (H) in Bladder Cancer

In 76 bladder tumors of various stage and grades examined with the SRCA technique for the presence of the ABO (H) cell surface antigen, 70% of the grade I lesions were positive for the cell surface antigen and

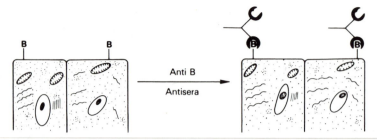

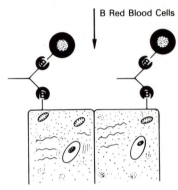

B Red Blood Cells

Figure 5–1. Schematic representation of SRCA

none of the 26 grade III tumors retained their antigens (Table 5–3). When correlated with clinical stage, no antigens were present on stages B to D tumors,[4,5] whereas 12 of 18 stage A lesions were positive for the antigen (Table 5–4). When stage A lesions were studied and the findings correlated with recurrence and metastasis/invasion rates, in only one lesion (which recurred at an invasive stage) was the cell

Table 5–3 Correlation of Grades and Cell Surface Antigens in 76 Patients with Bladder Cancer

	SRCA	
Pathologic grade	Positive	Negative
I	7	3
II	15	25
III	0	26

After Emmott and Javadpour.[5]

Table 5–4   Cell Surface Antigen in 76 Patients Correlated with the Stage of Tumor

	SRCA	
Clinical stages	Positive	Negative
A	12	16
B–D	0	48

After Emmott and Javadpour.[5]

surface antigen present on the initial tumor.[1,4,5] Therefore, it was concluded that ABO (H) cell surface antigens are helpful in predicting malignant potential in low-grade, low-stage cancer of the bladder. These antigens may offer the capability of selecting low-grade, low-stage bladder tumors destined to invade or metastasize while they are still at stages curable by cystectomy.

The findings of cell surface ABO (H) antigens in a limited number of various lesions examined for these antigens are included as controls. Squamous metaplasia in either neoplastic or non-neoplastic lesions consistently demonstrated the absence of the ABO (H) cell surface antigens. Conversely, cystitis cystica and cystitis glandularis were always positive for the presence of these cell surface antigens. Areas of carcinoma within lymph nodes were uniformly negative for the presence of ABO (H) antigens.

ABO (H) in Carcinoma *in Situ*

The recognition of carcinoma *in situ* has added a further dimension to the dilemma of the management of cancerous lesions.[15] Predicting the ultimate natural history of carcinoma *in situ* is of utmost importance in its management, but still remains controversial. The high incidence of its coexistence with infiltrative tumors in the bladder and the more ominous prognosis that this situation implies have encouraged onotologists toward more definitive early treatments. However, in the absence of gross lesions, carcinoma *in situ* may behave in a less aggressive manner. Mostofi has suggested that carcinoma *in situ* should be designated as intraepithelial tumor and separated into three grades: grade I (dysplasia), grade II (anaplasia), and grade III (carcinoma *in situ*).[5]

The findings of cell surface ABO (H) antigens in various grades are under study in an attempt to apply the conventional histopathologic examination and techniques for detecting cell surface antigens to help to grade these lesions. The treatment will then be designed accordingly.

In an ongoing study, our preliminary data indicate that most grade I and some grade II lesions retain their antigens. However, grade III (actual carcinoma *in situ*) lesions lose their ABO (H) antigen, which is indicative of their invasive and metastatic properties.

ABO (H) in Parathyroid Tumors

The histopathologic and clinical distinction between adenoma and hyperplasia of the parathyroid gland is a matter of debate.[16] There are no uniformly accepted criteria for adenoma, hyperplasia, or carcinoma of the parathyroid. Successful parathyroid surgery requires freedom from recurrence of persistent hyperparathyroidism. Utilizing histopathologic and clinical criteria, up to 5% of patients with nonfamilial hyperparathyroidism and up to 50% of patients with familial hyperparathyroidism or multiple endocrine neoplasms (MEN) syndrome have recurrent disease.

We have utilized SRCA to characterize the cell surface antigens in abnormal tissue from primary hyperparathyroidism in 42 patients at the National Institutes of Heath. The results are tabulated in Table 5–5.[6] The findings indicate that there is a loss of cell surface antigens in adenoma and carcinoma, but they are retained in normal and hyperplastic gland.

Table 5–5   Results of 42 Patients with SCRA and Histopathologic Diagnosis (CPD)

	Hyperplasia by SRCA	Adenoma by SRCA	Total
Hyperplasia by CPD	12	3	15
Adenoma by CPD	3	24	27
Total	15	27	42

Table 5–6 Quality Control and Improvements for SRCA

Convential H and E stain

Specificity controls
  Positive control
  Negative control
  Inflammatory lesions

Quality controls
  Fresh antisera and indicator RC
  Incubation—*Ulex* extract (30 min)
  pH of TBS (7.4)

The findings of ABO (H) cell surface antigens appear to be valuable additional means of providing a differentiation of adenoma and hyperplasia.

ABO (H) in Other Cancers

Cell surface antigens have been utilized successfully by Davidsohn and associates to diagnose carcinoma *in situ* from the infiltrating cervical cancers.

Perspective and Limitations

The development of SRCA to detect the presence or absence of blood group A, B, or O (H) antigens has been encouraging in predicting the natural history of pathologically low-grade, low-stage bladder cancer that may be transformed into high-grade and high-stage. Utilizing these markers, one may predict the natural history of a bladder cancer that would not be clear otherwise. A high-grade anaplastic tumor of the bladder will lose the antigen, although the low-grade, low-stages are immunologically well-differentiated. These findings by us and by other investigators have important implications in the management of bladder tumor. The need for the development of new markers such as steroid receptors needs no elaboration.

We have been making every effort to develop and utilize these markers in a number of prospective and/or randomized clinical protocols. Initially, we had several false-negatives, especially in

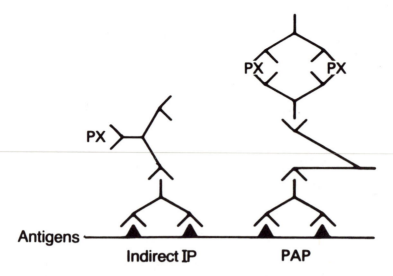

Figure 5–2. Schematic drawing of immunochemical techniques.

patients with type O blood groups. At the present time, the prolonged (30 min) incubation and preparation of fresh reagents with a pH of 7.4 has dramatically reduced the number of false-negatives. However, in patients receiving radiation therapy, a conversion from a negative to a positive reaction has been demonstrated in our laboratory and has also been reported by other investigators. In light of the lack of these isoantigens on the surface of squamous metaplastic cells of the bladder, the value of this reaction is limited. This limitation of SRCA does not affect the usefulness of the test since the majority of the bladder cancers in the western hemisphere are transitional cell carcinoma.

The use of immunocytochemical techniques in the testing of ABO (H) antigen has been encouraging. This technique is especially rewarding in the O (H) blood group where SRCA may yield false-negative results. There are a number of techniques (Fig. 5–2), including indirect immunoperoxidase and the avidin-biotin technique, with more sensitivity.[1,12]

TUMOR-ASSOCIATED ANTIGEN

Tumor-specific antigens have been demonstrated on a variety of animal tumors. Evidence that human tumors contain tumor-specific antigens comes from many sources, including the increased incidence of cancer in immune deficiency studies, the *in vitro* demonstration of cellular and humoral immune responses to tumor antigens, the positive skin-test reactivity of patients of autologous tumor extracts, and a variety of circumstantial clinical suggestions. Much has been learned about the basic immunobiology of the immune response to tumors in animals and humans. Many hypotheses exist to explain the continued growth of a tumor in the face of an active immunological response against it.

Immunological tests have been developed in a wide variety of tumor-associated antigens that may be of use in the immunodiagnosis and immunoevaluation of patients with cancer. Attempts to utilize the immune response for the treatment of malignant tumors are in their earliest stages. However, there are many reports that human bladder cancer may have a tumor-associated antigen.

Acute-phase proteins, such as plasminogen, hepatoglobulin, and immunoglobulin, have been reported to be associated with transitional carcinoma of the bladder. They are also seen in inflammatory lesions of the bladder and, therefore, are not specific. Onco-fetoproteins such as CEA and hCG have also been reported to be elevated in bladder cancer, but they are not consistent enough to serve as tumor markers. Other protein markers—including urinary polyamines, urinary fibrin degradation products, urinary aminoisobutyrate, urinary beta-glucuronidase, and urinary tryptophan metabolic products—have occasionally been found in bladder cancer, but they are not specific.

T ANTIGEN

The observation by Hubener, Thomsen, and Friedenreich that *in vitro* infection of blood specimens with certain bacteria made these specimens pan-agglutinable in any human sera lead to the initial discovery of the T antigen. This "T" effect was later noted to occur in blood samples infected with an influenza virus. It was found that treatment of uninfected red blood cells with neuraminidase, an enzyme secreted by the influenza virus, exposes the T antigen. This antigen is normally concealed in cell membranes of the urothelium.

The T antigen was further localized to the glycosphingolipids of the cell membrane in human epithelial cells. The observations by Springer and co-workers that the MN blood group antigens are inactivated with the appearance of the T antigen, and that *N*-acetylneuraminic acid was released upon treatment of RBC with

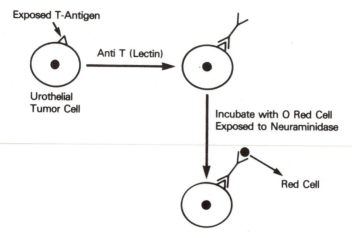

Figure 5–3. Schematic drawing of agglutination test to detect T-antigen.

neuraminidase, lead not only to the elucidation of the structure and location of the T antigen, but also to the discovery of the biosynethetic pathways of the MN blood group. The synthesis of the MN glyco-sphingolipids in the Golgi complex is thought to be similar to the synthesis of the A, B, O blood groups (Figure 5–3).

The lectin technique for detection of the T antigen is given in Table 5–7.

Table 5–7   Detection of T Antigen

The procedure for hydrating the section is the same as that described in Table 5–2 for the ABO (H) adherence technique. In the place of ABO (H) antibody, peanut lectin is used in this test:

1. Incubate the section with the peanut lectin for 30 min.
2. Wash the excess of lectin with phosphate buffer 5 min ×3.
3. Overlay the section with the cells previously activated by 50 units/ml neuraminidase for 5 min.
4. Centrifuge O blood, discard the supernantant, then add 50 units of neuraminidase per ml of this cell pack. Incubate for 4 h at 37°C, then wash with PBS and make 3% cell suspension in PBS.
5. Invert the slide and rest on two pieces of applicator stick in the petri dish, flood the petri dish with buffer, and let the unadhered cells settle down.
6. Move the slide to clear side of the petri dish, and examine under a low-powered microscope for the presence or absence of cell adherence.

The avidin-biotin technique appears to be a more sensitive method for detecting the presence or absence of the T antigen than the lectin method.

Also, in another study, we have demonstrated that a double-blind peroxidase antiperoxidase (PAP) correlates better with prognosis and invasiveness of bladder cancer in group O patients than SRCA. Furthermore, the convenience, permanence, and ready availability of the PAP technique should encourage its use in conventional histopathologic laboratories.

In a controlled study, we have shown that the lectin method, although simple, economical, and quick, has certain false-negative results. Coon and Weinstein and, later, McAlpine and Javadpour showed that lectin has decreased specificity as well as decreased reproducibility.

The avidin-biotin method, while more complex than the lectin method and requiring a greater understanding of the immunohistochemical mechanics, appears to be far more sensitive as well as specific and reproducible. Although this procedure requires more expensive and a greater variety of reagents, when performed on a large scale these disadvantages are off-set by the decrease in the amount of handling of slides.

With improved detection of the T antigen, the prediction of tumor behavior should also be enhanced.

CELL SURFACE ANTIGENS
WITH OTHER CELL MARKERS

Utilizing tumor markers, including T antigen, ABO isoantigens, and chromosomal abnormalities, will help to separate superficial bladder tumors with a good prognosis and low risk from superficial bladder tumors that will be invasive with a high rate of recurrence and a potential for metastases. This important clinical distinction will help to facilitate the selection of effective therapeutic modalities and lead to improved progress for patients with superficial bladder cancer.

Currently, we consider the presence of ABO antigens as strong consideration for conservation therapy of superficial bladder cancer, although loss of these antigens will put such patients into a high-risk group. Therefore, multiple cell markers, such as ABO isoantigens and T antigen, together with chromosomal analysis[10] and flow cytometry can distinguish those patients with high- or low-risk superficial bladder cancer and guide the clinician in selecting appropriate therapy

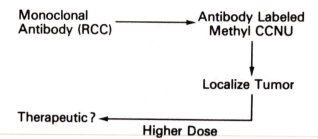

Figure 5–4. Monoclonal antibody to the tumor-associated antigen: a potential for tumor detection and therapy.

when these markers are taken into consideration with grade, stage, and other clinical findings. Cystectomy is not performed in these patients solely on the basis of low cell-surface antigens, but loss of those antigens serves as another parameter of future recurrence and invasiveness.

FUTURE PERSPECTIVES

The findings of varius tumor-associated antigens may be utilized as tumor markers to detect, stage, and monitor the cancer of a given organ.[2,11] The advent of monoclonal antibodies and the ability to tag these antibodies to various chemotherapeutic or radiotherapeutic agents may open an avenue for tumor localization and/or specific delivery of a cytotoxic agent and/or radioactive material to the tumor (Fig. 5–4).

REFERENCES

1. Bergman, S., and Javadpour, N. The cell surface antigen ABO (H) as an indicator of malignant potential in Stage A bladder carcinoma. Preliminary Report. J. Urol. 119: 49, 1978.

2. Diamond, B. A., Dale, E., Yelton, B. A., and Scharff, M. D. Monoclonal antibodies—a new technology for producing serologic reagents. N. Engl. J. Med. 304: 1344, 1981.

3. Davidsohn, I. Early immunologic diagnosis and prognosis of carcinoma. Am. J. Clin. Pathol. 57: 715, 1972.

4. Emmott, R. C., Javadpour, N., Bergman, S. M., and Soares, T. Correlation of the cell surface antigens with stage and grade in cancer of the bladder. J. Urol. 121: 37, 1979.

5. Emmott, C., Droller, M., and Javadpour, N. Studies of ABO (H) cell surface antigen specificity: Carcinoma *in situ* and nonmalignant lesions of the bladder. J. Urol. 125: 32, 1981.

6. Hicks, R. M. Carcinogenesis. A multiple stage process. In *Bladder Cancer*, edited by N. Javadpour. Baltimore: Williams & Wilkins, 1984.

7. Hsu, S., and Rane, L. Versatility of biotin-labeled lectins and avidin-biotin peroxidase complex for localization of carbohydrate in tissue sections. J. Histo. Cytochemistry 30: 157–161, 1982.

8. Javadpour, N. Biologic tumor markers in the management of testicular and bladder cancer. Urology 12: 177, 1978.

9. Javadpour, N. Tumor markers in urologic cancer. In *Principles and Management of Urologic Cancer*, edited by N. Javadpour, 2nd ed., p. 32. Baltimore: Williams & Wilkins, 1983.

10. Javadpour, N., Roy, J. B., Bottomly, R., and Dagg, K. Combined cell surface antigens and chromosomal studies in bladder cancer, Urology 19: 29, 1983.

11. Kohler, G., and Milstein, C. Continuous culture of fused cells secreting antibody of predefined specificity. Nature 256: 495–497, 1975.

12. McAlpine, R., and Javadpour, N. Comparison of specific red cell adherence and immunoperoxidase in detection of ABO (H) antigens in normal urothelium—A double blind study. Urology (in press).

13. Milstein, C., Adetugbo, K., and Cowan, N. J. Somatic cell genetics of antibody-secreting cells: Studies of clonal diversification and analysis by cell fusion. Cold Spring Harbor Symp. Quant. Biol. 41: 793, 1977.

14. Reddy, E. P. Nucleotide sequence analysis of T-24 human bladder carcinoma oncogen. Science 220: 1061, 1983.

15. Utz, D. W., Farrow, G. M., and Rife, C. C. Carcinoma *in situ* of the bladder. Cancer 45: 1842, 1980.

16. Woltering, E. A., Emmott, R. C., Javadpour, N., et al. ABO (H) cell surface antigens in parathyroid adenoma and hyperplasia. Surg. 90: 1–9, 1981.

6

Steroid Hormone Receptors as Tumor Markers

N. Bashirelahi, D. B. Ekiko, E. G. Elias,
S. Ganesan, H. Kohail, & J. D. Young, Jr.

Hormones have an important role in carcinogenesis and tumor growth in a variety of target tissues (47), but their exact role in this process is still under investigation. Biochemical studies on the mechanism of action of steroid hormones have led to the discovery that these hormones enter the cytoplasm of target cells, where they bind to specific receptor molecules. The receptor–steroid complex then translocates to the nucleus and stimulates transcription of mRNA, which then translates for the synthesis of a new protein. The protein formed is then responsible for the effects of the hormone on the cell, such as growth. The sensitivity to steroid hormones seems to be directly related to the receptor content in target cells. These receptors are specifically known to concentrate the steroids into target tissues (12). This physiological function has led to the pharmacological use of the receptor in the treatment of steroid-receptive neoplasia. The intention was that drugs with high affinity for the steroid receptor could be concentrated in the neoplastic tissues in the same manner as the steroid. Because of the basic role of these receptors, a series of studies have been undertaken by several groups to analyze the steroid receptor in malignant tissues known to respond to hormonal manipulations and to correlate the clinical responsiveness with their levels.

The most significant progress in this field of research has been made in human breast cancer (27,38,46), but the presence of steroid receptors has been well documented in other hormone-dependent malignancies such as acute leukemia (37,46) and endometrial cancer (50,63) and in malignant melanoma (20).

The determination of steroid receptor status to select cancer patients for endocrine therapy is of great importance. As mentioned above, responsiveness to endocrine therapy seems to be related to receptor content in target tissue; De Sombre and co-workers showed this for patients with low estrogen receptor (ER) levels (15). The detection of steroid receptors in tumors is achieved by several methods (23). Most of these employ the same basic principle of incubating tissue cytosol with radiolabeled steroids on their analogs and determining the amount of radioactivity bound to the receptor protein. Excess radioactive hormone is removed by a simple separation technique such as adsorption on dextran-coated charcoal (DCC) (35). Radioactivity bound specifically is distinguished from nonspecific binding to tissue macromolecules by a duplicate incubation containing, in addition to labeled hormone, a large excess of unlabeled hormone or antihormone which competitively binds the receptor; the difference between the two is due to specific binding to receptor. The receptor site and its affinity are then analyzed by a Scatchard (53) analysis of data obtained from binding studies.

The results obtained by these receptor assays can sometimes be false. Caution must be mustered in interpreting receptor assays, since there are occasions when they are falsely negative. Receptor assays can be falsely negative if a biopsy for receptor is obtained from a patient who has been treated with a steroid (specifically, estrogen in breast cancer). This is because the receptor will be in the nucleus instead of in the cytosol where it is assayed. Secondly, in premenopausal women, PgR may be difficult to detect during the luteal phase of the menstrual cycle, when endogenous hormone is high and could be blocking the binding site. Thirdly, there may be a false-negative PgR in postmenopausal women because of low levels of estrogen, which are insufficient to stimulate the synthesis of progesterone receptor (42).

ROLE OF ESTROGEN AND PROGESTERONE RECEPTORS IN BREAST CANCER

Hormonal therapy plays a very important role in the treatment of patients with breast cancer. It has been specifically effective in the treatment of recurrent and/or advanced breast cancer patients. It was first reported by Beatson (4) in 1896 that some human breast cancers will respond to endocrine manifestations; he induced tumor regression in patients with advanced breast cancer by oophorectomy.

The demonstration of ER by Toft and Gorski (61) in 1966, the proposal by Jensen et al. (28) in 1967 that this receptor may be found in mammary tumor cells, and the work of subsequent investigators (10,41) have clearly established the role of determining ER status of breast cancer in the selection of patients who may benefit from endocrine treatment (additive or ablative). The response rate to hormone therapy for estrogen receptor-positive tumors (ER+) is about 60%, and improved responses have been shown in patients who are also progesterone receptor-positive (PR+) (39,43).

Estrogen receptor status, however, does not always correctly predict the hormonal responsiveness of breast cancer, since at least 35% of women with tumors that have receptors will not benefit from endocrine therapy. A possible explanation for this finding is that in the process of differentiation some tumors may retain the ability to bind estradiol but may be unable to carry on subsequent steps of estrogen action, such as migration of the ER complex to the nucleus, stimulation of messenger-RNA, and initiation of mitogenesis. These tumors will, therefore, have receptors but will be hormone-resistant. If this hypothesis is correct, then the measurement of an end product of estrogen action is desirable. Progesterone receptor is one of the estrogen end products (25), and its determination in conjunction with ER could be a better predictor of response to endocrine therapy than the presence of ER alone. Many clinical trials have confirmed this hypothesis, and it is now well established that women with tumors possessing both receptors have an increased likelihood of responding to hormonal therapy, approaching 80% in some studies (42).

General Characteristics

Relationship to Age Most previous studies have reported that postmenopausal women have higher ER concentrations than premenopausal women. However, the relationship between age and ER levels has not been as clear. Clark et al. (11) have found that quantitative ER levels and the percentage of ER+ breast cancer tumors were directly related to the age of the patient. As a result of the strong correlation of ER to age, it was found that postmenopausal patients have a higher incidence of ER+ tumors than premenopausal patients. Age is more important than menopausal status in predicting the ER status of the patient (11). It is not clear why ER concentration should increase with age. One possible explanation might be that premenopausal women have higher concentrations of circulating estrogen that would bind to cytosol receptors, making them unavailable for routine assay.

A study was carried out at the University of Maryland Hospital on estrogen and progesterone receptors in 80 stage I and II breast cancer patients. It was found that the incidence of ER+ cases increased with age; the highest incidence was in patients over 60 years of age (42.3%), the lowest in those under 40 years (7.7%) (Table 6–1).

There are a few studies on the relationship between PR and either age or menopausal status; these studies concluded that no relationship exists between PR and age or menopausal status (1,21). However, none of these studies compared premenopausal and postmenopausal women of the same age. Clark et al. (11) have speculated that the level of PR might be a combined function of circulating estrogen, which stimulates PR synthesis, and the concentration of circulation progesterone, which might bind to and thereby mask receptors.

Relationship to Tumor Size   The relationship between the size of the primary tumor and the steroid receptor status is a matter of controversy among many researchers. Some investigators have found that there is no relationship between the size of the primary tumor and steroid receptor status (1,52). Others found a tendency for large tumors to be ER– (2,31). This may be due to the necrosis present in large tumors, which may result in destruction and lack of the steroid hormone receptors.

In the study done at the University of Maryland Hospital it was found that smaller tumors (less than 2 cm) were associated with high incidence of ER-positivity (Table 6–2).

Relationship to Axillary Lymph Nodes   Because the axillary nodal status has a very significant prognostic effect on the disease-free and

Table 6–1.   Estrogen Receptors and Age

ER status*	No. of patients	Age (years)			
		≤ 40	41–50	51–60	> 60
ER+	52	4(7.7%)	9(17.3%)	17(32.7%)	22(42.3%)
ER–	28	4(14.3%)	9(32.1%)	8(28.6%)	7(25%)

*ER+ = more than 10 fmol/mg cytosol protein.
Data from Kohail et al.[33]

Table 6–2 Size of the Primary Tumor in Relation to Axillary Lymph Node (L.N.) Pathology and ER status

Lymph node status	L.N. −ve		L.N. +ve		
	< 2 cm	≥ 2–5 cm	< 2 cm	≥ 2–5 cm	Total
Er+	5(71%)	8(47%)	12(80%)	27(60%)	52
ER−	2(29%)	9(53%)	3(20%)	14(43%)	28
Total	7	17	15	41	80

Data from Kohail et al.[33]

overall survivals, one might anticipate a possible relationship between ER, PR, and nodal status. Many investigators failed to identify any correlation between steroid receptors and lymph node status (21,31,52). However, even in a large series of patients studied by Clark et al. (11) these variables were independent. This was also found in the study at the University of Maryland, although patients with involved axillary lymph nodes were more likely to have positive hormone receptors in their primary tumor (Table 6–2). This was statistically nonsignificant.

Relationship between Estrogen and Progesterone Receptors It has been noted in several laboratories that PR positivity is mostly present in ER+ tumors (7,48). This is consistent with their estrogen-dependent synthesis, where progesterone receptors are induced by estrogen in estrogen target issues (26). It was found that 65% of patients were ER+. Of these patients, 85% were PR+. On the other hand, 86% of ER− cases were also PR−. The presence of PR was rare in the absence of ER (Table 6–3) (33).

Receptor Status and Prognosis There are differing views on the association between receptor status and prognosis. Some reports have shown that ER status helps to predict disease-free survival (DFS) (13,34) as well as overall survival (5). On the other hand, others have reported that ER status is unhelpful in those respects (54). Considering the PR status, again controversy still exists with regard to its prognostic significance. PR has been reported to be a better indicator of DFS and overall survival (49) than ER, while other reports have shown no significant effect of PR status on DFS (57).

Table 6–3   Correlation of ER to PR

ER status	PR+	PR−	Total
ER+	44(85%)	8(15%)	52(65%)
ER−	4(24%)	24(86%)	28(35%)
Total	48(60%)	32(40%)	80

The DFS was significantly higher in patients with ER+ than in those with ER− ($p < 0.005$) as well as in patients with PR+ than in those with PR− ($p < 0.005$). When combining both receptors together, it became clear that the ER+/PR+ group had a significantly higher DFS than the ER−/PR− group ($p < 0.005$) (33).

When overall survival was observed, the situation was nearly the same as for DFS except that the difference between the PR+ and PR− groups was not significant. ER status affected the survival; i.e. the difference between the ER+ and ER− groups was statistically significant ($p < 0.025$) and the difference between the ER+/PR+ and ER−/PR− groups was also significant ($p < 0.025$).

The study done at the University of Maryland Hospital analyzed the influence of lymph node state on prognosis and its relation to ER status. ER+ patients had significantly better DFS regardless of the state of axillary lymph nodes. The worst prognosis was seen in the group showing no receptors in their primary tumor with tumor involvement of axillary lymph nodes. This result makes the ER and lymph node status synergistic in the assessment of prognosis in breast cancer patients (33).

ENDOMETRIAL CARCINOMA

Endometrial carcinoma is at present the most common malignancy of the female genital tract, and together with breast carcinoma it is the most important target for endocrine cancer therapy. Hormone therapy is widely used for advanced and recurrent disease and is also used prophylactically after the initial therapeutic measures. At present there are encouraging results that indicate that the use of ER, and especially PR, determination could help the selection of proper therapeutic regimens for individual patients with endometrial carcinoma (62).

A recent study demonstrates a significantly increased survival time for women with ER+ adenocarcinoma of the endometrium when compared with that of those with ER− tumors ($p < 0.05$) (39). Another study indicates that ER+ and more particularly PR+ tumors frequently responded to progestin treatment, whereas the opposite was true for receptor-poor tumors (63). It has also been shown that receptor-poor tumors tended to behave more aggressively than receptor-rich tumors in relation to survival time (62). Collectively, the data available imply that measurement of cytosol female sex steroid receptors could serve as a practical indicator for selecting effective treatment for patients with endometrial carcinoma at least in advanced or recurrent cases.

OVARIAN CARCINOMA

Effective management of ovarian cancer is the outstanding problem facing gynecological oncology today, and any potential predictive index in ovarian cancer will merit careful evaluation, particularly if hormonal therapy is to be of any value. Several studies have reported the presence of estrogen, progesterone, and androgen receptors in varying concentrations and combinations in ovarian cancer (64). The detection of estrogen and progesterone receptors, alone or in combination, in approximately two-thirds of ovarian cancer tissues is similar to that described for breast cancer (64). This pattern of receptors in ovarian cancers is significantly different from the pattern found in normal tissues and in benign tumors and suggests that a majority of ovarian carcinomata may be hormonally sensitive (64).

On the basis of several studies it is likely that ER and PR measurements may give additional information that is not always obtainable by conventional histologic and staging characterization of ovarian carcinomas. The available data indicate that not only the presence of ER and PR but also their concentrations should be used in evaluating ovarian malignancies (30). Hormonal chemotherapy has not been used in the treatment of advanced ovarian carcinoma, understandably, due to the poor efficacy of progestins, with response rates varying from 10% to 24%. An anti-estrogen, tamoxifen, has been found to be effective in some ovarian carcinomas. The frequent presence of steroid hormone receptors in ovarian carcinoma tissue and the inhibitory action of steroid hormones on nucleic acid synthesis of cultured ovarian carcinoma tissue calls for studies employing combination hormonal chemotherapy and for the introduction of hormonal agents to complement cytotoxic chemotherapy (30).

PROSTATIC CANCER

Prostatic cancer affects about 50% of men over 80 years of age and primarily involves epithelial elements in the peripheral region of the prostate (51). The prostatic gland depends on androgens for its function and normal development. Androgens are of importance also for abnormal development of the human prostate since with few exceptions neither prostatic cancer nor hyperplasia have been reported in males castrated before the age of 40 (51).

Several investigations have established the presence of androgen, estrogen, and progesterone receptors in human prostate. Assays for steroid receptor concentrations in human prostate have been beset with difficulties (51), such as normal prostatic tissue not being available for comparison (16), the presence of endogenous androgens and plasma proteins (SHBG) (3), and the proportion of stromal to epithelial elements in any given piece of prostatic tissue (16).

Based on preliminary findings in our laboratory it appears that patients who demonstrate absence or insignificant amounts of estrogen receptor protein and/or high cytosol androgen receptor content fail to respond to additive or ablative endocrine therapy for any significant interval (66). An 80% correlation between nuclear steroid receptors and response to hormonal treatment has been reported. Different cut-off points have been used by different laboratories to distinguish between receptor-rich and receptor-poor tumors, which eventually determine the observed response rates (16).

Diethylstilbestrol (DES) has been widely used for the conservative treatment of prostatic cancer. Although 75–80% of all prostatic carcinomas respond to estrogen therapy, many relapses eventually occur. Castration seems to be at least as effective as estrogen treatment in controlling the growth of prostatic carcinoma. The current opinion is that estrogen effectively suppresses circulating testosterone levels. However, a direct action of estrogen on tumor cells should also be considered. Thus, reports of the presence of estrogen receptors in human BPH and prostatic cancer has evoked considerable interest (51).

Although encouraging results have been recorded, clinical correlations between androgen and/or estrogen receptors and the response to prostatic cancer are few, and many more cases have to be studied.

STEROID HORMONE RECEPTORS AND MENINGIOMA

The possibility that some meningiomas might be hormone dependent has been suggested following the observations that (a) women with breast cancer have a higher likelihood of also having a meningioma than do a matched group of women without breast cancer (44); (b) meningiomas occur more commonly in women than in men (17); (c) symptoms may develop or worsen with increasing levels of sex hormones during pregnancy; (d) and increased tumor growth with puberty has been observed in some meningiomas.

Therefore to test the possibility that steroid receptors might be involved in the pathogenesis or in the modulation of growth of meningiomas, some investigators have tried to measure specific binding of these steroids in such tumors (6,40). One group of investigators reported the presence of specific estradiol binding in about 70% of meningioma patients tested; also, the receptor concentrations proved to be too low (43). Others found lower levels of ER and PR in meningiomas studied, and this was thought to be due to the use of preoperative glucocorticoid therapy (9). On the other hand, the absence of estradiol receptor and the presence of progesterone receptor has been documented (6,60). The levels of PR were as high as those found in breast carcinoma, and the levels for female and male patients were identical (8).

Therefore, the presence of PR in meningiomas might be an indication of the possible use of antiprogestin therapy in cases where complete surgical resection is not possible.

STEROID RECEPTORS AND MELANOMA

The role of hormones in malignant melanoma remains a question with conflicting answers. The state of understanding is that the clinical course of melanoma often changes with the onset of puberty, with pregnancy, and with the inception of contraceptive estrogens. Moreover, regression of a melanoma following delivery has been observed, and all this seems to support the notion that this disease is steroid hormone-dependent (36,55). Biochemical studies have shown substantial numbers of melanomas to contain variable numbers of estrogen and progesterone receptors.

However, some patients have had responses to the administration of tamoxifen that appear to be independent of ER levels (29), and a study of a melanoma patient, during and after pregnancy, did not correlate very well in that the tumor was more aggressive at a time when ER levels were low or absent (58). Another study seems to show that the presence of an estradiol-binding component in melanoma is an artifact (67). Data presented so far for the role of steroid receptor in melanoma clearly indicate the need for a large, well-controlled study for the relationships among hormone receptors, stage of disease, clinical course, and response to endocrine manipulation in patients with malignant melanoma.

LEUKEMIA AND GLUCOCORTICOID RECEPTOR

Immunological and cytochemical classification of subgroups in acute leukemia has in the past few years raised the hope of more accurate diagnosis and differentiated treatment. Moreover, biochemical studies have identified several marker enzymes that will aid an exact diagnosis and, as a corollary, a more precise therapy (18,24). Of all the steroid hormones, glucocorticoids have the widest range of biological actions in mammals, and most of their metabolic actions are initiated by the binding of the hormone to soluble cytoplasmic receptors (19,59). The distribution of glucocorticoid receptors (GR) is universal; thus, by altering the amount of circulating glucocorticoids either by endocrine ablation or exogenous hormone administration, one can modify a variety of important regulatory systems. In this light it is not surprising that these hormones have unlimited therapeutic uses, although their mechanism of action remains a mystery.

Some investigators ask the question whether the information obtained by tissue GR determination can be applied to the steroid treatment of leukemias (34); i.e., can GR levels be used as a biochemical marker for prediction of prognosis and response to endocrine therapy? Glucocorticoid receptor determinations in acute lymphoblastic leukemia (ALL) have shown a correlation between high receptor levels and response to cytotoxic drug combinations containing glucocorticoids (65) or glucocorticoid alone (8,14). The receptor sites per cells have been determined to be about 8,000, and patients with less than 4,500 receptor sites per cell have failed to respond to hormone therapy (8,14). The correlation between response to therapy and GR levels has not always been positive where other types of leukemias are concerned (34), e.g. acute nonlymphoblast leukemia and chronic lymphocytic leukemia (56), although the receptor levels have not been found to be different in these patients (8,14).

It appears that the types of leukemia are heterogeneous in terms of cellular identity as well as glucocorticoid responsiveness and can be placed in subclasses, which reflect sequential stages of early lymphocyte differentiation and show a rank order of good prognosis in the sequence:* ALL > null ALL > T-ALL > B-ALL (22).

CONCLUSIONS AND FUTURE CONSIDERATIONS

Steroid hormones regulate the normal growth and development of their target organs by binding to specific cytosolic receptors. When abnormal growth results, the hyperplastic/neoplastic cells might retain their ability to respond to hormonal stimulation. This fact is then used to design hormone manipulation therapy to control neoplastic growth. The presence or absence of steroid receptors in the neoplastic tissue is thus thought to be a prognostic indicator of response to hormonal therapy. Breast cancer is the most extensively studied neoplasm and is the only neoplasm where a good correlation exists between ER+/PR+ tumors and response to estrogen deprivation. Mere presence of ER in breast tumors is not a sufficient prognostic indicator, since some other step in the mechanism of steroid hormone action might be aberrant. The presence of PR, which is one of the end-products of estrogen action, along with ER significantly increases the observed correlation with prognosis. Presence of ER and PR has also been correlated with response to endometrial and ovarian carcinoma. Some correlations have also been observed between nuclear androgen receptors and cytoplasmic estrogen receptors and response to hormonal manipulation in prostatic carcinoma. Presence of glucocorticoid receptors has been reported in leukemia, and estrogen and progesterone receptors have been reported in malignant melanoma. However, only breast cancer shows a good correlation with the presence of ER and PR, and further controlled clinical studies are necessary before receptor levels can be routinely used as prognostic indicators in malignancies other than breast cancer.

---

*ALL—acute lymphoblastic leukemia; null ALL—unclassified acute lymphoblastic leukemia; B-ALL—a rare variant acute lymphoblastic leukemia; T-ALL—thymic acute lymphoblastic leukemia.

REFERENCES

1. Allegra, J. C., Lippman, M. E., and Thompson, E. B. Distribution, frequency, and quantitative analysis of estrogen, progesterone, androgen, and glucocorticoid receptors in human breast cancer. Cancer Res. *39*, 1447–1454 (1979).

2. Antoinnaides, K., and Spector, H. Quantitative estrogen receptor values and growth of carcinoma of the breast before surgical intervention. Cancer *50*, 793–796 (1982).

3. Bashirelahi, N., Young, J. D., Jr., S. M. Sidh, and Sanefugi, H. Androgen, oestrogen and progestogen and their distribution in epithelial and stromal cells of human prostate. In *Steroid Receptors, Metabolism and Prostatic Cancer*, edited by F. H. Schroeder and H. J. de Voogt. Amsterdam: Excerpta Medica, pp. 240–256 (1980).

4. Beatson, G. T. On the treatment of inoperable cases of carcinoma of the mammary. Suggestions for a new method of treatment with illustrative cases. Lancet *2*, 104–107 (1896).

5. Blamey, R. W., Bishop, H. M., Blake, T. R. S., Doyle, P. J., Elston, C. W., Haybittle, J. L., Nicholson, R. R., and Griffiths, K. Relationship between primary breast tumour receptor status and patient survival. Cancer *46*, 2765–2769 (1980).

6. Blankenstein, M. A., Blaauu, G., Lamberts, S. W. J., and Mulder, E. Presence of progesterone receptors and absence of oestrogen receptors in human intracranial meningioma cytosols. Eur. J. Cancer Clin. Oncol. *19*, 365–370 (1983).

7. Bloom, N., Tobin, E., and Degenshein, G.A. Clinical correlation of endocrine ablation with estrogen and progesterone in advanced breast cancer. In *Progesterone Receptors in Normal and Neoplastic Tissues*, edited by W. L. McGuire, J. P. Raynaud, and E. E. Baulieu. New York: Raven Press, pp. 125–139 (1976).

8. Bloomfield, D. C., Smith, K. A., Peterson, B. A., and Munck, A. GR in acute lymphoblastic leukemia. Cancer Res. *41*, 4857–4860 (1981).

9. Cahill, D. W., Bashirelahi, N., Solomon, L. W., Dalton, T., Salcman, M., and Ducker, T. B. Estrogen and progesterone receptors in meningiomas. J. Neurosurg *60*, 985–993 (1984).

10. Clark, G. M., McGuire, W. L., Hubay, C.A., Pearson, O. H., and Marshall, J. S. Progesterone receptor as a prognostic factor in stage II breast cancer. New Engl. J. Med. *309*, 1343–1347 (1983).

11. Clark, G. M., Osborne, D. K., and McGuire, W. L. Correlations between estrogen receptors, progesterone receptors, and patient characteristics in human breast cancer. J. Clin. Oncol. *2*(10), 1102–1109 (1984).

12. Clark, J. H., and Peck, Jr., E. J. *Female Sex Steroid Receptors and Function: Monographs on Endocrinology*, Vol. 14. Berlin: Springer Verlag (1979).

13. Cooke, T., George, D., Shields, R., Maynard, P. and Griffiths, K. Estrogen receptors and prognosis in early breast cancer. Lancer, *1*, 995–997 (1979).

14. Crabtree, G. R., Bloomfield, C. D., Smith, K. A., McKenzie, R. W., Peterson, B. A., Hilderbrandt, L., and Munck, A. Glucocorticoid receptors and *in vitro* responses to glucocorticoid in acute nonlymphocytic leukemia. Cancer Res. *41*, 4853–4856 (1981).

15. De Sombre, E. R., Carbone, P. P., Jensen, E. V., McGuire, W. L., Wells, S. A., Jr., Wittliff, J. L., and Lipsett, M. B. Special report: Steroid receptor in breast cancer. New Engl. J. Med. *301*, 1011–1012 (1979).

16. De Voogt, H. J., and Rao, B. R. Present concept of the relevance of steroid receptors for prostatic cancer. J. Steroid Biochem. *19*, 845–849 (1983).

17. Donnell, M. S., Meyer, G., and Donegan, W. L. Estrogen-receptor protein in intracranial meningiomas. J. Neurosurg. *50*, 499–502 (1979).

18. Ellis, R. B., Rapson, N. T., Patrick, A. D., Greaves, M. F., and Path, M. R. C. Expression of hexogaminidase isoenzymes in childhood leukemia. New Eng. J. Med. *298*, 476–480 (1978).

19. Feldman, D. The role of hormone receptors in the action of adrenal steroids. Ann. Rev. Med. *26*, 83–90 (1975).

20. Fisher, R. I., Neifield, M. E., and Lippman, M. E. Estrogen receptor in human malignant melanoma. Lancet *2*, 337–338 (1976).

21. Fisher, B., Wickerham, D. L., Brown, A., and Redmond, C. K. Breast cancer estrogen and progesterone receptor values: Their distribution, degree of concordance, and relation to number of positive axillary nodes. J. Clin. Oncol. *1*, 349–358 (1983).

22. Greaves, M. F. Analysis of the clinical and biological significance of lymphoid phenotypes in acute leukemias. Cancer Res. *41*, 4752–4766 (1981).

23. Hawkins, R. A., Roberts, M. M., and Forest, A. P. H. Oestrogen receptors and breast cancer: Current status. Br. J. Surg. *67*, 153–159 (1980).

24. Hoffbrand, A., Ganeshaguru, K., Janossy, G., Greaves, M. F., Catsvsky, D., and Woodroff, R. K. Terminal deoxynucleotidyl-transferase levels and membrane phenotypes in diagnosis of active leukemia. Lancet, Sept. 10, 520–523 (1977).

25. Horwitz, K. B., and McGuire, W. L. Nuclear mechanisms of estrogen action effects of estradiol and anti-estrogens on estrogen receptors and nuclear estrogen receptor processing. J. Biol. Chem. *253*, 8188–8191 (1978).

26. Janne, O., Kontula, K. Lunkkainen, T., and Vihko, R. Estrogen induced progesterone receptors in human uterus. J. Steroid Biochem. *6*, 501–509 (1975).

27. Jensen, E. V., Block, G. E., Smith, S., and De Sombre, E. R. Hormonal dependency of breast cancer: Recent results. Cancer Res. *42*, 55–62 (1973).

28. Jensen, E. V., De Sombre, E. R., and Jungblut, P. W. Estrogen receptor in hormone responsive tissues and tumours. In *Endogenous Factors Influencing Host–Tumour Balance*, edited by R. W. Wissler, T. L. Dae, and S. Wood, Jr. Chicago: University of Chicago Press, pp. 15–30 (1967).

29. Karakousis, C. P., Lopez, R. E., and Bhakoo, H. S. Estrogen and progesterone receptors and tamoxifen in malignant melanoma. Cancer Treatment Rev. *64*, 819–827 (1980).

30. Kauppila, A., Vierikko, P., Kivinen, S., Stenback, F., and Vihko, R. Clinical significance of estrogen and progestin receptors in ovarian cancer. Obstetrics and Gynecology *61*(3), 320–326 (1983).

31. Kern, W. H. Morphologic and clinical aspects of estrogen receptors in carcinoma of the breast. Surg. Gynecol. Obstet. *148*, 240–242 (1979).

32. Knight, W. A., Livingston, R. V., George, E. J., and McGuire, W. L. Estrogen receptors as an independent prognostic factor for early recurrence in breast cancer. Cancer Res. *37*, 4669–4671 (1977).

33. Kohail, H. M., Elias, E. G., El-Nowiem, S. A., Bashirelahi, N., Dodolkar, M. S., and Reed, W. P. A multifactorial analysis of steroid hormone receptors in stage I and II breast cancer. Ann. Surgery (in press).

34. Kontula, K. Glucocorticoid receptors and their role in human disease. Ann. Clin. Res. *12*, 223–235 (1980).

35. Korenman, S. G., and Duke, B. A. Specific estrogen binding by cytoplasm of human breast carcinoma. J. Clin. Endocrin. Metals *30*, 639–645 (1970).

36. Lerner, A. B., Norlund, J. J., and Kirkwood, J. M. Effects of oral contraceptives and pregnancy on melanomas. New Engl. J. Med. *301*, 47 (1979).

37. Lippman, M. E., Halterman, R. H., Leventhal, B. C., Perry, S., and Thompson, E. B. Glucocorticoid binding proteins in human acute lymphoblastic leukemia blast cells. J. Clin. Invest. *52*, 1715–1721 (1973).

38. Lippman, M. E., Bolan, G., and Huff, K. The effects of estrogen and antiestrogens on hormone receptive human breast cancer in long term tissue culture. Cancer Res. *36*, 4595–4601 (1976).

39. Maass, H., and Jonat, W. Steroid receptors as a guide for therapy of primary and metastatic breast cancer. J. Steroid Biochem. *19*, 833–837 (1983).

40. Martuza, R. L., MacLanghlin, D. T., and Ojemann, R. G. Specific estradiol binding in schwannomas, meningiomas, and neurofibromas. Neurosurgery *9*, 665–671 (1981).

41. McGuire, W. L., Carbone, P. P., and Sears, M. E. Estrogen receptors in human breast cancer: An overview. In *Estrogen Receptors in Human Breast Cancer*, edited by W. L. McGuire, P. O. Carbone, and E. P. Volmer. New York: Raven Press, pp. 1–7 (1975).

42. McGuire, W. L., Horwitz, K. B., Pearson, O. H., and Segaloff, A. Current status of estrogen and progesterone receptors in breast cancer. Cancer *39*, 2934–2947 (1977).

43. McGuire, W. L. Hormone receptors: Their role in predicting prognosis and response to endocrine therapy. Semin. Oncol. *5*, 428–433 (1978).

44. Mehta, D., Khatib, R., and Patel, S. Carcinoma of the breast and meningioma: Association and management. Cancer *51*, 1937–1940 (1983).

45. Mockus, M. B., Lessey, B. A., Bower, M. A., and Horwitz, K. B. Estrogen-insensitive progesterone receptor in a human breast cancer line. Characterization of receptors and of a ligand exchange assay. Endocrinology *110*, 1564–1571 (1982).

46. Mouriquand, J., Jacrot, M., Louis, J., Mermet, M., Saez, S., Sage, J., and Mouriquand, C. Tamoxifen-induced fluorescence as a marker of human breast tumor cells: Responsiveness to hormonal manipulations: Correlation with progesterone receptor content and ultrastructure alterations. Cancer Res. *43*, 3948–3954 (1983).

47. Nobel, R. L. Tumors and hormones. In *The Hormones*, edited by G. Pincus, K. V. Thiamann, and E. B. Astwood, Vol. 5, pp. 559–695. Academic Press: New York (1964).

48. Pichon, M. F., and Milgram, E. Characterization and assay of progesterone receptors in human mammary carcinoma. Cancer Res. *37*, 464–471 (1971).

49. Pichon, M. F., Pallud, C., Brunet, M., and Milgram, E. Relationship of presence of progesterone receptors to prognosis in early breast cancer. Cancer Res. *40*, 3357–3360 (1980).

50. Pollow, K., Lubbert, H., Broquoi, E., Krenzer, G., and Pollow, B. Characterization and comparison of receptor for 17β-estradiol and progesterone in human endometrial carcinoma. Endocrinology *96*, 319–329 (1975).

51. Robel, P. Sex steroid hormone receptors and human prostatic hyperplasia and carcinoma. Ann. Clin. Res. *12*: 216–222 (1980).

52. Rosen, P. P. Mendez-Botef, C., Nisselbaum, J. S., Urban, J. A., Mike, V., Fracchia, A., and Schwartz, M. K. Pathologic review of breast lesions analyzed for estrogen receptor protein. Cancer Res. *35*, 3187–3194 (1975).

53. Scatchard, G. The attraction of proteins for small molecules and ions. Ann N.Y. Acad. Sci. *51*, 660–672 (1949).

54. Shapiro, C. M., Schifeling, D., Bitran, J. D., Desser, R. K., Rockman, H., Michel, A., Shapiro, R., Evans, R., Kozloff, M. F., Recant, W., and Billings, A. A. Prognostic value of estrogen receptor level in pathologic stage I and II adenocarcinoma of the breast. J. Surg. Oncol. *19*, 119–121 (1982).

55. Shaw, H. M., Milton, G. W., Farago, G., and McCarthy, W. H. Endocrine influences on survival from malignant melanoma. Cancer *42*, 669–677 (1978).

56. Simonsson, B., Terenius, L., and Nilsson, K. Glucocorticoids receptors: Clinical characteristics and implications for prognosis in chronic lymphocytic leukemia. Cancer *49*, 2493–2496 (1982).

57. Stewart, J. F., Rubens, R. D., Millis, R. R., King, R. J. B., and Hayward, J. L. Steroid receptors and prognosis in operable (stage I & II) breast cancer. Sur. J. Cancer. Clin. Oncol. *19*, 1381–1387 (1983).

58. Sutherland, C. M., Wittliff, J. L., Fuchs, A., and Mabie, W. C. The effect of pregnancy on hormone levels and receptors in malignant melanoma. J. Surg. Oncol. *22*, 191–192 (1983).

59. Thompson, F. B., and Lippman, M. E. Mechanism of action of glucocorticoids. Metabolism *23*, 159–202 (1974).

60. Tilzer, L. L., Plapp, F. V., Evans, J. P., Stone, D., and Alward, K. Steroid receptor proteins in human meningiomas. Cancer *49*, 633–636 (1982).

61. Toft, D., and Gorski, J. A receptor molecule for estrogens: Isolation from the rat uterus and preliminary characterisation. Proc. Natl. Acad. Sci. USA *55*, 1574–1580 (1966).

62. Vihko, R., Janne, O., and Kauppila, A. Steroid receptors in normal, hyperplastic and malignant human endometria. Ann. Clin. Res. *12*, 208–215 (1980).

63. Vihko, R., Isotalo, H., Kauppila, A., and Vierikko, P. Female sex steroid receptors in gynecological malignancies: Clinical correlations. J. Steroid Biochem. *19*, 827–832 (1983).

64. Willcocks, D., Toppila, M., Hudson, C. N., Tyler, J. P. P., and Baird, P. J. Estrogen and progesterone receptors in human ovarian tumors. Gynecol. Oncol. *16*, 246–253 (1983).

65. Yarbo, G. S. K., Lippman, M. E., Johnson, G. E., and Leventhal, B. G. Subpopulation of childhood acute lymphocytic leukemia. Cancer Res. *37*, 2688–2695 (1977).

66. Young, Jr., J. D., Sidh, S. M., and Bashirelahi, N. The role of estrogen, androgen and progestogen receptors in the management of carcinoma of the prostate. Trans. Amer. Assoc. Genito-Urinary Surgeons *71*, 23–25 (1979).

67. Zava, D. T., and Goldhirsch, A. Estrogen receptor in malignant melanoma: Fact or artefact? Eur. J. Cancer Clin. Oncol. *19*, 1151–1159 (1983).

7

Carbohydrate Antigens Associated with Gastrointestinal Tumors

Magdalena Blaszczyk, Zenon Steplewski,
& Hilary Koprowski

INTRODUCTION

One of the biochemical approaches to the study of human tumors is based on elucidating the tumor cell surface composition and searching for antigenic tumor markers that might be used for diagnostic and therapeutic purposes. The purpose of this chapter is to present an overview of the human gastrointestinal tract (GI) tumor-associated antigens that might be considered as useful markers of the carcinogenic process. Regardless of the initiating transforming agent, alterations in carbohydrate composition associated with glycolipids and glycoproteins which frequently accompany oncogenic transformation have been detected. Carbohydrate determinants coexist as glycolipids and glycoproteins in most of the endothelial tissues and express most of the tumor-associated antigenic activities. The best studied examples of glycosphingolipid-associated GI-tumor antigens are blood group (BG) and related substances extensively studied and reviewed by Hakomori (1–9). The glycoproteins bearing the same tumor-related determinants are mostly associated with extensively studied CEA and mucin-type antigens (for review, see 10–15).

The authors wish to thank Mrs. Marina Hoffman for her excellent editorial assistance.

This chapter concentrates on the examples of tumor-associated carbohydrate antigens that result from transformation-dependent changes in specific glycosyltransferase activity. Specific biochemical differences may be exploited with the recent advances in the field of structural analysis of glycosphingolipids and oligosaccharides and the immunochemical analysis with monoclonal antibody technology.

AB BLOOD GROUP ANTIGENS

The differential expression of major blood group (ABH) and related antigens on normal vs. tumor tissue has been exploited in screening populations at high risk of developing gastrointestinal cancers. The terminal structures of the A, B, and H antigens are:

A: $GalNAc\alpha 1 \rightarrow 3Gal\beta 1 \rightarrow 4GLcNAc\beta 1 \rightarrow$
$$2$$
$$\uparrow$$
$$Fuc\alpha 1$$

B: $Gal\alpha 1 \rightarrow 3Gal\beta 1 \rightarrow 4GLcNAc\beta 1 \rightarrow$
$$2$$
$$\uparrow$$
$$Fuc\alpha 1$$

H: $\qquad Gal\beta 1 \rightarrow 4GLcNAc\beta 1 \rightarrow$
$$2$$
$$\uparrow$$
$$Fuc\alpha 1$$

The presence of blood group substances, which have been demonstrated on various epithelial cells throughout the human body, and the changes in expression of these substances (16–18) assume importance in light of the epithelial origin of most human gastrointestinal cancers. Still controversial, however, is the extent to which loss of these allogeneic antigens or change in the original phenotype with respect to the normal tissue isoantigens are useful markers of malignant change. The availability of monospecific antisera, lectins, and especially monoclonal antibodies to detect blood group substances (BGS) has recently enabled such antigenic comparisons between tumor cells and normal adjacent tissue. In adenocarcinomas of the gastrointestinal tract, alterations in normal BGS expression have been demonstrated both by the examination of glycoprotein-rich extracts (19–21), and more directly with the use of a variety of immunohistochemical techniques (22–24), specific red blood cell adherence tests with conventional polyclonal antisera (25–28), and chemical analysis (29–32). Monoclonal antibodies as blood group reagents seem to confer special advantages in all types of investigations (33–38).

Blood group substances ABO have been studied extensively in fetal (16,39–41) and normal adult epithelium (27,42). BGS are present in the stomach, cecum, and proximal colon, with smaller quantities in the transverse colon and only trace amounts in the distal colon and rectum. However, in various epithelial malignancies, the BGS distribution is altered as compared with normal tissues of the same region (for review see 7–9). Early studies, in which blood group glycoproteins from tumors and normal mucosa were compared chemically and immunologically (19,43), revealed a marked depletion and deletion of blood group A and B antigens in glycoprotein-rich extracts of human gastric carcinoma. Blood group AB activities of glycolipid fractions obtained from colonic tumors were also markedly decreased or absent compared to normal tissue as measured by hemagglutination inhibition (31). In that study, no concomitant increase of the H glycolipid, the immediate precursor of blood group A and B substances, was detected.

Loss of blood group A or B haptens in gastric adenocarcinoma tissue regardless of the blood type of the donor (29,32,44,45) has been demonstrated. The absence of A and B antigens has also been associated with premalignant dysplasia of oral epithelium (46,47) and malignant oral lesions (35). Loss of A antigen in premalignant lesions of oral epithelium was accompanied by an accumulation of H antigen, as detected in all cell layers by monoclonal antibodies (46,47). It was suggested that the loss of AB antigens in stomach and pancreas tumors occurs in a progressive manner from primary to invasive and metastatic carcinoma (48–50). The absence of ABH antigens in primary carcinomas has been taken as an indication of ability to metastasize (34,49), and the value of BGS determination in predicting tumor invasiveness has been noted (48). Reports on BGS expression in metastases of gastric cancer are conflicting. Some studies (48,49) have noted that lymph node metastases of gastric cancer were negative in 80–100% of patients, regardless of the BGS expression in the primary tumor, whereas in other studies (34) with the use of monoclonal antibodies, these metastases were found to express BGS and to reflect the isoantigen status of the primary tumor. Ernst et al. (38), also using monoclonal antibodies, reported that half of all gastric, proximal colon, and pancreatic carcinomas lacked AB antigens, and that antigen expression in the metastases matched that of the primary tumors expressing the antigens.

In patients with intestinal metaplasia, which is considered a precancerous state, loss of BGS antigens was more striking (51,52). Intestinal sucrases, which appear focally in the gastric mucosae of patients with intestinal metaplasia, lacked blood group activities, unlike the sucrases of normal small intestine, which express blood group activities in accord with the individual's blood group and secretor status (53).

The distal colon is unique with respect to BGS expression since normal mucosal epithelium of distal colon and rectum, unlike that in small intestine and colonic epithelium of the cecum and proximal colon, show no BGS reactivity (16,17,26,42,54). By contrast, primary adenocarcinomas of the distal colon and rectum and the liver metastases do express BGS (25,26,38,42,54,55), usually of the type consistent with the patient's blood group. It was suggested that the presence of BGS in carcinomas of the transverse or distal colon characterizes tumors with a lower incidence of metastases or recurrences; carcinomas of the transverse, descending, and rectosigmoid colon, which express no BGS, frequently develop metastases or recurrences (24).

It has been proposed that carcinomas of the large intestine progress through a polyp–cancer sequence (56–58). Adenomas and adenocarcinomas represent two common forms of colonic neoplasia. Hyperplastic polyps do not express BGS and are thus not considered precursors of malignancies (42,59). By contrast, polyps with adenomatous epithelium, which do express BGS, are thought to develop colonic adenocarcinoma. In most patients with both polyps and carcinoma of the distal colon, BGS activity is detected in both tissues (42).

The appearance of BGS in mucosal cells of colon polyps has been related to the histologic degree of differentiation, and BGS activity has been detected in well-differentiated polyps. Polyps tend to reflect the antigenic characteristics of adenocarcinomas (42,59) and, as such, are considered precancerous lesions in humans (60).

The change in BGS expression may be an early biochemical abnormality in the mucus cells of gastrointestinal metaplasias and may be useful in identifying a premalignant state. There is some evidence for a deficiency in *N*-acetylgalactosaminyltransferase activity in epithelium of gastric adenocarcinoma as compared with gastrointestinal mucosal epithelium (61). Selective reduction in galactosyltransferase activity in cancerous colonic tissue of patients with blood type B (62) and a marked reduction in *N*-acetylgalactosaminyltransferase activity (63), which are the enzymes encoded by A and B genes, was observed. The lack of precursor substance for biosynthesis of A and B (H type 2 substance), which might result from an impaired regulatory function of the secretor gene, may also account for the reduced level of antigen. This hypothesis is supported by the observation that Ii structures instead of ABH accumulated in human adenocarcinomas (64). The deletion of ABH activity in tumors has been traced to low activity of the enzymes responsible for synthesis of A, B, and H substances instead of a high glycosidase activity (63).

Decreased levels of BGS in adenocarcinomas of the stomach, small intestine, and ascending colon, and BGS reappearance in the distal colon, consistent with the high BGS levels found during the period of greatest epithelial maturation in fetal and neonatal colon (13,39,41), suggest that these neoplastic cells express certain characteristics of early fetal gastrointestinal tract epithelium. If true, this might suggest a genetic regulatory mechanism by which certain genes encoding glycosyltransferase are suppressed in adenocarcinomas of the stomach, small intenstine, and ascending colon, whereas embryonic gene function is derepressed during carcinogenesis of the distal colon and rectum.

INCOMPATIBLE BLOOD GROUP ANTIGENS

ABH

Among various incompatible blood group antigens in tumors, the most frequently detected in human cancer is A-like antigen. Early studies on the presence of A-like antigen in carcinomas of blood group O or B patients have been reviewed extensively (6). Heterologous BG-A activity has been demonstrated immunohistochemically in patients of B and O blood group in carcinomas of the stomach and colon (45,65–68). In most patients with polyps and distal colon cancers, blood group antigen is expressed in both tissues, the particular type corresponding to the patient's blood group. However, expression of A antigen in colon carcinomas as well as in colon polyps of a blood group B patient was also found (42). In rare cases, the opposite is possible: Denk et al. (25) reported B antigen expression in carcinomas of the stomach and colon in blood group A patients. Inappropriate A expression was detected in pancreatic but not in gastric or colon carcinoma with the use of monoclonal antibodies. Inappropriate expression of B substance was not detected in any tissue, and one out of three polyps from a blood group B patient showed the presence of A antigen (38). Inappropriate A-like antigen expression was further confirmed with chemical analysis in which A-active glycolipids were isolated from gastric adenocarcinomas of blood group O patients (29,69). Recently, an A-like heptaglycosylceramide with an additional fucose at the glucosamine was detected (30). The fraction containing this structure reacted with some anti-A antisera, which probably contained a population of antibodies directed against A-7, but did not react with anti-Forssman antisera, which are known to cross-react with the ordinary blood group A antigen (30,70).

A ceramide pentasaccharide that was A-active but contained no detectable fucose was isolated from a colonic cancer patient with BG-A activity. In this tumor, the major fucose-containing A-active glycolipid was depleted. The unfucosylated structure may not be considered as an appropriate antigen since the tumor tissue was derived from a BG-A patient (31). Finan et al. (34) did not detect expression of any of the A-like inappropriate isoantigens in gastric adenocarcinoma from blood group O patients using monoclonal antibodies and the immunoperoxidase method. The failure to detect A-like antigens is probably due to the specificity of the anti-A monoclonal antibody which is restricted to the A-6 monofucosylated determinant and does not detect the A-7 difucosylated structure, assuming that the latter represents the tumor-specific A-active structure (34). A-like glycolipid, which inhibits A hemagglutination, was isolated from the hepatocarcinoma of a blood group O patient and was also precipitated with the *Rana catesbiana* lectin, which reacts with GalNAcα1→03Galβ1→4GlcNAcβ1→4 but not with the Forssman structure (71). The absence of the fucose residue that characterizes the normal A-determinant suggested a structure similar to that reported by Siddiqui et al. (31); however, it is possible that the A-like antigen is a ceramide hexasaccharide with an altered internal structure since digestion with α-N-acetylgalactosaminidase yields a glycolipid with a slower migration than paragloboside on TLC gels. Mass spectrometry of the fraction indicated the presence of GalNAcα→Hex→HexN→R but the absence of a tetrasaccharide A determinant with a fucosyl residue. The structure did not contain the characteristic fucose residue of the A-determinant and contained no Forssman activity. However, the same tumor did express the Forssman determinant in a short carbohydrate chain (71).

The inappropriate expression of BGS-A in tumors may explain the increased incidence of stomach carcinoma in blood group A patients, i.e. the immunological system of these patients may fail to recognize the tumor cells because of the structural similarity and cross-reactivity of the tumor glycolipid with the A substance.

It is as yet difficult to postulate about the mechanism of these changes. Since biosynthesis of these alloantigens is genetically controlled, somatic mutation might be the basis for A-like antigen expression. Again, assuming that A-7 (30) or defucosylated A-like structures determine the activity (31,71) of tumor cells, it would be interesting to determine whether glycosyltransferases with different specificity are derepressed or simply show broader specificity than their normal counterparts. For example, GalNAc may be attached to a difucosylated structure, or fucosyltransferase might act on an A-6 structure as an acceptor to form A-7 tumor-associated antigen. Human adenocarcinoma may produce an unusual glycosyl transferase with less restricted substrate specificity so that an unusual difucosylated A-7 structure (30) or the A-determinant without a fucosyl residue (31,71) are formed. On the other hand, loss of A-antigen accompanied by accumulation of H antigen in premalignant and malignant oral lesions (35), of I antigen in gastric carcinoma of secretors (45), and of the precursor structure LN_3 in colon carcinoma (64), suggest a decreased activity of *N*-acetylgalactosyltransferase in the first case, and of galactosyltransferase in the latter two cases.

H-Type-2 Blood Group Antigen

Other changes in expression of ABH alloantigens have been detected by immunoperoxidase and immunofluorescence methods (35,45). Loss of A and B epithelial cell membrane-bound BG-A in premalignant and malignant oral lesions with epithelial dysplasia is accompanied by an accumulation of BG precursors. The H antigen has been detected by immunohistochemical staining with monoclonal antibody to H antigen only in basal and suprabasal cells of normal mucosa, independent of the patient's blood group. The antigen was found in 90% of premalignant lesions and was present in cell membranes in all layers of the epithelium (35). This change in expression in cell surface antigens may be due to an arrest of cells at a stage of differentiation comparable to that of the basal layers of normal epithelium. The difference in distribution of H antigen in oral premalignant lesions and in normal epithelium may be useful in the early diagnosis of epithelial cancer (35). Tumor tissue of nonsecretor individuals of blood group A showed A and H or only H staining (25). Glycolipids isolated from human gastric and cecal adenocarcinoma lacked BG-A and BG-B activities but weakly expressed BG-H and Le[a] specificities (29). Similarly, "secretor-like" areas with strong H antigen staining appear in nonsecretor gastric mucosa of chronic benign gastric ulcer patients (45).

The H-type-2 blood group antigen was found by an immunohistochemical technique with lectins and monoclonal antibody to be expressed on adenocarcinomas and adenomas of distal large bowel, whereas it is usually not found in normal adult epithelium (72–74). However, the H-type-2 antigen is found in adenomas much less frequently than Y antigen, a H-type-2-related, α3-linked fucosylated (Fucα1→3GlcNAc) structure (75). The H-type-2 antigen was found only in the proximal colon of adults, whereas it is expressed throughout the large bowel of the fetus (76). Thus again, expression of H-type-2 antigen in colorectal carcinomas (72–74) might be considered an oncofetal marker in human tumors of distal colon. The H-type-2 molecule is the structural precursor for A, B, and Y substances. All these antigens are of oncofetal character in large bowel tumors. It can be postulated that the biosynthesis of blood group carbohydrates, which involves a step-by-step elongation, is blocked during oncogenesis. The level of H-type-2 antigen in tumors also might be modulated by activation of α1→3 fucosyltransferase, β1→4 galactosyltransferase, or β1→4 N-acetyl galactosyltransferase to form Y, B, and A antigens, respectively.

Ii Antigens

Normal mucosa of secretor individuals expresses A, B, and H antigens, whereas normal nonsecretor type mucosa expresses the I determinant (77), as detected by anti-I (Ma) antibody which recognizes the oligosacharride structure:

Galβ1→4GlcNAcβ1→6

Expression of the i determinant has not been correlated with the secretor/nonsecretor status of the normal mucosa. The majority of gastric carcinomas from secretors show intense staining with anti-I (Ma) antibody, in contrast to normal secretors (21,45,77,78). Only weak staining with anti-I (Ma) was observed in nonsecretor tumors (45). Remarkable quantitative differences were observed between the intestinal tumors and normal intestinal mucosa in the levels of the precursor I structure:

GlcNAcβ1→3Galβ1→4Glcβ1→1CER

Tumor tissue characteristically had an accumulation of the first amino sugar-containing precursor structure of synthesis of components of various blood group chains, including an extended and branched structure (64).

The accumulation of precursor structures Ii and the amino structures involved in blood group antigen biosynthesis in tumor tissue probably results from a block of BG chain synthesis. Similar precursor structures were detected immunologically in appreciable quantity in erythrocytes of fetuses and neonates, whereas these structures were less abundant in adult erythrocytes (64).

PP$_1$ Antigen

Another example of the expression of incompatible blood group antigens in human adenocarcinoma was found in the P blood group system (79,80). The patient, who had gastric cancer, was blood group O and a very rare variant of the P system identified as pp. Prior to subtotal gastrectomy, this patient was transfused with incompatible blood, which caused a severe hemolytic reaction and an increase in her initial anti-PP$_1$Pk antibody titer from 8 to 512. The patient died 22 years later of brain hemorrhage without any evidence of metastases. Chemical analysis of the patient's tumor showed that the adenocarcinoma expressed inappropriate determinants of the PP$_1$Pk complex (81). The major glycolipid isolated is a pentasaccharide ceramide with the same terminal structure as the globoside (P antigen) and an internal structure identical to paragloboside,

$$\text{GalNAc}\beta 1 \rightarrow 3\text{Gal}\beta 1 \rightarrow 4\text{GlcNAc}\beta 1 \rightarrow 3\text{Gal}\beta 1 \rightarrow 4\text{Glc}\beta 1 \rightarrow 1\text{CER}$$

designated P-like antigen. Glycolipid with P$_1$ activity was also demonstrated. Globo-series glycolipids (Pk-ceramide trihexoside and P-globoside) are not synthesized in normal tissues of these individuals due to the lack of α-galactose transferase, which converts lactosylceramide to ceramide trihexoside. The lack of synthesis of major globo-series glycolipids results in an accumulation of lactosylceramide and increased synthesis of paragloboside and sialosylparagloboside. The conversion of paragloboside to the P$_1$ structure is defective also because of the lack of α-galactose transferase. Breimer (82) obtained similar results in an analysis of normal gastric mucosa of pp phenotype individuals. P and P-like antigens are found in normal tissue of pp individuals but at much lower levels than in tumor tissue. Tumor tissues of pp individuals also do not synthesize Pk and P antigens, although the conversion of paragloboside to P$_1$ is activated and the conversion of paragloboside to P-like antigen is greatly enhanced. Consequently, the levels of paragloboside and sialylparagloboside become lower than in normal tissues. Globo-series structures have been detected in teratocarcinomas using a monoclonal antibody that reacts with an internal structure of these compounds (83).

Recently it was shown that the "extended" GL-5,6,7 globo-series structures are unique to human teratocarcinoma and embryos and may display previously uncharacterized antigens in the P blood group system (84). It is possible that all of the antigens in the P blood group system function as developmental antigens in human embryogenesis and oncogenesis and represent an oncofetal type of antigen. Although, in the case of the gastric cancer from the pp individual, globo-series antigens were not detected, the major component was a lacto-series glycolipid with the same terminal structure as globoside (81).

Forssman Antigen

The Forssman antigen is a glycosphingolipid whose structure was identified (85,86) as:

$$GalNAc\alpha1 \rightarrow 3GalNAc\beta1 \rightarrow 3Gal\alpha1 \rightarrow 4Gal\beta1 \rightarrow 4Glc1 \rightarrow CER$$

Most individuals do not express Forssman antigen. Although the Forssman glycolipid may not be synthesized by human erythrocytes, this glycolipid was identified in 20–30% of gastrointestinal normal mucosa of a Taiwanese population (F^+ population). The possible role of the Forssman antigen as a tumor antigen was suggested based on its presence in gastric and colon tumors derived from F^- mucosa and its absence in tumors originating in F^+ individuals (70,87,88). On the other hand, Forssman antigen synthetic activity was observed in the majority of normal and neoplastic lung tissue samples examined. This discrepancy with the data for gastrointestinal mucosa might rest in tissue differences (89).

Forssman antigen was isolated and chemically identified in one case of metastasized biliary duct carcinoma, but the glycolipid composition of normal tissue was not examined (90). A short-chain Forssman determinant, which was not the normal ceramide pentasaccharide structure, was found in a blood group O individual with hepatocarcinoma (71). Approximately 70–80% of sera from normal donors contain anti-Forssman antibody. The anti-Forssman antibody titer in the sera of the Taiwanese cancer patients was generally lower than that of the control group, i.e. Taiwanese gastric ulcer patients. This observation suggests that Forssman-positive tumors might affect serum anti-Forssman antibody levels (91). Levine showed that only 38% of patients with adenocarcinomas had serum anti-Forssman activity as compared with 79% of normal sera (92,93). However, anti-Forssman antibody levels are age-related in normal populations; i.e. 90% of sera in younger age groups are positive for anti-Forssman antibody, whereas only 59% in the age group of 60–80 years are positive (92,93).

Forssman antigen has been demonstrated on the surface membrane of SV-40 and polyoma virus-transformed BHK fibroblastic cells but has not been detected on nontransformed control cells (94). The W4-3 cell line is oncogenic in syngeneic newborn mice and possesses tumor-specific transplantation antigens (95), and thus the expression of Forssman antigen is clearly associated with the malignant nature of the cells resulting from infection with the viral DNA or its fragments.

T, Tn ANTIGENS

Another example of carcinoma-associated antigens is given by the blood group precursor antigens T and Tn, with structures, respectively,

$$\text{Gal}\beta1{\rightarrow}3\text{GalNAc}\alpha1{\rightarrow}0\text{-Ser/Thr}$$

and

$$\text{GalNAc}\alpha1{\rightarrow}0\text{-Ser/Thr}$$

A recent excellent review by Springer (96) describes their relevance as an adenocarcinoma-associated antigen. T and Tn antigens in normal tissues represent immediate precursor structures for human blood group MN antigens, though they are present on most normal tissues as penultimate carbohydrates, in a masked form by covalently linked αNANA residues (97). T and Tn antigens are expressed throughout human embryonal life (98) and occur as a surface antigen on most primary carcinomas and their metastases (99,100) in a glycoprotein or glycolipid form (101,102). The recent development of a monoclonal antibody specific for the T structure should enable further studies on the role of T as an oncofetal antigen (103,104). All human sera contain anti-T antibodies (100,105). In patients with metastatic gastrointestinal cancer, however, serum levels of anti-T were shown to be depressed as compared to normal controls, and there was inverse correlation between the level of circulating anti-T and tumor burden (99,100). The anti-T antibodies in these patients may be depleted through immune complex formation.

Based on the structural interrelationship between MN antigens and their precursors, it seems likely that expression of T and Tn antigens in tumor tissues results from defective sialyltransferase and N-acetylgalactosyltransferase activity, respectively.

LEWIS ANTIGENS

The Lewis blood group antigens offer another system with potential diagnostic usefulness, since the distribution of Lewis antigen, like that in the ABH system, differs in normal and tumor tissues. The structures of the Lewis a and b antigens are:

$$Le^a:\quad Gal\beta1\rightarrow3GlcNAc\beta1\rightarrow4Gal\beta1\rightarrow4Glc\beta1\rightarrow1CER$$
$$2$$
$$\uparrow$$
$$Fuc\alpha1$$

$$Le^b:\quad Gal\beta1\rightarrow3GlcNAc\beta1\rightarrow4Gal\beta1\rightarrow4Glc\beta1\rightarrow1CER$$
$$4\qquad\qquad\qquad 2$$
$$\uparrow\qquad\qquad\qquad\uparrow$$
$$Fuc\alpha1\qquad\qquad Fuc\alpha1$$

Normal human intestines reflect the same phenotype as erythrocytes and express Le^a or Le^b antigens (106).

In an analysis of the glycolipid composition of normal human gastric mucosa, both Le^a and Le^b activity was detected and glycolipids were represented by Le^a −5 and the Le^b −6 and Le^b −8 species (107). Gastric tumors contained higher levels of Le^a-active glycolipid and lower levels of Le^b-active glycolipid than found in uninvolved tissue. It was postulated (69) that blood group A-active glycolipids may be present in the form of hybrid types with Lewis activity or that A-active glycolipids may coexist with Lewis-active glycolipids in these gastric adenocarcinomas. The Le^b active structures of Le^b −6 and Le^b −8 were found to be among the dominant glycosphingolipids isolated from human gastric carcinoma (30). The glycosphingolipid fraction isolated from gastric and cecal adenocarcinomas expressed weak Le^a but no AB activity (29). A similar deletion of ABH antigens was in some cases found to result in an increase in the amount of Lewis-active glycolipid antigens and more frequent instances of Lewis antigen coexpression (32).

The immunohistologic profile of these antigens in gastrointestinal adenocarcinomas and normal mucosa has been characterized with anti-Le^a and Le^b monoclonal antibodies and an immunoperoxidase technique (108). Le^a antigen was expressed in 40% of normal and 80% of malignant tissue, and coexpression of Le^a and Le^b was more frequent in tumor tissue. There was no significant difference in the percentage of Le^b positive normal (80%) and malignant (73%) specimens. Thus exclusive or predominant expression of Le^a in gastric carcinomas may be considered abnormal. Le^a and Le^b coexisted in normal mucosa of proximal colon, as they do in some gastric mucosae (17). Proximal colon adenocarcinoma showed the Lewis phenotype of its normal counterpart, i.e. Le^{a-b+}, of a Lewis-positive patient. However, all distal colon adenocarcinoma specimens coexpressed Le^a and Le^b antigens, whereas normal tissue expressed only Le^a (108). The same results were obtained by immunochemical analysis (109). Isolated neutral glycosphingolipids from normal colonic mucosa showed Le^a activity only, and the antigen was represented by Le^a -5 and Le^a -7 isomers. Expression of Le^b antigens was demonstrated in isolated glycolipids from colon adenocarcinomas and in all cell lines derived from gastrointestinal adenocarcinomas (39,109). Le^b antigen may be considered as a marker antigen of distal colonic adenocarcinomas. It is possible that in distal colon carcinomas, the transformation process either induces $\alpha1\rightarrow4$ fucosyltransferase, which is a product of the *H* gene, or activates a regulatory function of the secretor gene over the *H* gene. Either mechanism would result in the biosynthesis of Le^b substance since $1\rightarrow2$ fucosyltransferase, a product of the *Le* gene, is presumably active in light of the presence of Le^a in both normal and tumor tissue.

Pompecki et al. (110) demonstrated high levels of anti-Le^{ab} antibodies in serum of cancer patients, as measured by the CEA BP-160 binding assay which detects H, Le^b, and MN determinants. The antibodies are likely to result from sensitization to embryonic proteins or from incomplete biosynthesis of blood group substances expressed in tumor tissue. In colon cancer patients, a correlation has been observed between binding activity of anti-Le^{ab} antibodies and serum CEA levels, and a possible relationship exists between CEA BP-160 binding activity and tumor burden (110).

The histologic distribution of blood group ABH and Le antigens during fetal development of several tissues has been studied by immunofluorescence techniques (111). Lewis antigens have been found to be present in fetal gut, but those of the distal colon disappear after birth. An important source of fetal antigens (112) may be meconium since, during fetal development, epithelial cells lining the intestine are extruded into the intestinal lumen. Because meconium is produced during most of the fetal period, the glycolipids might be an important source of transiently expressed fetal antigens (113). The presence of Le^a and Le^b glycolipids as major fucolipids, consistent with blood group phenotype, in meconium from humans has been reported (114, 115), although Le^b-active glycosphingolipids have been identified in meconium of a phenotypically A,Le^{a+b-} nonsecretor individual (116).

X Antigen

The X or Lewis^X glycolipid was first isolated from human adenocarcinomas, where it was shown to accumulate (117):

$$Gal\beta1\rightarrow4GLcNAc\beta1\rightarrow3Gal\beta1\rightarrow4Glc\beta1\rightarrow1CER$$
$$3$$
$$\uparrow$$
$$Fuc\alpha1$$

A series of monoclonal antibodies derived from mice immunized with human adenocarcinomas of the stomach and liver metastasis of a colon adenocarcinoma were found to be directed to the same antigen described as the X structure (118). Another series of monoclonal antibodies, derived from mice immunized with human small lung carcinoma, displayed the same specificity (119). Although this antigen, also referred to as stage-specific embryonic antigen (SSEA-1), was described as a marker of murine embryos and murine embryonal carcinoma cells, it is not expressed by human embryonal carcinoma stem cells (120). However, the expression of X antigen may be useful as an *in vitro* differentiation marker in the human embryonal carcinoma system (121).

Recently, an extensive chemical study on the X-hapten glycolipids was undertaken to define the structures of the antigen in normal and tumor cells. The major glycolipids containing the X determinant in normal tissues are characterized by an unbranched type 2 chain with a fucosyl $\alpha1\rightarrow3$ linkage at the penultimate GlcNAc (122,123). In contrast, tumor tissue and particularly adenocarcinoma showed a large accumulation of novel, polyfucosylated structures of glycolipids, in addition to lactofucopentaosyl ceramide accumulating in human adenocarcinoma (123–126). One is difucosyl neolactonorhexaosylceramide and the other is trifucosyl neolactonoroctaosylceramide. Both glycolipids are based on a type 2 polylactosamine backbone and a fucosyl residue linked to every GlcNAc through an $\alpha1\rightarrow3$ linkage, i.e. multimeric X-hapten. These structures are not detected in normal erythrocytes, granulocytes, normal colonic mucosa, or normal liver (123). All structures which accumulate exclusively in tumors have the common fucosylated unit at the internal GlcNAc:

$$R\rightarrow4GlcNAc\beta1\rightarrow3Gal\beta1\rightarrow4Glc\beta1\rightarrow Cer$$

$$\underset{Fuc\alpha1}{\overset{3}{\uparrow}}$$

Since difucosyl neolactonorhexaosylceramide and trifucosyl neolacto-noroctaosylceramide—structures that contain this unit—characteristically accumulate in membranes of various human cancer cells, murine monoclonal antibodies that recognize internal fucosyl residues but not external X determinants were established (126). Such reagents are extremely useful in detecting tumor cells that are enriched for di- or trifucosylated type 2 chain structures. The proposed synthetic pathway for polyfucosylated polylactosaminyl lipids with a type 2 chain involves the active elongation of type 2 chain and a simultaneous fucosylation of the GlcNAc residues. It is possible that a specific fucosyltransferase for synthesis of the internal R-4GlcNAc[3←1Fuc]$\beta1\rightarrow$3Gal structure is greatly enhanced in human adenocarcinomas. On the other hand, the fucosyltransferase for synthesis of the terminal X determinant may not be affected by cancer since the X determinants at the long type 2 chain terminus are present in normal tissue (122,123). The synthetic pathway in normal tissues and cells proceeds through branching and chain elongation but without GlcNAc fucosylation (125).

Recent studies using a monoclonal antibody to SSEA-1 have shown that the X determinant is present in normal colon in much lower amounts than in tumor sections (127). A faint positive reaction was seen only in the lower crypts, suggesting that X-antigen expression as detected with anti-SSEA monoclonal antibody decreases during the maturation process. Also, in human fetal colon, the number of crypts and the intensity of staining increased drastically. The X-5 determinant appears earlier during embryonic development than multimeric X structures and is expressed after birth (128). Furthermore, transitional mucosa adjacent to human colon adenocarcinoma expresses this antigen. Thus, the X and poly-X glycolipids represent an onco-developmental marker of human colonic adenocarcinoma and characterize a premalignant state of colonic mucosa.

Y Antigen

The Y glycolipid is another Lewis isomeric difucosylated structure based on a type 2 chain involving the sequence $Fuc\alpha1\rightarrow2Gal$, the product of a fucosyltransferase specified by the H blood group gene:

$$Gal\beta1\rightarrow4GLcNAc\beta1\rightarrow3Gal\beta1\rightarrow3Glc\beta1\rightarrow1CER$$
$$\begin{array}{cc} 2 & 3 \\ \uparrow & \uparrow \\ Fuc\alpha1 & Fuc\alpha1 \end{array}$$

This antigen was detected by immunoperoxidase techniques and monoclonal antibody in luminal surfaces of the majority of adenocarcinomas of the human colon and rectum (96%) and in all colorectal adenomas (100%) (129,130). In normal mucosa, the Y hapten was consistently found in secretors, in mucosa of the esophagus, stomach, small intestine, and proximal colon. In normal mucosa of the distal colon, Y antigen was found irrespective of secretor status but only in immature cells of crypt bases. These results suggest that the Y hapten, like the Le^b antigen, might represent an antigenic marker of distal colon carcinomas. Furthermore, the presence of this antigen in adenomas and ulcerative colitis lesions, which are considered to be premalignant stages, support the notion of an adenoma–carcinoma sequence in adenocarcinoma development (75).

LACTOSYLCERAMIDE

The lactosylceramide glycolipid is a normal membrane constituent of most mammalian cells and is accumulated in gastrointestinal tract tumors (131,132). It was shown that the sera of gastric and colonic cancer patients contain lactosylsphingosine-reactive antibodies (132,133), as detected by reactivity with an artificial lactosylsphingosine–polyacrylamide conjugate (134). This test seems to be more sensitive than assays of CEA titer and is valuable for the detection of colorectal cancer and monitoring in these patients (135). The availability of monoclonal antibody to lactosylceramide (136) should provide another useful tool for analysis of expression of this antigen in tumor tissues.

GANGLIOSIDES

The ganglioside content in colon and pancreatic tumors, as well as in metastases, has been shown to be much higher than in normal colon mucosa (137,138). A significant increase in the amount of GD_3 and GM_3, as well as complex mono- and disialogangliosides, was observed (137). Several recent findings suggest that monosialogangliosides of gastrointestinal adenocarcinomas are characteristic of the tumor state and contain several gastrointestinal tumor-associated antigens. The monosialoganglioside fraction of primary colorectal adenocarcinomas and the metastases of colonic and pancreatic adenocarcinomas contain "tumor-associated" undefined antigens recognized by monoclonal antibodies (139). Analysis of human cancer gangliosides using a monoclonal antibody that detects a sialosyl $\alpha2\rightarrow6$ galactosyl residue revealed accumulation of two major gangliosides in human colonic and liver adenocarcinoma. These gangliosides were represented by a sialosyl $\alpha2\rightarrow6$ lacto-neotetraosylceramide and lactonorhexaosylceramide internally fucosylated at GlcNAc (140). Also, an abundance of an $\alpha2\rightarrow3$ sialosyl derivative of difucosyllactonorhexaosylceramide was detected in tumor tissue, whereas normal tissue contained only trace amounts of these gangliosides (140,141). Of particular interest is the accumulation of the latter fucoganglioside, with a fucose substitution at the internal GlcNAc residue (see section on X antigen). Similar monosialogangliosides, which after desialylation coincide with the X structure, were detected in a human colon carcinoma cell line and in meconium (142).

The Hanganutziu-Deicher (HD) antigen was identified as a ganglioside containing the N-glycolylneuraminosyl $\alpha\rightarrow3$ galactosyl residues in various types of human cancers using heterophile HD antibodies and antibodies to N-glycolylhematoside (143,144). Of particular interest is the absence of N-glycolylneuraminic acid from normal human tissues.

Gastrointestinal Cancer Antigen

The monoclonal antibodies NS 19-9 and NS 52a produced against colon carcinoma cell line SW 1116 were found to detect an antigen not only in colorectal adenocarcinoma tissue, but also on gastric and pancreatic cancer cell lines (145). The gastrointestinal cancer antigen (GICA) defined by these monoclonal antibodies was found in the monosialoganglioside fraction of human adenocarcinoma cell line SW 1116, human pancreatic carcinoma, and meconium, but not in extracts of normal intestinal mucosa, normal spleen, erythrocytes, a melanoma cell line, or in human brain gangliosides (146,147). Intestinal epithelial cells of human adults contain practically no gangliosides, which are instead preferentially located in nonepithelial stroma (148,149). GICA was identified as a monosialoganglioside (146), and the structure of the antigen was determined as sialosyl-Le^a (147):

$$NeuAc\alpha2\rightarrow3Gal\beta1\rightarrow3GlcNAc\beta1\rightarrow3Gal\beta1\rightarrow4Glc\beta1\text{-}1CER$$
$$2$$
$$\uparrow$$
$$Fuc\alpha1$$

The ceramide is composed mainly of phytosphingosine and 16-24 carbon 2-hydroxy fatty acids (150). Both monoclonal antibodies NS 19-9 and NS 52a detected a specific determinant, since no reactivity was observed with the isomeric structures (146).

Extensive immunohistochemical studies with the immunoperoxidase (IP) method and monoclonal antibody NS 19-9 revealed that the monosialo-Le^a antigen (GICA) was not exclusively tumor-specific, since it was detected in differentiated normal adult glandular epithelia such as endocervix, gall bladder, pancreas, and salivary glands (151). However, the antigen appears to be abundant in most colorectal and endometrial primary adenocarcinomas and their metastases (152). The presence of the GICA antigen in colorectal cancer cells might be associated with more aggressive tumor behavior (153), although GICA immunoreactivity did not correlate with other diagnostic parameters such as stage or histological grade (154). GICA also was demonstrated in colorectal tissue from patients with chronic ulcerative colitis, although the pattern and intensity of staining did not correlate with the degree of dysplasia, i.e. mild to moderate epithelial dysplasia was often GICA-positive, whereas severely dysplastic areas were GICA-negative (155). This antigen was virtually absent in normal or hyperplastic epithelium, although single cells scattered throughout the mucosa adjacent to the tumor were stained (152,155).

GICA has been identified in some colonic polyps, including both tubular and villous adenomas (152). The presence of 19-9 may indicate a premalignant alteration and is related to the level of differentiation of gastrointestinal tract adenocarcinomas. A similar observation was made for blood group substances AB, Le^b, and Y antigens which might be considered as markers of early premalignant changes in distal colon. Since GICA represents a sialylated-Le^a antigen and is not detected in normal tissues such as colon, the "abnormal" sialyltransferase that synthesizes GICA is presumably absent in this organ.

Thus, GICA synthesis in colon carcinomas may involve the induction of sialyltransferase.

The relative percentages of tumors derived from colon, pancreas, and stomach that express Le^a and GICA are similar. Le^a expression is also enhanced in adenocarcinomas (108); however, further studies are necessary to establish the relationship of GICA to the Le antigens in the same tumor.

The presence of the NS 19-9 antigen in human gastrointestinal tract adenocarcinomas and meconium suggests that the molecule represents a gastrointestinal tumor-associated embryonic antigen. This observation is supported by the data of Roux et al. (156) and Olding et al. (157), showing that human embryonic tissues at certain stages of ontogenesis express sialosyl-Le^a antigen. Olding et al. (157) consistently detected GICA in the mucosal epithelium of the small intestine, especially in the duodenum and jejunum, but was unable to demonstrate it in the mucous membrane of the colon–rectum either by immunohistological techniques or by analysis of glycolipid extracts from the large intestine. This observation contrasts with the results of Roux et al. (156), who detected GICA in the colon–rectum by immunofluorescence and concluded from biochemical experiments that the 19-9 epitope exists as a glycoprotein and not as a glycolipid.

Arends et al. (151) reported that goblet cells of intestinal mucosa of 12-week embryos were positive for the 19-9–defined antigen. In later stages of gestation, the antigen was also expressed on the brush border of the columnar epithelium in the small and large bowels (151). Surface cells of human bowel specimens of 14–17 weeks' gestation showed focal staining for GICA (152). The oncofetal nature of this antigen implies that the enzyme is re-expressed in tumor cells of the gastrointestinal tract. However, Paulson et al. (unpublished) observed that normal purified fucosyltransferase does not add fucose to the LS-tetrasaccharide a structure, nor does purified sialyltransferase add a sialic acid residue to lacto-N fucopentaose II (Le^a) to form sialylated-Le^a. Those authors suggested that glycosyltransferases of tumor origin express a different specificity toward acceptors than the mature form of the enzymes.

Several observations suggest that $\alpha2 \rightarrow 3$ sialyltransferase is an enzyme re-expressed in tumor tissue and responsible for biosynthesis of GICA using Le^a substance as the precursor. Approximately 5% of the population is phenotypically Le^{a-b-}, and such individuals are unable to synthesize either Le^a or Le^b antigen because they lack the fucosyltransferase specified by the *Le* gene. These Le^{a-b-} individuals also do not express GICA in their sera, tumor tissues, or normal saliva (158–160). Thus, it is possible that Le^{a-b-} individuals have a different susceptibility to gastrointestinal tract malignancies and that the distribution of Le^{a-b-}, Le^{a+b-}, and Le^{a-b+} phenotypes differs among patients with gastric and pancreatic cancer (158,159).

A positive correlation has been demonstrated between the presence of GICA in resected colonic carcinomas and in the sera of these patients (152). Antigen detected with antibody NS 19-9 was found in 70% of the sera from patients with colorectal adenocarcinomas, 80% with gastric adenocarcinomas, and 90% with pancreatic carcinomas (161–163). Kuusela et al. (164), using the CA-19-9® test, detected the 19-9 antigen in the sera of 46% and 45% of patients with advanced (Dukes C or D) carcinoma and verified recurrences, respectively. Similarly, Del Villano et al. (165) found elevated CA-19-9 values in 46% of patients with advanced carcinomas. Sears et al. (166), also using this assay, were able to predict the recurrence of colorectal cancer 3–18 months prior to the development of any clinical or laboratory signs. Some individuals with no detectable 19-9 antigen in their sera showed the presence of this antigen in immunoperoxidase assay of their tumor specimen, although the presence of 19-9 antigen in tumor tissue does not preclude its absence in the serum (152). Some tissue culture cell lines express membrane and cytoplasmic antigens detectable in RIA but do not shed the antigens into tissue culture medium (167). On the other hand, the antigen might circulate in the form of an immune complex(es), escaping detection in inhibition assay (RIA) or double-determinant immunoassay (DDIA). The latter possibility seems unlikely since the 19-9 antigen is present in serum as a multi-determinant, high molecular weight mucin molecule and not as a monovalent monosialoganglioside (168). The DDIA technique, which was developed as an immunodiagnostic test for detection of cancer antigens in serum, was based on the assumption that the antigenic determinant detected by the monoclonal antibody is repeatedly present on the molecule (161).

CARCINOEMBRYONIC ANTIGEN

The carcinoembryonic antigens (CEA) are a group of glycoprotein cell surface markers that have been extensively studied in carcinomas of the gastrointestinal tract (169–171). Serum CEA levels have been used to monitor the response of gastrointestinal and pancreatic carcinoma patients to therapy (169,172,173) and in the early detection of recurrences (174,175). However, not all patients with carcinomas of these organs have abnormal serum CEA levels (173). CEA was first isolated by Gold and Freedman (176,177) in 1966 as a 180-kd molecular weight glycoprotein and defined as an antigenic substance found exclusively in adenocarcinomas arising from endodermally derived epithelia of the digestive system and in fetal gut epithelia during the first trimester (176,177). Several subtypes of CEA have subsequently been identified, and several CEA-related normal adult tissue components have been identified in fetal adult epithelium, feces, bile, and some non-neoplastic gastrointestinal diseases (178–185). NCA is one of the relatively well characterized CEA-related antigens (186–191). This antigen shares antigenic determinants with CEA and is frequently detected in normal tissues as well as in malignant tissues. Since the pioneer work, CEA has been the subject of many reviews that provide a guide to the literature on this marker (10–12).

CEA consists of a single polypeptide chain, six disulfide bridges, and a carbohydrate content of 50% with asparagine-linked oligosaccharide chains that occur with an average spacing of about 1 chain per 10 amino acid residues (192). Considerable heterogeneity has been observed in the carbohydrate composition of CEA isolated in various studies, despite the similarity in amino acid compositions of the different preparations used (192–196).

Extensive homology was demonstrated between the NH_2 terminal sequences of CEA and NCA, which differed at only 1 of 26 residues (alanine 21 of NCA is valine in CEA) (196–198). The carbohydrate chains are linked to asparagine residues of the protein through N-acetylglucosamine. The synthesis of N-asparagine-linked carbohydrate specifically requires the sequence Asn-X-Ser/Thr in a polypeptide chain to effect the transfer of precursor oligosaccharides from dolichol phosphate intermediates to the nascent polypeptide chain. Glycopeptides isolated from CEA have been shown to contain at least 120 of the amino acids involved in this sequence (199). Protein sequence studies on CEA are technically difficult since CEA contains over 50% carbohydrate and over 600 amino acids. Nevertheless, it has been possible to determine the amino terminal sequences of several tryptic peptides (200,201).

Progress in determining the carbohydrate structure of CEA, however, has been considerable, although the total carbohydrate and fucose content as well as the extent of sialylation have been variably reported depending on the preparation used (189–191). The structure of the carbohydrate unit of CEA has been proposed (202) as:

GlcNAc→Man→Man→GlcNAc→GlcNAc→Asn
  ↑   ↑   ↑
           GlcNAc
           ↑
        Gal←Fuc or NANA

Recent studies by Chandrasekaran et al. (199) have indicated three different types of N-asparagine-linked oligosaccharide chains in CEA. About 80% of the oligosaccharide chains in CEA are tetra-antennary, while the remaining chains are triantennary (15–20%) or diantennary. The sialic acids in CEA are α-linked to the 3 and 6 positions of the penultimate galactose units. Most of the tetra-antennary chains also contain one or two fucose residues α-linked to the 3 position of penultimate GlcNAc units. About half of the triantennary chains contain 1 or 2 residues of sialic acid α-linked at positions 3 and 6 of the terminal galactosyl units, and most of these chains also contain one fucose residue α-linked to the 3 position of a penultimate GlcNAc unit. Only 5–10% of the chains are diantennary (199). The presence of some GalNAc units suggests the presence of additional O-serine-linked glycoproteins (203).

The problems associated with immunological heterogeneity of CEA have been minimized by the use of monoclonal antibodies. The exquisite immunospecificity of monoclonal antibodies has enabled the identification of CEA antigenic markers that have been associated with the tumor state. Monoclonal antibodies that react with antigenic determinants on CEA have been reported (204–213). Some of these anti-CEA monoclonal antibodies have proven useful in immunohistochemical localization of CEA in tissue sections to distinguish normal or benign cells from malignant ones. In colon carcinoma, the CEA content increases as a function of tumor differentiation, with poorly differentiated carcinomas staining only weakly (214–216). However, Wiley et al. recently reported an increased incidence of metastases from tumors of the transverse and distal colon that were negative for both CEA and blood group antigens, irrespective of tumor histology (24).

Direct sensitive immunoassays and the ability to distinguish tumor-specific from cross-reactive determinants of CEA should prove valuable in the prognosis and monitoring of the therapy of human gastrointestinal tumors (217).

MUCINS

The mucins are high molecular weight glycoproteins synthesized and secreted by epithelial cells of the underlying mucosa. Mucines are present along the entire length of the gastrointestinal tract and are structurally (62,218,219), functionally, and antigenically (220,221) heterogeneous, depending on the segment of GI tract (for review, see

222). Many of the carbohydrate structures of these mucins also occur on certain membrane glycoproteins and glycolipids of cells that express blood group antigens A, B, H, Lewis, Ii (223), SSEA-1, and sialylated structures (for review, see 13,14).

The malignant change in gastrointestinal mucosa is characterized by a decrease in or absence of sulfomucins, which are predominant in the normal mucosa of the large intestine, and by an increase in sialylated mucins (224). Carbohydrate analysis of mucoproteins from colon adenocarcinoma has shown that the sialic acid content is much greater than that in mucins of normal colon from the same patient (225). Neoplastic tissue also produces relatively less O-acetyl substituted sialic acid (226). The increase in sialomucins is directly related to increased invasiveness of a carcinoma (according to Dukes' classification) but not to its degree of differentiation or its histologic pattern (227). A positive relationship has been reported between sialic acid content and metastatic properties of the tumor (228). The presence of sialylated antigens in tumor cells may not only mask these antigens from the host, but also shield them from immunocompetent cells. This hypothesis may explain why sialic acids are most abundant in the most invasive cases (227). Transitional mucosa adjacent to carcinoma of the large intestine is also characterized by an increase in sialomucins as compared with normal mucosa where sulfomucins predominate (227,229). These changes may represent an early stage of malignant transformation. Filipe (230) has demonstrated in rat colon that sialomucins predominate in areas of experimentally induced early dysplasia. This shift from sulfomucins to sialomucins has not been observed in nonmalignant, pathologic conditions of the large bowel, e.g. ulcerative colitis, Crohn's disease, or diverticular disease (224). However, the predominance of sialomucins over sulfated ones does characterize the mucus secretion patterns of the fetal gut (231). Thus, mucin changes might reflect a transformation to a fetal type of epithelium and indicate an early stage of carcinogenesis (221,231,232).

Kim and Isaacs (62), however, reported a decrease in the sialyltransferase activity involved in the addition of sialic acid to mucinous glycoproteins in tumor tissue. Similarly, analysis of glycopeptide fractions have demonstrated chemical alterations in mucin-type glycoproteins of colorectal adenocarcinoma, i.e. the tumor glycopeptide fraction contained less acidic glycopeptides and less sialic acid (227,233). The membrane glycoprotein fraction of human colonic carcinoma also has a lower sialic acid, glactosamine, and fucose content than that of normal colonic mucosa (63).

Colonic mucoprotein antigen is probably the major secretory product of the large bowel epithelium (234). The protein core, comprising about 25% of the molecule's mass, is rich in threonine and proline. The carbohydrate chains containing sialic acid, fucose, galactose, glucosamine, and galactosamine are linked to the peptide core via a galactosamino-O-glycosialic bond to threonine (234). The mucoprotein obtained from colonic adenocarcinomas, however, differs chemically (225) and immunologically from that in normal colon (235): the threonine and proline content is greatly diminished while the aspartic acid content is increased; fewer sugar residues are present, suggesting a lower density of carbohydrate moieties on the peptide core (225); and the activity of polypeptidyl:N-acetylgalactosaminyl transferase, which catalyzes the addition of N-acetylgalactosamine to threonine and/or serine, is lower (62).

Alterations in the carbohydrate structure of colonic mucin during cellular differentiation and malignant transformation have also been analyzed using lectins (236). The binding of two GalNAc-binding lectins, DBA and SBA, to goblet cell mucins increased as a function of the extent of differentiation of these cells, but neither lectin bound to the mucin secreted by the majority of colon cancers. The Gal-binding agglutinin PNA, on the other hand, did not bind to the goblet-cell mucin of any normal colonic mucosa, but did bind to the mucin of all colonic cancers, of all transitional mucosa (227,236), and of benign colonic polyps (237,238). The presence of a similar mucin in benign colonic polyps and in colon carcinomas suggests that biochemical manifestations of malignancy may precede morphological changes (238). Although only adenomatous but not hyperplastic polyps are considered to be precursors of colon cancers (58,229), both types of lesions contain the cancer-associated antigen (238,239,240). The disaccharide Galβ1→3GalNAc is often found in the inner portion of oligosaccharide chains in the normal mucin-type glycoprotein (241). The high binding levels of PNA to this structure in tumor tissue suggest that this disaccharide is recognized as a terminal structure and thus that oligosaccharide chains in these mucins are incompletely glycosylated. Decreased activities of an N-acetyl-galactosaminyltransferase and galactosyltransferase in human cancer as compared with normal colon have been demonstrated (63), which result in incompletely glycosylated side chains of mucin molecules. ConA binding with mucins has been shown in rats to be a good marker for gastric adenocarcinomas induced experimentally (242).

In secretor individuals, the superficial gastric mucosal cells and glycoproteins extracted from them strongly express blood group ABH antigens in accord with the type found on the red blood cells of that individual (223). In nonsecretors, instead, the I antigen is strongly expressed (21). These antigens are totally or regionally deleted in most gastric carcinomas, as discussed in the section on ABH blood groups. These changes have been documented by immunochemical analysis of mucins extracted from tumor tissues (21,243). The normal distal colon, however, also does not express blood group antigens. The blood group I (Ma) determinant has been detected in glycoprotein extracts of metastases of certain colonic cancers (244). Analyses of mucins extracted from non-neoplastic mucosa of the distal colon have shown that Le^a antigen is strongly expressed irrespective of secretor status and that Le^b and H antigens are strongly expressed on tumor mucins (for review, see 13). This observation is in agreement with the Lewis status of tumor tissues as determined by immunohistochemical methods (108) and by chemical analyses of glycolipid and glycoprotein antigens (109).

The mucin-type cancer antigen, Ca, recognized by monoclonal antibody, is expressed specifically by the majority of human epithelial malignant tumors and not by tumors of neural crest origin or by normal tissues. This antigen is represented by two glycoproteins of 350- and 390-kd molecular weight (245,246). Major oligosaccharides, which are O-glycosialically linked to the polypeptide chain, consist of the tetra-, tri-, and disaccharides with the general structure:

$$(SA)_n\text{-}Gal \rightarrow GalNAc$$

where n = 0, 1, or 2 (247). An anti-Ca monoclonal antibody discriminates between malignant and nonmalignant cells and also between the malignant and nonmalignant segregants of isogenic human hybrid cells. Those results suggest that the reappearance of the Ca antigen is associated with the malignant state of the cell.

The antigenicity of the Ca antigen is destroyed by neuraminidases and certain endoglycosidases, suggesting the structural variations of the mucous glycoproteins in normal and malignant cells. It has been suggested that synthesis of the Ca antigen can be induced by high concentrations of lactate. The high glycolytic activity of malignant cells generates large amounts of lactate, which accumulate in tumor cells (248,249).

SUMMARY

Gastrointestinal tract tumors, like all tumor cells, are characterized by alterations in carbohydrate composition and structure as compared to their normal counterparts irrespective of the mechanism of oncogenic transformation. All these alterations involve shifts in activity of enzymes, which, in a programmed manner, are involved in the biosynthetic pathway. Blocked synthesis and accumulation of precursor structures is due to suppressed glycosyltransferase(s) activity, and *de novo* synthesis of carbohydrate structure depends on expression (or re-expression) of an inappropriate enzyme or one with less restricted specificity. If transformation is assumed to be a multi-step process, the expression of *onc* genes may be a critical initiating event in the acquisition of the malignant phenotype and may be reflected in an altered glycosyltransferase activity. These types of changes are usually associated with an expression of oncofetal molecules specific for malignancy of the gastrointestinal tract epithelium and its premalignant states. Since tumor-associated antigens represent oncodevelopmental markers, the activation of retrodifferentiation mechanism results in expression of masked host-genomic information (for review, see 1). How this mechanism starts and the control of expression of normal phenotypic expression is lost is fundamental to an understanding of cancer phenomena.

REFERENCES

1. Hakomori S-i, Kannagi R. Glycosphingolipids as tumor-associated and differentiation markers. J. Natl Cancer Inst 71: 231–251, 1983.

2. Hakomori S-i. Glycolipids of tumor cell membrane. Adv Cancer Res 18: 265–315, 1973.

3. Hakomori S-i. Tumor-associated carbohydrate antigens. Ann Rev Immunol 2: 103–126, 1984.

4. Hakomori S-i. Tumor-associated glycolipid markers in experimental and human cancer. Membrane alteration in cancer. In *Gann Monograph on Cancer Research.* Makita A, Tsuiki S, Fujii S, Warren L, eds. Tokyo: Japanese Cancer Association, 1983, pp 113–27.

5. Hakomori S-i. Structures and organization of cell surface glycolipids. Dependency on cell growth and malignant transformation. Biochim Biophys Acta 417: 55–89, 1975.

6. Hakomori S-i, Young WW. Tumor-associated glycolipid antigens and modified blood group antigens. Scand J Immunol (Suppl.) 6: 97–117, 1978.

7. Young W Jr, Hakomori S-i. Status of blood group carbohydrate chains in human tumors. In *Glycoproteins and Glycolipids in Disease Processes.* Wallborg, EF, ed. Washington: American Chemical Society, 1978, pp 357–371.

8. Hakomori S-i, Kobata A. Blood group antigens. In *The Antigens.* Sela M, ed. New York: Academic Press, 1974, pp 79–140.

9. Hakomori S-i. Fucolipids and blood group glycolipids in normal and tumor tissue. Prog Biochem Pharmacol 10: 167–196, 1975.

10. Burtin P, Gold B. Carcinoembryonic antigen. Scand J Immunol 8, Suppl 8: 27–38, 1978.

11. Shively JE, Todd SW. Carcinoembryonic antigen. Scand J Immunol 7, Suppl 6: 19–31, 1978.

12. Hammarström S, Svenberg T, Hedin A, Sundblad G. Antigens related to carcinoembryonic antigen. Scand J Immunol 7, Suppl 6: 33–46, 1978.

13. Hounsell EF, Feizi T. Gastrointestinal mucins. Rev Med Biol 60: 227–236, 1982.

14. Feizi T. Blood group antigens and gastric cancer. Med Biol 60: 7–11, 1982.

15. Yageeswaran G. Surface glycolipid and glycoprotein antigens. In *Cancer Markers*. Sell S, ed. New York: The Humane Press, 1980, pp 371–401.

16. Szulman AE. The histological distribution of blood group substances A and B in man. J Exp Med 111: 785–807, 1960.

17. Szulman AE. The histological distribution of blood group substances in man as disclosed by immunofluorescence. II. The H antigen and its relation to A and B antigens. J Exp Med 115: 977–1005, 1962.

18. Holborow EJ, Brown PC, Glynn LE, Hawes, MD, Gresham, GH, O'Brien, TF, Coombs RRA. The distribution of the blood group A antigen in human tissues. Br J Exp Pathol 41: 430–437, 1960.

19. Kawasaki H. Molish-positive mucopolysaccharides of gastric carcinoma as compared with the corresponding components of gastric mucosae. Tohoku J Exp Med 68: 119–137, 1958.

20. Schrager Y, Oates MD. A comparative study of the major glycoprotein isolated from normal and neoplastic gastric mucosa. Gut 14: 324–329, 1973.

21. Picard J, Waldron-Edward D, Feizi T. Changes in the expression of the blood group A,B,H,Le^e and Le^b antigens and the blood group precursor associated I(Ma) antigen in glycoprotein-rich extracts of gastric carcinomas. J Clin Lab Immunol 1: 119–128, 1978.

22. Glynn, LE, Holborow EJ. Distribution of blood-group substances in human tissues. Br Med Bull 15: 150–153, 1959.

23. Eckland AE, Gullbring B, Lagerlof B. Blood group specific substances in human gastric carcinoma study with fluorescent antibody technique. Acta Pathol Microbiol Scand 59: 447–455, 1963.

24. Wiley EL, Mandelsohn G, Eggeleston JC. Distribution of carcinoembryonic antigens and blood group substances in adenocarcinoma of the colon. Lab Invest 44: 507–513, 1981.

25. Denk H, Tappeiner G, Davidovits A, Eckerstorfer R, Holzner JH. Carcinoembroyonic antigen and blood group substances in carcinomas of the stomach and colon. J Natl Cancer Inst 53: 933–942, 1974.

26. Cooper HS, Haesler WE. Blood group substances as tumor antigens in distal colon. Am J Clin Pathol 69: 594–598, 1978.

27. Davidsohn I, Kovarik S, Lee CL. A, B and O substance in gastrointestinal carcinomas. Arch Pathol 81: 381–390, 1966.

28. Davidsohn I, Ni LY, Steljskal R. Tissue isoantigens of the stomach. Arch Pathol 92: 456–464, 1971.

29. Hakomori S-i, Koscielak J, Bloch KJ, Jeanloz RW. Immunologic relationship between blood group substances and a fucose containing glycolipid of human adenocarcinoma. J Immunol 98: 31–38, 1967.

30. Breimer ME. Adaptation of mass spectrometry for the analysis of tumor antigens as applied to blood group glycolipids of a human gastric carcinoma. Cancer Res 40: 897–908, 1980.

31. Siddiqui B, Whitehead YS, Kim YS. Glycosphingolipids in human colonic adenocarcinoma. J Biol Chem 253: 2168–2175, 1978.

32. Hakomori S-i, Andrews HD. Sphingoglycolipids with Le^b activity, and the co-presence of Le^e-, Le^b-glycolipids in human tumor tissue. Biochim Biophys Acta 202: 225–228, 1970.

33. Hansson GC, Karlsson K-A, Larson G, McKibbin JM, Blaszczyk M, Herlyn M, Steplewski L, Koprowski H. Mouse monoclonal antibodies against human cancer lines; site specificities for blood group and related antigens. J Biol Chem 258: 4091–4097, 1983.

34. Finan PJ, Wight DGD, Lennox ES, Sacks SH, Bleehen NM. Human blood group isoantigen expression on normal and malignant gastric epithelium studied with anti-A and anti-B monoclonal antibodies. J Natl Cancer Inst 70: 679–685, 1983.

35. Dabelsteen E, Vedtofte P, Hakomori S-I, Young W. Jr. Accumulation of a blood group antigen precursor in oral premalignant lesions. Cancer Res 43: 1451–1454, 1983.

36. Voak D, Lennox ES, Sacks S, Milstein C, Darnborough YD. Monoclonal anti-A and anti-B antibodies: Principles and development as cost effective reagents. Med Lab Sci 39: 109–122, 1982.

37. Lennox ES, Voak D, Sacks SH. Monoclonal antibodies as new blood typing reagents. In: *New Approaches to Laboratory Medicine*, Rosalli SB, ed. Darmstadt: GIT Verlag, 1981, pp 105–112.

38. Ernst C, Atkinson B, Wunzel H, Herlyn M, Thurin J, Civin C, Koprowski H. Monoclonal antibody localization of A and B isoantigens in normal and malignant fixed human tissue. Lab Invest (in press).

39. Szulman AE. The histological distribution of blood group substances in man, as disclosed by immunofluorescence. III. The A, B and H antigens in embryos and fetuses from 18 mm in length. J Exp Med 119: 503–516, 1964.

40. Szulman AE. The A, B and H blood-group antigens in human placentae. N Engl J Med 286: 1028–1031, 1972.

41. Szulman AE. The histological distribution of the blood group substances in man as disclosed by immunofluorescence. IV. The ABH antigens in embryos of the fifth week post fertilization. Hum Pathol 2: 575–585, 1971.

42. Cooper HS, Cox Y, Patchefsky AS. Immunohistologic study of blood group substances in polyps of distal colon. Expression of a fetal antigen. Am J Clin Pathol 73: 345–350, 1980.

43. Masamone H, Kawasaki H, Sinohara H, Abe S, Abe S-I. Molish-positive mucopolysaccharides of gastric cancers as compared with the corresponding components of gastric mucosae. Tohoku J Exp Med 72: 328–337, 1960.

44. Hakomori, S-i. Glycosphingolipids having blood-group ABH and Lewis specificities. Chem Phys Lipids. 5: 96–115, 1970.

45. Dabelsteen E, Fulling JH. A preliminary study of blood substances A and B in oral epithelium exhibiting atypia. Scand J Dent Res 79: 387–393, 1971.

46. Dabelsteen E, Fayerskov O. Distribution of blood group antigen A in human oral epithelium. Scand J Dent Res 82: 206–211, 1974.

47. Dabelsteen E, Roed-Petersen B, Pindborg JJ. Loss of epithelial blood group antigens A and B in oral premalignant lesions. Acta Pathol Microbiol Scand Sect A 83: 292–300, 1975.

48. Davidsohn I. Early immunologic diagnosis and prognosis of carcinoma. Am J Clin Pathol 57: 715–730, 1972.

49. Sheanan DG, Horowitz SA, Zamcheck N. Deletion of epithelial ABH isoantigens in primary gastric neoplasm and in metastatic cancer. Am J Dig Dis 16: 961–969, 1971.

50. Davidsohn I. Early immunologic diagnosis and prognosis of carcinoma. Am J Clin Pathol 57: 715–730, 1972.

51. Ming S-C, Goldman H, Freiman DG. Intestinal metaplasia and histogenesis of carcinoma in human stomach. Light and electron microscopic study. Cancer 20: 1418–1429, 1967.

52. Morson BC. Carcinoma arising from areas of intestinal metaplasia in the gastric mucosa. Br J Cancer 9: 377–385, 1955.

53. Kurisu M, Numanyu N, Kawachi T, Sigimura T. Blood group activity of human sucrase from intestinal metaplasia. J Biol Chem 252: 3277–3280, 1977.

54. Sheanan DG. Epithelial ABH isoantigen loss in adenomatous polyps and carcinoma of the colon. Gastroenterology 68: 984 (abstract), 1975.

55. Denk H, Tappeiner G, Holzner JH. Blood group substances (BG) as carcinofetal antigens in carcinomas of the distal colon. Eur J Cancer 10: 487–490, 1974.

56. Bockus HL, Tachdjian V, Ferguson LK, et al. Adenomatous polyp of colon and rectum: Its relation to carcinoma. Gastroenterology 41: 225–232, 1961.

57. Morson BC. Evolution of cancer of the colon and rectum. Cancer 34: 845–849, 1974.

58. Fenoglio CM, Lane N. The anatomical precursor of colorectal carcinoma. Cancer 34: 819–823, 1974.

59. Denk H, Holzner JH, Obiditsch-Maur I. Epithelial blood group antigens in colon polyps. I. Morphologic distribution and relationship to differentiation. J Natl Cancer Inst 54: 1313–1317, 1975.

60. Skinner JM, Whitehead R. Tumor-associated antigens in polyps and carcinoma of the human large bowel. Cancer 47: 1241–1245, 1981.

61. Stellner K, Hakomori S-I, Warner GA. Enzymic conversion of "H1-glycolipid" to A- or B-glycolipid and deficiency of these enzyme activities in adenocarcinoma. Biochem Biophys Res Commun 55: 439–445, 1973.

62. Kim YS, Isaacs R. Glycoprotein metabolism in inflammatory and neoplastic diseases of the human colon. Cancer Res 35: 2092–2097, 1975.

63. Kim YS, Isaacs R, Perdomo JM. Alterations of membrane glycopeptides in human colonic adenocarcinoma. Proc Natl Acad Sci USA 71: 4869–4873, 1974.

64. Watanabe, K, Hakomori, S-i. Status of blood group carbohydrate chains in ontogenesis and in oncogenesis. J Exp Med 144: 644–654, 1976.

65. Häkkinen IP, Virtanen S. The blood group activity of human gastric sulfoglycoproteins in patients with gastric cancer and normal controls. Clin Exp Immunol 2: 669–675, 1967.

66. Häkkinen IP, Raunio V, Virtanen S, Kohanen, G. Blood group activities in water-soluble glycoproteins and in microsomal fractions of gastric mucosa in peptic ulcer and gastric cancer patients. Clin Exp Immunol 4: 149–157, 1969.

67. Häkkinen I. A-like blood group antigen in gastric cancer cells of patients in blood groups O or B. J Natl Cancer Inst 44: 1183–1193, 1970.

68. Denk H, Tappeiner G, Davidovits A. Independent behaviour of blood group A- and B-like activities in gastric carcinomata of blood group AB individuals. Nature 248: 428–420, 1974.

69. Hattori H, Uemura K, Taketomi T. Glycolipids of gastric cancer. The presence of blood group A-active glycolipids in cancer tissues from blood group O patients. Biochim Biophys Acta 666: 361–369, 1981.

70. Hakomori S-i, Wang S-M, Young W Jr. Isoantigenic expression of Forssman glycolipid in human gastric and colonic mucosa: Its possible identity with a "A-like antigen" in human cancer. Proc Natl Acad Sci USA 74: 3023–3027, 1977.

71. Yokota M, Warner GA, Hakomori S-i. Blood group A glycolipid and a novel Forssman antigen in the hepatocarcinoma of blood group O individual. Cancer Res 41: 4185–4190, 1981.

72. Yonezawa, S., Nakamura, T., Tanaka, S., Sato, S. Glycoconjugate with Ulex europaens Agglutinin I-binding sites in normal mucosa, adenoma and carcinoma of the human large bowel. J Natl Cancer Inst 69: 777–785, 1982.

73. Yonezawa, S., Nakamura, T., Tanaka, S., Maruta, K., Nishi, H., Sato, E. Binding of Ulex europaens Agglutinin I in polyposis coli: Comparative study with solitary adenoma in the sigmoid colon and rectum. J Natl Cancer Inst 71: 19–24, 1983.

74. Brown A, Ellis IO, Embleton MJ, Baldwin RW, Turner DR, Hardcastle JD. Immunochemical localization of Y hapten and the structurally related H-type-2 blood-group antigen on large bowel tumors and normal adult tissues. Int J Cancer 33: 727–736, 1984.

75. Muto T, Bussey M Jr, Morson BC. The evolution of cancer of the colon and rectum. Cancer 36: 2251–2270, 1975.

76. Szulman EA. The histological distribution of the blood-group substances in man as disclosed by immunofluorescence. J Exp Med 115: 977–996, 1962.

77. Feizi T. The blood group Ii system: A carbohydrate antigen system defined by naturally monoclonal or oligoclonal autoantibodies of man. Immunol Commun 10: 127–165, 1981.

78. Kapadia A, Feizi T, Yewell D, Keeling J, Slavin G. Immunocytochemical studies of blood group A,H,I and i antigens in gastric mucosae of infants with normal gastric histology and of patients with gastric carcinoma and chronic benign peptic ulceration. J Clin Pathol 34: 320–337, 1981.

79. Marcus DM, Kundu SK, Suzuki A. The P blood group system: Recent progress in immunochemistry and genetics. Semin Hematol 18: 63–71, 1981.

80. Marcus DM, Naiki M, Kundu SK. Abnormalities in the glycosphingolipid content of human Pk and p erythrocytes. Proc Natl Acad Sci USA 73: 3263–3267, 1976.

81. Kannagi R, Levine P, Watanabe K, Hakomori S-i. Recent studies of glycolipids and glycoprotein profiles and characterization of the major glycolipid antigen in gastric cancer of a patient of blood group genotype pp ($T_i{}^a$) first studied in 1951. Cancer Res 42: 5249–5254, 1982.

82. Breimer M, Cedergren B, Karlsson K-A, Nilsson K, Samuelsson BE. Glycolipid pattern of stomach tissue of a human with the rare blood group A. FEBS Lett 118: 209–211, 1980.

83. Andrews PW, Goodfellow PN, Schevinsky LH, Bronson DL, Knowles BB. Cell-surface antigens of a clonal human embryonal carcinoma cell line: Morphological and antigenic differentiation in culture. Int J Cancer 29: 523–531, 1982.

84. Kannagi R, Levery SB, Ishigami F, Hakomori S-i, Shevinsky LH, Knowles BB, Solter D. New globoseries glycosphingolipids in human teratocarcinoma reactive with the monoclonal antibody directed to a developmentally regulated antigen, stage-specific embryonic antigen 3. J Biol Chem 258: 8934–8942, 1983.

85. Siddiqui B, Hakomori S-i. A revised structure for the Forssman glycolipid hapten. J Biol Chem 246: 5766–5769, 1971.

86. Stellner K, Saito H, Hakomori S-i. Determination of amino sugar linkages in glycolipids by methylation: Amino sugar linkages of ceramide pentasaccharides of rabbit erythrocytes and of Forssman antigen. Arch Biochem Biophys 155: 464–472, 1973.

87. Kawanami J. The appearance of Forssman hapten in human tumor. J Biochem (Tokyo) 72: 783–785, 1972.

88. Mori T, Sudo T, Kano K. Expression of heterophil Forssman antigen on cultured malignant cell lines. J Natl Cancer Inst 70: 811–818, 1983.

89. Taniguchi N, Yokosawa N, Narita M, Mitsuyama T, Makita A. Expression of Forssman antigen synthesis and degradation in human lung cancer. J Natl Cancer Inst 67: 577–583, 1981.

90. Kawanami J. The appearance of Forssman hapten in human tumor. J Biochem 72: 783–785, 1972.

91. Young WW Jr, Hakomori S-i, Levine P. Characterization of anti-Forssman (anti-F_s) antibodies in human sera: Their specificity and possible changes in patients with cancer. J Immunol 123: 92–96, 1979.

92. Levine P. Tissue familiar genetic markers in adenocarcinomas. Semin Oncol 5: 28–34, 1978.

93. Levine P. Self-nonself concept for cancer and autoimmune disease. Proc Natl Acad Sci USA 75: 5697–5701, 1978.

94. Makita A, Seyama Y. Alteration of Forssman-antigenic reactivity and of monosaccharide composition in plasma membrane from polyoma-transformed hamster cells. Biochim Biophys Acta 241: 403–411, 1971.

95. Shiroki K, Shimojo H, Maeta Y, Yamada C. Tumor-specific transplantation and surface antigen in cells transformed by the adenovirus 12 DNA fragments. Virology 99: 188–191, 1979.

96. Springer GF. T and Tn general carcinoma autoantigens. Science 224: 1199–1206, 1984.

97. Springer GF, Desai PR, Yang HJ, Schachter H, Nanasimhan S. Interrelation of blood group M and precursor specificities and their significance in human carcinoma. In *Human Blood Groups, 5th Int Convoc Immunol, Buffalo, NY, 1976*. Mohn JF, ed. Basel: Karger, 1977, pp 179–187.

98. Springer GF, Tegtmeyer H, Cromer DW. Are T and Tn differentiation antigens? Fed Proc Fed Am Exp Biol 43: 1750, 1984.

99. Bray J, Maclean GD, Dusel FJ, McPherson TA. Decreased levels of circulating lytic anti-T in the serum of patients with metastatic gastrointestinal cancer: A correlation with disease burden. Clin Exp Immunol 47: 176–182, 1982.

100. Springer GF, Desai PR, Murthy MS, Tegtmeyer H, Scanlon EF. Human carcinoma-associated precursor antigens of blood group MN system and the host immune response to them. Prog Allergy 26: 42–96, 1979.

101. Rauvala H, Finne J. Structural similarity of the terminal carbohydrate sequences of glycoproteins and glycolipids. FEBS Lett 97: 1–8, 1979.

102. Desai PR, Springer GF. Tn-, T-, N- and M-blood group specific glycolipids in L-10 guinea pig carcinoma. Fed Proc 43: 1949, 1984.

103. Metcalfe S, Springer GF, Svvennsen R, Tegtmeyer H. Anti-T and -Tn monoclonal antibodies specific for human carcinoma associated T and Tn antigens. Fed Proc 43: 1682, 1984.

104. Rahman AFR, Longenecker BM. A monoclonal antibody specific for the Thomsen-Freidenreich cryptic T antigen. J Immunol 129: 2021–2024, 1982.

105. Boccardi V, Attina D, Girelli G. Influence of orally administered antibiotics on anti-T agglutinin of normal subjects and of cirrhotic patients. Vox Sang 27: 268–272, 1974.

106. McKibbon JM, Spencer WA, Smith EL. Lewis blood group fucolipids and their isomers from human and canine intestine. J Biol Chem 257: 755–760, 1982.

107. Hattori H, Uemura K-I, Taketomi T. Glycolipids of human gastric mucosa, the coexistence of Le^a and Le^b fucolipids. Japan J Exp Med 50: 145–148, 1980.

108. Ernst C, Atkinson BB, Wysocka M, Blaszczyk M, Herlyn M, Sears H, Steplewski Z, Koprowski H. Monoclonal antibody localization of Lewis antigens in fixed tissue. Lab Invest 50: 394–399, 1984.

109. Blaszczyk M, Pak KY, Sears HH, Steplewski Z, Koprowski H. Characterization of Lewis antigens in normal colon and gastrointestinal adenocarcinomas. Proc Natl Acad Sci USA (submitted).

110. Pompecki R, Shively JE, Todd CW. Demonstration of elevated anti-Lewis antibodies in sera of cancer patients using a carcinoembryonic antigen-polyethylene glycol immunoassay. Cancer Res 41: 1910–1915, 1971.

111. Szulman AE. The ABH and Lewis antigens of human tissues during prenatal and postnatal life. In: *Human Blood Groups*. JF Mohn, RW Plunkett, RK Cunningham, RH Lambert, eds. Basel: Karger, 1977, pp 426–436.

112. Karlsson K-A, Larson G. Molecular characterization of cell-surface antigens of human fetal tissue: Meconium, a rich source of epithelial blood-group glycolipid. FEBS Lett 87: 283–287, 1978.

113. Coggin JH Jr, Anderson NG. Cancer differentiation and embryonic antigens: Some central problems. Adv Cancer Res 19: 105–165, 1974.

114. Karlsson K-A, Larson G. Molecular characterization of cell surface antigens of fetal tissue. Detailed analysis of glycosphingolipids of meconium of human O (Le^{a-b+}). J Biol Chem 256: 3512–3524, 1981.

115. Karlsson K-A, Larson G. Potential use of glycosphingolipids of human meconium for blood group chemotyping of single individuals. FEBS Lett 128: 71–74, 1981.

116. Larson G. Glycosphingolipids of human meconium. Ph.D. thesis, Dept of Medical Biochemistry, University of Goteborg, Sweden.

117. Yang HJ, Hakomori S-i. H sphinigolipid having a novel type of ceramide and lacto-*N*-fucopentaose III. J Biol Chem 246: 1192–1200, 1971.

118. Brockhaus M, Magnani JL, Herlyn M, Blaszczyk M, Steplewski Z, Koprowski H, Ginsburg V. Monoclonal antibodies directed against the major sequence of lacto-*N*-fucopentaose III are obtained from mice immunized with human tumors. Arch Biochem Biophys 217: 647–651, 1982.

119. Huang LC, Brockhaus M, Magnani JJL, Cuttitta SR, Minna JD, Ginsburg V. Many monoclonal antibodies with an apparent specificity for certain lung cancers are directed against a sugar sequence found in lacto-*N*-fucopentaose III. Arch Biochem Biophys 220: 518–520, 1983.

120. Solter D, Knowles BB. Monoclonal antibody defining a stage-specific mouse embryonic antigen SSEA-1. Proc Natl Acad Sci USA 75: 5565–5569, 1978.

121. Andrews PW, Goodfellow PN, Schevinsky LH, Bronson DL, Knowles BB: Cell-surface antigens of a clonal human embryonal carcinoma cell line: Morphological and antigenic differentiation in culture. Int J Cancer 29: 523–531, 1982.

122. Kannagi R, Nudelman E, Levery SB, Hakomori S-i. A series of human erythrocyte glycosphingolipids reacting to the monoclonal antibody directed to a developmentally regulated antigen SSEA-1. J Biol Chem 257: 14865–14874, 1983.

123. Hakomori S-i, Nudelman E, Kannagi R, Levery SB. The common structure in fucosylactosaminolipids accumulating in human adenocarcinomas and its possible absence in normal tissue. Biochem Biophys Res Commun 109: 36–44, 1982.

124. Hakomori S-i, Nudelman E, Levery S, Solter D, Knowles BB. The hapten structure of a developmentally regulated glycolipid antigen (SSEA-1) isolated from human erythrocytes and adenocarcinoma: A preliminary note. Biochem Biophys Res Commun 100: 1578–1586, 1981.

125. Hakomori S-i, Nudelman E, Levery SB, Kannagi R. Novel fucolipids accumulating in human adenocarcinoma. I. Glycolipids with di- or trifucosylated type 2 chain. J Biol Chem 259: 4672–4680, 1984.

126. Fukushi Y, Hakomori S-i, Nudelman E, Cochran N. Novel fucolipids accumulating in human adenocarcinoma. II. Selective isolation of hybridoma antibodies that differentially recognize mono-, di- and trifucosylated type 2 chain. J Biol Chem 259: 4681–4685, 1984.

127. Shi ZA, McIntyre LJ, Knowles BB, Solter D, Kim YS. Expression of a carbohydrate differentiation antigen, stage-specific embryonic antigen-1 in human colonic adenocarcinoma. Cancer Res 44: 1142–1145, 1984.

128. Fukushi Y, Hakomori S-i, Shepard T. Localization and alteration of mono-, di- and trifucosyl $\alpha1\rightarrow3$ type chain structures during human embryogenesis and in human cancer. J Exp Med 160: 506–519, 1984.

129. Brown A, Feizi T, Gooi HC, Embleton MJ, Picard JK, Baldwin RW. A monoclonal antibody against human colonic adenoma recognizes difucosylated type-2 blood group chains. Biosci Rep 3: 163–170, 1983.

130. Brown A, Ellis IO, Embleton MJ, Baldwin RW, Turner DR, Hardcastle JD. Immunohistochemical localization of Y hapten and the structurally related H-type-2 blood-group antigen on large-bowel tumors and normal adult tissues. Int J Cancer 33: 727–736, 1984.

131. Pacuszka T, Jozwiak W, Miller-Podraza H, Koscielak J. Neutral glycolipid composition in human cancer. Cancer Biochim Biophys 5: 1–6, 1980.

132. Koscielak J, Jozwiak W, Pacuska T, Miller-Podraza H. Glycolipid composition of human cancer and a positive role of lactosylceramide as tumor antigen. In *Glycoconjugates, Proc. Fifth Int. Symp. Kiel*. Schauer R, Boer P, Buddecke E, Kramer MF, Vliegenthart JFG, Wiegandt H, eds. Stuttgart: Georg Thieme, 1979, pp 619–620.

133. Jozwiak W, Koscielak Y. Possibility of using antibodies to lactosylsphingosine in diagnosis of neoplasm. Acta Haematol Pol 10: 307–310, 1979.

134. Jozwiak W, Koscielak J. Occurrence of lactosphingosine-reactive antibodies in sera of cancer patients. Acta Haematol Pol 11: 173–179, 1980.

135. Jozwiak W, Koscielak J. Lactosylsphingosine-reactive antibody and CEA in patients with colorectal cancer. Eur J Cancer Clin Oncol 18: 617–621, 1982.

136. Symington FW, Bernstein ID, Hakomori S-i. Monoclonal antibody specific for lactosylceramide. J Biol Chem 259: 6008–6012, 1984.

137. Keränen A, Lempinen M, Puro K. Ganglioside pattern and neuraminic acid content of human gastric and colonic carcinoma. Clin Chim Acta 70: 103–112, 1976.

138. Fredman P, Nilsson O, Suennerholm L, Myrvold H, Persson B, Petterson S, Holmgren J, Lindholm L. Colorectal carcinomas have a characteristic ganglioside pattern. Med Biol 61: 45–48, 1983.

139. Lindholm L, Holmgren J, Svenerhohm L, Fredman P, Nilsson O, Persson B, Myrvold H. Monoclonal antibodies against gastrointestinal tumor-associated antigens isolated as monosialogangliosides. Int Archs Allergy Appl Immun 71: 178–181, 1983.

140. Hakomori S-i, Nudelman E, Levery SB, Patterson CM. Human cancer-associated gangliosides defined by a monoclonal antibody (1B9) directed to sialosyl $\alpha2\rightarrow6$ galactosyl residue: A preliminary note. Biochem Biophys Res Commun 113: 791–798, 1983.

141. Fukushi Y, Nudelman E, Levery SB, Hakomori S-i, Rauvala H. Novel fucolipids accumulating in human adenocarcinoma. III. A hybridoma antibody (FH6) defining a human cancer-associated difucoganglioside. J Biol Chem 259: 10511–10517, 1984.

142. Blaszczyk M, Ross A, Ernst C, Marcusio M, Atkinson B, Pak KY, Steplewski Z, Koprowski H. A fetal glycolipid expressed on adenocarcinomas of the colon. Int J Cancer 33: 313–318, 1984.

143. Nishimaki T, Kano K, Milgrom F. Hanganutziu-Deicher antigen and antibody in pathological sera and tissues. J Immunol 122: 2314–2318, 1979.

144. Ikuta K, Nishi Y, Shimizu Y, Higashi H, Kitamoto N, Kato S, Fujita M, Nakano Y, Taghuchi T, Naiki M. Hanganutziu-Diecher type heterophile antigen-positive cells in human cancer tissues demonstrated by membrane immunofluorescence. Biken J 25: 47–50, 1982.

145. Kiprowski H, Steplewski Z, Mitchell KF, Herlyn M, Herlyn D, Fuhrer P. Colorectal carcinoma antigens detected by hybridoma antibodies. Somat Cell Genet 5: 957–972, 1979.

146. Magnani JL, Brockhaus M, Smith DF, Ginsburg V, Blaszczyk M, Mitchell KF, Steplewski Z, Kiprowski H. A monosialoganglioside is a monoclonal antibody-defined antigen of colon carcinoma. Science 212: 55–56, 1981.

147. Magnani JL, Nilsson B, Brockhaus M, Zopf D, Steplewski Z, Koprowski H, Ginsburg V. A monoclonal antibody-defined antigen associated with gastrointestinal cancer is a ganglioside containing sialylated lacto-N-fucopentaose II. J Biol Chem 257: 14365–14369, 1982.

148. Falk KE, Karlsson KA, Leffler H, Samuelsson BE. Specific pattern of glycosphingolipids enriched in mucosa scraping of human small intestine. FEBS Lett 101: 2 3–276, 1979.

149. Holmgren J, Lönnroth I, Mansson JE, Svennerholm L. Interaction of cholera toxin and membrane G_M, a ganglioside of small intestine. Proc Natl Acad Sci USA 72: 2520–2524, 1975.

150. Falk KE, Karlsson KA, Larson J, Thurin J, Blaszczyk M, Steplewski Z, Koprowski H. Mass spectrometry of human tumor glycolipid antigen being defined by mouse monoclonal antibody NS 19-9. Biochem Biophys Res Commun 110: 383–391, 1983.

151. Arends, JW, Verstynen C, Bosman FT, Hilgers J, Steplewski Z. Distribution of monoclonal antibody-defined monosialoganglioside in normal and cancerous human tissues: An immunoperoxidase study. Hybridoma 2: 219–229, 1983.

152. Atkinson B, Ernst C, Herlyn M, Steplewski Z, Sears H, Koprowski H. Gastrointestinal cancer-associated antigen in immunoperoxidase assay. Cancer Res 42: 4820–4823, 1982.

153. Arends JW, Wiggers T, Verstijnen C, Hilgers J, Bosman FT. Gastrointestinal cancer-associated antigen (GICA) immunoreactivity in colorectal carcinoma in relation to patient survival. Int J Cancer 34: 193–196, 1984.

154. Arends JW, Wiggers T, Schuffe B, Thijs CT, Verstijnen C, Hilgers J, Blijham GH, Bosman FT. Monoclonal antibody (1116 NS 19-9) defined monosialoganglioside (GICA) in colorectal carcinoma in relation to stage, histopathology and DNA flow cytometry. Int J Cancer 32: 289–293, 1983.

155. Olding LB, Ahren C, Svalander C, Karlsson K-A, Thurin J, Koprowski H. Gastrointestinal carcinoma-associated antigen detected by a monoclonal antibody in dysplasia and adenocarcinoma associated with chronic ulcerative colitis (in press).

156. Roux H, Labbe T, Fondanecke M-C, Koprowski H, Burtin PH. Study of gastrointestinal cancer-associated antigen (GICA) in human fetal organs. Int J Cancer 32: 315–319, 1983.

157. Olding LB, Thurin J, Svalander C, Koprowski H. Expression of gastrointestinal carcinoma-associated antigen (GICA) detected in human fetal tissues by a monoclonal antibody NS 19-9. Int J Cancer 34: 187–192, 1984.

158. Koprowski H, Brockhaus M, Blaszczyk M, Magnani JL, Steplewski Z, Ginsburg V. Lewis blood-type may affect the incidence of gastrointestinal cancer. Lancet 1 (8285): 1332–1333, 1982.

159. Brockhaus M, Wysocka M, Magnani J, Steplewski Z, Koprowski H, Ginsburg V. The gastrointestinal and pancreatic cancer-associated antigen detected by monoclonal antibody 19-9 in the serum mucin of patients also occurs in normal salivary mucin. Vox Sanqui (in press).

160. Pak KY, Blaszczyk M, Steplewski Z, Koprowski H. Identification and isolation of Lewis blood group antigens from human saliva using monoclonal antibodies. Hybridoma 3: 1–10, 1984.

161. Herlyn M, Sears HF, Steplewski Z, Kiprowski Z. Monoclonal antibody

detection of a circulating tumor-associated antigen. I. Presence of antigen in sera of patients with colorectal, gastric, and pancreatic carcinoma. J Clin Immunol 2: 135–140, 1982.

162. Sears HF, Atkinson B, Mattis J, Ernst C, Herlyn D, Steplewski Z, Häyry P, Koprowski H. Phase-I clinical trial of monoclonal antibody in treatment of gastrointestinal tumors. Lancet: 762–765, 1982.

163. Koprowski H, Herlyn M, Steplewski Z, Sears HF. Specific antigen in serum of patients with colon carcinoma. Science 212: 53–55, 1981.

164. Kuusela P, Yalanko H, Roberts P, Sippanen P, Mechin J-P, Pitkänen R, Mäkelä O. Comparison of CA 19-9 and carcinoembryonic antigen (CEA) levels in the serum of patients with colorectal diseases. Br J Cancer 49: 135–139, 1984.

165. Del Vilano BC, Brennan S, Brock P, Bucher C, Liv V, McClevre M, Rake B, Space S, Westric B, Schomaker H, Zurawski Vr Jr. Radioimmunometric assay for a monoclonal antibody-defined tumor marker CA 19-9. Clin Chem 29: 549–552, 1983.

166. Sears HF, Herlyn M, Del Vilano B, Steplewski Z, Kiprowski H. Monoclonal antibody detection of a circulating tumor-associated antigen. II. Longitudinal evaluation of patients with colorectal cancer. J. Clin Immunol 2: 141–149, 1982.

167. Steplewski Z, Chang TH, Herlyn M, Koprowski H. Release of monoclonal antibody defined antigens by human colorectal carcinoma and melanoma cells. Cancer Res 41: 2723–2727, 1982.

168. Magnani JL, Steplewski Z, Koprowski H, Ginsburg V. Identification of the gastrointestinal and pancreatic cancer-associated antigen detected by monoclonal antibody 19-9 in the sera of patients as a mucin. Cancer Res 43: 5489–5492, 1983.

169. Ellis DJ, Speirs C, Kingston RD, Brookes VS, Leonard J, Dykes PW. Carcinoembryonic antigen levels in advanced gastric carcinoma. Cancer 42: 623–625, 1978.

170. Goldenberg DM, Sharkey RM, Primus FJ. Carcinoembryonic protein in histopathology: Immunoperoxidase staining in conventional tissue sections. J Natl Cancer Inst 57: 11–22, 1976.

171. O'Brien MJ, Zamcheck N, Burke B, Kirkham SE, Saravis CA, Gottlieb LS. Immunocytochemical localization of carcinoembryonic antigen in benign and malignant colorectal tissues. Assessment of diagnostic value. Am J Clin Pathol 75: 783–790, 1981.

172. Jubert AV, Talbott TM, Maycroft TM. Characteristic of adenocarcinomas of the colorectum with low levels of postoperative plasma carcinoembryonic antigen (CEA). Cancer 42: 635–639, 1978.

173. Gold P, Shuster J, Freedman SO. Carcinoembryonic antigen (CEA) in clinical medicine. Cancer 42: 1399–1405, 1978.

174. Kalser MH, Barkin JS, Redlhammer D, Heal A. Circulating carcinoembryonic antigen in pancreatic carcinoma. Cancer 42: 1468–1471, 1978.

175. Neville AM, Patel S, Capp M, Laurence DJR, Cooper EH, Turberville C, Coombes RC. The monitoring role of plasma CEA alone and the association with other tumor markers in colorectal and mammary carcinoma. Cancer 42: 1448–1451, 1978.

176. Gold P, Freedman SO. Purification and characterization of carcinoembryonic antigen of the human digestive system: Nature 215: 67, 1967.

177. Gold P, Freedman SO. Demonstration of tumor-specific antigens in human colonic carcinomata by immunological tolerance and absorption techniques. J Exp Med 121: 439–459, 1966.

178. Burtin P, Quan P, Sabine MC. Nonspecific crossreacting antigen as a marker for human polymorphs, macrophages and monocytes. Nature 255: 714–716, 1975.

179. Fritsche R, Mach J-P. Isolation and characterization of carcinoembryonic antigen (CEA) extracted from normal colon mucosa. Immunochemistry 14: 119–127, 1977.

180. Svenberg T, Hammarström S, Hedin A. Purification and properties of biliary glycoprotein I (BGPI). Immunochemical relationship to carcinoembryonic antigen. Mol Immunol 16: 245–252, 1979.

181. Isaacson P, Judd, A. Immunochemistry of carcinoembryonic antigen in small intestine. Cancer 42: 1554–1559, 1978.

182. Lowenstein HS, Zamcheck, N. Carcinoembryonic antigen (CEA) levels in benign gastrointestinal disease states. Cancer 42: 1412–1418, 1978.

183. Martin F, Martin M. Demonstration of antigens related to colonic cancer in the human digestive system. Int J Cancer 6: 352, 1971.

184. Hammarström S, Svenberg T, Sundblad G. Immunochemical studies on carcinoembryonic antigen (CEA): Number of antigenic determinants and relationship to a glycoprotein from normal human bile. In: *Oncofetal Development Gene Expression.* Fishman WH, Sell S, eds. New York: Academic Press, 1976.

185. Rule AH, Kirsch ME. Gene activation of molecules with carcinoembryonic antigen determinants in fetal development and in adenocarcinoma of the colon. Cancer Res 36: 3503–3509, 1976.

186. Von Kleist S, Chavanel G, Burtin P. Identification of a normal antigen that crossreacts with the carcinoembryonic antigen. Proc Natl Acad Sci USA 69: 2492–2494, 1972.

187. Burtin P. The carcinoembryonic antigen of digestive system (CEA) and the antigen crossreactive with it. Ann Immunol Inst Past 129C: 185–198, 1978.

188. Darcy DA, Turberville G, James R. Immunological study of carcinoembryonic antigen (CEA) and a related glycoprotein. Br J Cancer 28: 147–160, 1973.

189. Kessler MJ, Shively JE, Pritchard DG, Toold CW. Isolation, immunological characterization, and structural studies of a tumor antigen related to carcinoembryonic antigen. Cancer Res 38: 1041–1048, 1978.

190. Mach J-P, Pusztacheri G. Carcinoembryonic antigen (CEA): Demonstration of a partial identity between CEA and a normal glycoprotein. Immunochemistry 9: 1031–1034, 1972.

191. Turberville C, Darcy DA, Laurence DJR, Johns EW, Neville AM. Studies on carcinoembryonic antigen (CEA) and a related glycoprotein CCEA-2 preparation and clinical characterization. Immunochemistry 10: 841–863, 1973.

192. Wang AC, Banjo C, Fuks H, Shuster J, Gold P. Heterogeneity of the protein moeity of carcinoembryonic antigens. Immunol Comm 5: 205–210, 1976.

193. Terry WD, Henkart PA, Coligan JE, Tooloe CW. Carcinoembryonic antigen characterization and clinical applications. Transplant Rev 20: 100–129, 1974.

194. Terry WD, Henkart PA, Coligan JE, Todd CV. Structural studies of the major glycoprotein in preparation with carcinoembryonic antigen activity. J Exp Med 136: 200–204, 1972.

195. Banjo C, Shoster J, Gold P. Proceeding: Intermolecular heterogeneity of the carcinoembryonic antigen. Cancer Res 34: 2114–2121, 1974.

196. Shively JE, Toold CW, Go VLW, Egan M. Amino-terminal sequence of carcinoembryonic antigen-like glycoprotein isolated from the colonic lavages of healthy individuals. Cancer Res 138: 503–505, 1978.

197. Engvall E, Shively JE, Wrann M. Isolation and characterization of the normal crossreacting antigen: Homology of its NH_2-terminal amino acid sequence with that of carcinoembryonic antigen. Proc Natl Acad Sci USA 75: 1670–1674, 1978.

198. Egan ML, Pritchard DG, Todd CW, Go VW. Isolation and immunochemical and chemical characterization of carcinoembryonic-like substances in colon lavages of healthy individuals. Cancer Res 37: 2638–2643, 1977.

199. Chandrasekaran EV, Davila M, Nixon DW, Goldfarb M, Mendicius J. Isolation and structures of the oligosaccharide units of carcinoembryonic antigen. J Biol Chem 258: 7213–7222, 1983.

200. Shively JE, Wessler MJ, Toold CW. Amino-terminal sequences of the major tryptic peptides obtained from carcinoembryonic antigen by digestion with trypsin in the presence of Triton X-100. Cancer Res 38: 2199–2208, 1978.

201. Glassman JNS, Todd CS, Shively J. Chemical deglycosylation of carcinoembryonic antigen for amino-acid sequence studies. Biochem Biophys Res Commun 85: 204–216, 1978.

202. Coligan JE, Britchard DG, Schnute WC Jr, Toold CW. Methylation analysis of the carbohydrate portion of carcinoembryonic antigens. Cancer Res 36: 1915–1917, 1976.

203. Egan ML, Coligan JE, Pritchard DG, Schnute WC Jr, Todd CW. The chemistry of carcinoembryonic antigen. Cancer Res 36: 3487–3485, 1976.

204. Acolla RS, Carrel S, Mach JP. Monoclonal antibodies specific for carcinoembryonic antigen and produced by two hybrid cell lines. Proc Natl Acad Sci USA 77: 563–566, 1979.

205. Rogers GT, Rawlings GA, Bagshawe KD. Monoclonal antibodies against carcinoembryonic antigen (CEA). In: *Proteins and Related Subjects.* Peeters, M, ed, Vol. 28. New York: Plenum Press, 1980, pp 517–522.

206. Rogers GT, Rawlines GA, Bagshaw KB. Somatic cell hybrids producing antibodies against CEA. Br J Cancer 41: 1–4, 1981.

207. Kupchik ML, Zurawski VR Jr, Hurrell JGR, Zamcheck N, Black PM. Monoclonal antibodies to CEA produced by somatic cell fusion. Cancer Res 41: 3306–3310, 1981.

208. Grunert F, Wank K, Luckenbach GA, Von Kleist S. Monoclonal antibodies against CEA. Comparison of the immunoprecipitates by fingerprint analysis. Oncodevelop Biol Med 3: 191–200, 1982.

209. Mitchell KF. A carcinoembryonic antigen (CEA) specific monoclonal hybridoma antibody that reacts only with high molecular weight CEA. Cancer Immunol Immunother 10: 1–5, 1980.

210. Blaszczyk, M, Pak KY, Herlyn P, Lindgren J, Pessano S, Steplewski Z, Kiprowski H. Characterization of gastrointestinal tumor-associated carcinoembryonic antigen-related antigens defined by monoclonal antibodies. Cancer Res 44: 245–253, 1984.

211. Lindgren J, Hang B, Hurme M, Mäkelä O. Monoclonal antibodies to carcinoembryonic antigen (CEA) characterization and use in a radioimmunoassay for CEA. Acta Pathol Microbiol Immunol Scand 90: 159–162, 1982.

212. Hedin A, Hammarström S, Larsson A. Specificities and binding properties of eight monoclonal antibodies against carcinoembryonic antigen. Mol Immunol 19: 1641–1648, 1982.

213. Stähli C, Miggiano V, LeDain M, Ianelli D, Fessler R, Häring P, Schmidt J, Staehelin T. Distinction and characterization by monoclonal antibodies of epitopes on four proteins of clinical interest. Res Monogr Immunol 3: 201–208, 1981.

214. O'Brien MJ, Zamcheck N, Burke B, Kirkham SE, Saravis CA, Gottlieb LS. Immunocytochemical localization of carcinoembryonic antigen in benign and malignant colorectal tissues. Assessment of diagnostic value. Am J Clin Pathol 75: 283–290, 1981.

215. Primus FJ, Clark GA, Goldenberg DM. Immunohistochemical detection of carcinoembryonic antigen. In *Diagnostic Immunochemistry.* DeLellis, RA, ed. New York: Messon Publishing, 1981, pp 263–276.

216. Primus JF, Kuhns WJ, Goldenberg DM. Immunological heterogeneity of carcinoembryonic antigen: Immunohistochemical detection of carcinoembryonic antigen determinants in colonic tumors with monoclonal antibodies. Cancer Res 43: 693–701, 1983.

217. Buchegger F, Phan M, Rivier D, Carrel S, Accola RS, Mach J-P. Monoclonal antibodies against carcinoembryonic antigen (CEA) used in solid-phase enzyme immunoassay: First clinical results. J Immunol Meth 49: 129–139, 1982.

218. Pearson J, Allen A, Venables CV. Gastric mucus: Isolation and polymeric structure of the undegraded glycoprotein: Its breakdown by pepsin. Gastroenterology 78: 709–715, 1980.

219. Mantle M, Mantle D, Allen A. Polymeric structure of pig small-intestinal mucus glycoproteins. Biochem J 195: 277–285, 1981.

220. Ma J, DeBoer WGRM, Nayman J. Intestinal mucinous substances in gastric intestinal metaplasia and carcinoma studied by immunofluorescence. Cancer 49: 1664–1667, 1982.

221. Bara J, Loisillier F, Burtin P. Antigens of gastric and intestinal mucous cells in human colonic tumors. Br J Cancer 61: 209–221, 1980.

222. JR Clamp, ed. Mucus. Br Med Bull 34: 5–41, 1978.

223. Watkins WM. Biochemistry and genetics of the ABO, Lewis and P blood group system. In *Advances in Human Genetics*. Harris H, Hirschorn K, eds, Vol. 10. New York: Plenum Publishing, 1980, pp 1–136, 379–385.

224. Filipe MI. Value of histochemical reactions for mucosubstances in the diagnosis of certain pathological conditions of the colon and rectum. Gut 10: 577–586, 1969.

225. Gold DV, Miller F. Comparison of human colonic mucoprotein antigen from normal and neoplastic mucosa. Cancer Res 38: 3704–3211, 1978.

226. Rogers CM, Cooke KB, Filipe MI. Sialic acids of human large bowel mucosa: O-acetylated variants in normal and malignant states. Gut 19: 587–592, 1978.

227. Filipe MI, Branfoot, AC. Abnormal patterns of mucus secretion in apparently normal mucosa of large intestine with carcinoma. Cancer 34: 282–290, 1974.

228. Yogeeswaran G, Salk PL. Metastatic potential is positively correlated with cell surface sialylation of cultured murine tumor cell lines. Science 212: 1514–1516, 1981.

229. Dawson PA, Filipe MI. An ultrastructural and histochemical study of the mucous membrane adjacent to and remote from carcinoma of the colon. Cancer 37: 2388–2398, 1976.

230. Filipe MI. Mucous secretion in rat colonic mucosa during carcinogenesis induced by dimethylhydrazine. A morphological and histochemical study. Br J Cancer 32: 60–77, 1975.

231. Lev R. A histochemical study of glycogen and mucin in developing human fetal epithelia. Histochemistry 7: 152–165, 1968.

232. Bara J, Burtin P. Mucus associated gastrointestinal antigens in transitional mucosa adjacent to human colonic adenocarcinomas: Their "fetal type" association. Eur J Cancer 16: 1303–1310, 1980.

233. Isemura M, Sato M, Kikuchi H, Munakata H, Ototani, Goto K, Yosizawa Z. Sialoglycopeptides obtained from a transplantable rat colorectal adenocarcinoma: A comparison with those from normal colonic mucosa. Gann 74: 373–381, 1983.

234. Gold DV, Miller F. Characterization of human colonic mucoprotein antigen. Immunochemistry 11: 369–375, 1974.

235. Gold D, Miller F. Chemical and immunological differences between normal and tumoral colonic mucoprotein antigen. Nature 255: 85–87, 1975.

236. Boland CR, Montgomery CK, Kim YS. Alteration in human colonic mucin occurring with cellular differentiation and malignant transformation. Proc Natl Acad Sci USA 79: 2051–2055, 1982.

237. Dawson PA, Filipe MI. An ultrastructural feature of the colonic epithelium in familiar polyposis coli. Histopathology 1: 105–113, 1978.

238. Boland CR, Montgomery CK, Kim YS. A cancer-associated mucin alteration in benign colonic polyps. Gastroenterology 82: 664–672, 1982.

239. Lane N. The precursor tissue of ordinary large bowel carcinoma. Cancer Res 31: 2669–2672, 1976.

240. Bara J, Languille O, Gendron MC, Daher N, Martil E, Burtin P. Immunohistological study of precancerous mucus modification in human distal colonic polyps. Cancer Res 43: 3885–3891, 1983.

241. Allen A. Structure of gastrointestinal mucus glycoproteins and the viscous and gel-forming properties of mucus. Br Med Bull 34: 28–33, 1978.

242. Tatematsu T, Katsuyama T, Fukushima S, Takahashi M, Shirai T, Ito N, Nasu T. Mucin histochemistry by paradoxical concanavalin A staining in experimental gastric cancers induced in Wistar rats by N-methyl-N'-nitrosoguanine or 4-nitroquinoline 1-oxide. J Natl Cancer Inst 64: 835–844, 1980.

243. Schrager J, Oates MDG. Human gastrointestinal mucus and disease states. Br Med Bull 34: 79–82, 1978.

244. Feizi T, Turberville C, Westwood MM. Blood group precursors and cancer-related antigens. Lancet 2: 391–393, 1975.

245. Ashall F, Bramwell ME, Harris H. A new marker for human cancer cells. I. The Ca antigen and the Ca1 antibody. Lancet: 1–6, 1982.

246. McGee JO'D, Woods JC, Ashall F, Bramwell ME, Harris H. A new marker for human cancer cells. 2. Immunohistochemical detection of the Ca antigen in human tissues with Ca1 antibody. Lancet: 7–10, 1982.

247. Bramwell ME, Bhavanandan VP, Weisman G, Harris H: Structure and function of the Ca antigen. Br J Cancer 48: 177–183, 1983.

248. Hirst DG, Denekamp J, Hobson B. Proliferation kinetics of endothelial and tumour cells in three mouse mammary carcinomas. Cell Tissue Kinet 15: 251–261, 1982.

249. Vaupel PW, Frinak S, Bicher HI. Heterogeneous oxygen partial pressure and pH distribution in C3H mouse mammary adenocarcinoma. Cancer Res 41: 2008–2013, 1981.

8

Flow Cytometry in the Search for Cancer Markers

Jose V. Ordonez

INTRODUCTION

Flow cytometry—the study of single cells when presented in a liquid stream—constitutes a powerful analytical tool with applications in many fields of biology. It is performed with sophisticated instruments such as cell sorters or cell analyzers. Since the introduction of the first flow cytometer by Fullwyler in 1965, the capabilities of the instrument have been substantially improved, with the result of better analysis and data presentations. Applications of flow cytometry include hematology, oncology, cell biology, biochemistry, enzymology, and microbiology, to mention only the more common ones. In addition to surface marker determination, flow cytometry has made a great contribution to the study of the DNA content of cells, cell cycle analysis, and DNA synthesis, and sophisticated theoretical models have been proposed for estimating the rate of DNA synthesis (33). The areas of endeavor that have received the impact of flow cytometry seem sometimes far removed from the conventional applications. In searching for plants that produce fuel materials, cell sorting has been used to select for high-yield hybrids after transfer of the desired gene (3). This illustrates how versatile the technique is and how far its applications can reach. Figure 8–1 shows a schematic representation of a cell sorter.

Readers interested in the historical aspects and detailed description of the principles and operation of these instruments are referred to several comprehensive publications (12,23,24).

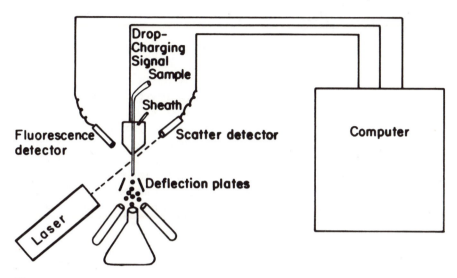

Figure 8–1. Schematic representation of a cell sorter.

PRINCIPLES OF FLOW CYTOMETRY

.Flow cytometers are computer-based instruments capable of making multiple measurements on single cells simultaneously, when the cells are presented in a fluid stream. The stream of cells is surrounded by a sheath of fluid that isolates the cells from the walls of a nozzle and in this laminar form exits from the flow chamber through an orifice 50–200 μm in diameter. The stream of cells is focused so that they can be illuminated by a light beam, usually from a laser or a mercury arc lamp. When a cell is illuminated, two types of signals are generated: light scatter and fluorescence. The signals so generated are collected by appropriate detectors and converted into electrical impulses, which are then processed by the computer. Large numbers of cells can be analyzed in seconds (3,000–5,000 per sec), a characteristic that accounts for the speed of the technique. Measurements from single cells are temporarily stored in the memory of the computer in a cumulative manner and can be displayed for analysis in a variety of ways, including profile histograms and bi- or tridimensional displays. The data can be permanently stored on magnetic discs or tapes and manipulated or analyzed in different ways. For this purpose most machines are equipped with built-in programs, and several investigators and manufacturers are developing new software to improve machine performance and data analysis.

ANALYTICAL PARAMETERS

Light Scattering

Light scattering is a characteristic of any particle struck by a light beam. Light scattering by cells occurs in all directions, but the amount of light scattered at any angle varies and is a complex phenomenon related to size, refractive index, and reflective properties of the cell. For a review on the subject the reader is referred to a paper by Salzman et al. (p. 105 in ref. 24). Most of the light scattered by the cell is in the forward direction around 0° where diffraction is the major contributory factor, and the measurements correlate well with cell size. Reflection from the nucleus and cytoplasm contributes more for the amount of light scattered at 90°, giving information on the characteristics of such structures. Most flow cytometers are equipped or can be equipped to register both types of light scatter. The pattern of light scatter is commonly used to identify different cell populations. Correlating the cell populations defined by light scatter with the fluorescence profile of a sample specifically stained for the marker of interest allows for the identification of subpopulations. Correlating light scatter at two different wave lengths has been proposed as a method for determining cell viability (22). Figure 8–2 shows examples of light scatter profiles (histograms).

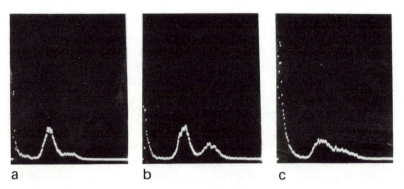

a   b   c

Figure 8–2. Scatter histograms of Ficoll-Hypaque lymphocyte preparations. The main peak represents the lymphocyte population; erythrocytes appear to the left, monocytes to the right, and cell debris far to the left of the lymphocyte peak. (*a*) Normal person; (*b*) patient with cancer of the larynx prior to surgery and radiation therapy; (*c*) the same patient as in (*b*) after surgery and radiation therapy. Changes in scatter pattern are frequent in such patients.

Fluorescence Measurements

The emission of light at a higher wavelength (color) than the wave length of the light used to excite a substance is called fluorescence. Fluorescence in a cell can be of one or two types: autofluorescence, present in varying degrees depending on the type of cell but usually of low intensity and susceptible to discrimination by the instruments; or artificial fluorescence, dependent upon a fluorescent probe applied to the cells under study. Various fluorochromes with different absorption and emission characteristics are in common use in biological determinations. By the use of appropriate filters or filter combinations one can eliminate unwanted signals and identify a cell on the basis of its specific reaction with the reagent applied. Some instruments are equipped with tuneable lasers, allowing the investigator to choose between different wavelengths from the ultraviolet to the visible light range. By the use of dichroic mirrors in the fluorescence path one can split the signal and measure fluorescence from two fluorochromes at the same time. Also, the parallel and vertical polarization of the fluorescence can be measured by the use of appropriate polarizing filters. Table 8–1 lists some of the most commonly used fluorochromes.

APPLICATIONS OF FLOW CYTOMETRY

Cell Surface Markers Determination

The availability of a wide variety of fluorescent probes has stimulated the application of flow cytometry to a wide variety of problems. The hybridoma technology and the monoclonal antibodies so produced have given a new dimension to the field of immunology and when used in conjunction with flow cytometry constitute the most rapid, reproducible, and semi-automated procedure for the detection of cell surface antigens used as markers for the identification of normal or neoplastic cells. The heterogeneity of the cells of the immune system was known before the widespread use of flow cytometry. However, the advent of this technology has greatly expanded the study of such cells. Information is rapidly accumulating on the status of the different lymphoid cell subpopulations in disorders ranging from infectious diseases to chronic diseases, disorders of the immune mechanisms, and organ transplant-related problems. Flow cytometry is especially suited for the study of the hematopoietic cells since this tissue naturally meets the first requirement for flow cytometric analysis—a single-cell suspension. Apart from determination of lymphocyte subsets, this technology has been applied to the study of such problems as quantification of malaria parasitized red cells (33) and detection of rare events in the blood such as the presence of fetal red cells in the mother's blood (6). Although flow cytometry has also been used for the detection of surface markers in other types of cells, hematology is the area that has received by far the most attention. Cells can be stained and analyzed immediately, or fixed and analyzed later. Formaldehyde

Table 8–1   Common Fluorescent Probes Used in Flow Cytometry

Type of assay	Reagent
Cell surface markers	Fluoroescein Rhodamine B Phycobiliproteins (Phycoerytrin)
Mitochondrial staining	Rhodamine 123
Phagocytosis	Fluorescent microspheres
Measure of membrane potential	Lipophilic cationic dyes
Oxidative burst	Dichlorofluorescin diacetate
Transfer of water-insoluble agents across cell membrane	Boronic acid derivatives (FluoroBoras)
DNA determination	Propidium iodide Ethidium bromide Acridine orange Acriflavine Auramine-O Proflavine 4'-6 Diamidino-2-phenylindole (DAP1) 4'-6 Bis(2'-imidazolinyl-4H, 5H)-2-phenylindole (DIPI) Mithramycin Chromomycin A3 Olivomycin
DNA (vital staining)	Bisbenzimidazole dyes (Hoechst dyes)
Enzyme analysis	Fluorogenic substrates
Receptors	Fluorescent labeled ligands

Adapted from refs. 14, 20, 21, 23, 26, 30, 32.

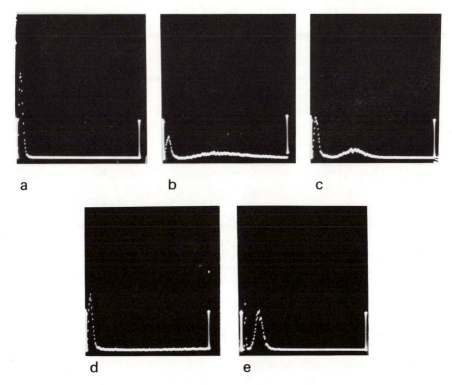

Figure 8–3. Fluorescence pattern of human lymphocytes. *(a)* Unstained control; *(b)* sample stained for total lymphocytes; *(c)* proportion of helper cells; *(d)* proportion of suppressor cells; *(e)* cells from a patient with B-cell lymphoma stained for B cells.

and paraformaldehyde fixation are commonly used for this purpose. Techniques have been developed for the simultaneous determination of surface markers and DNA content. Fixation with ethanol preserves the surface structures well, rendering the cell permeable to nucleic acid stains. Care must be taken to eliminate staining due to binding of the fluorochrome by RNA. This is easily accomplished by treatment of the cells with RNAase (5). By the use of two lasers it is possible to stain a cell sample for three different markers and define subpopulations by multiparameter analysis. Figure 8–3 shows a sequence of histograms obtained from peripheral blood lymphocytes separated by Ficoll Hypaque gradient and stained with monoclonal antibodies specific for the different markers. The analysis was performed in a FACS IV flow cytometer.

Analysis of Cell Physiology

Conventional biochemical techniques for the study of cell physiology are carried out in heterogeneous cell populations analyzed as a unit, and the results are usually expressed as average values per cell. This procedure has obvious disadvantages since cell populations are rarely homogeneous and differences among subpopulations cannot be determined. Measurements on individual cells, in the other hand, enable the investigator to define such subpopulations and to study, for example, their response to different stimuli. The range of physiologic processes that can be investigated by flow cytometry is ample. One can assume that once a fluorescent probe can be included in the process and appropriate filters for collecting the emitted fluorescence are available, the phenomenon is appropriate for flow cytometric analysis. The expanding applications of flow cytometry to the study of cell physiology include: studies on cell activation, changes in cell membrane potential, changes in cellular calcium distribution, oxidative product formation, transfer of water-insoluble agents across the cell membrane, identification of mitogen-responding lymphocytes, detection of infected cells, phagocytosis, and determination of intracellular pH (2,14,15,21,30). This list is by no means complete, and new applications constantly appear in the literature.

DNA and Cell Life-Cycle Analysis

Cell division is preceded by a series of events that include nucleic acid synthesis. DNA synthesis occupies a discrete period of the cell life cycle, and not all cells in a population necessarily undergo DNA synthesis and division. The current concept of the cell cycle considers cells in a population to be in one of four phases: G1, S, G2, or M. The G1 phase is composed of cells that have gone through mitosis but have yet to start DNA synthesis for a new round of division. This phase also contains a portion of noncycling or quiescent cells (Go) unable to incorporate DNA precursors. The S phase contains cells actively engaged in DNA synthesis. Their DNA content increases according to how far along the S phase they are. The G2 phase is the period between the end of DNA synthesis and the start of mitosis. The M phase contains cell in mitosis when their DNA content is twice as high as that of cells in G1. For more details on the different aspects of the cell life cycle, the interested reader is referred to recent publications (7,24).

Flow cytometry has been one of the principal elements in the current understanding of the cell life cycle. Several fluorescent dyes with different binding characteristics are available for this purpose. Techniques have been developed for staining nuclei after hypotonic cell burst (19), and a semi-permanent staining procedure enables the investigator to analyze together samples taken at different times (8). Staining of nuclei with preservation of the cell membranes permits the simultaneous analysis of DNA and components of the cell surface, making possible the correlation of cell surface marker expression and cell cycle phase (5). Accurate determination of the proportion of cells in each phase of the life cycle is not always easy. One major problem is the overlap between two contiguous phases, making it difficult to decide, from a histogram, which cells (within the overlapping zones) correspond to each phase. Computer programs have been developed to apply mathematical curve-fitting techniques to deal with this problem. However, no generally acceptable technique has been found, since some programs work only for undisturbed cell populations and are therefore of no use in cell kinetic studies of cell populations subjected to drug treatments that alter the life cycle. However, even in such cases, visual analysis of the DNA profiles and quantitation of the cells in the different areas of the histogram provides valuable information. Figure 8–4 shows a series of histograms obtained with a sample of the K562 cell line derived from a patient with chronic myelogenous leukemia and cells from a patient with acute lymphoblastic leukemia. The cells were stained with propidium iodide in a hypotonic solution, and the kinetics after synchronization with methotrexate were studied.

Incorporation of DNA precursors detected by autoradiography has been the only available technique for quantitating cells actively synthesizing DNA. More recently, a flow-cytometric technique that makes use of the suppression of fluorescence of DNA-bound achridine orange as a result of incorporation of the thymidine analog, bromody-oridinc (BrdU) was developed by Darzynkiewicz and collaborators (7). With the development of a monoclonal antibody specific of BrDU (9) it is now possible not only to measure total DNA content, but also to identify cells that move into the S phase and are therefore actively synthesizing DNA. This will undoubtedly facilitate cell kinetic studies, and comparison of results between different laboratories will be possible.

Karyotyping and the study of chromosome abnormalities is usually hampered by the low number of cells that go into mitosis. Synchronization with different drug treatments is used to increase the proportions of cells that progress to mitosis (13), but the number of mitotic cells does not always increase substantially. The quantitative capabilities of flow cytometry and the availability of instruments with high resolution make possible the determination of individual chromo-

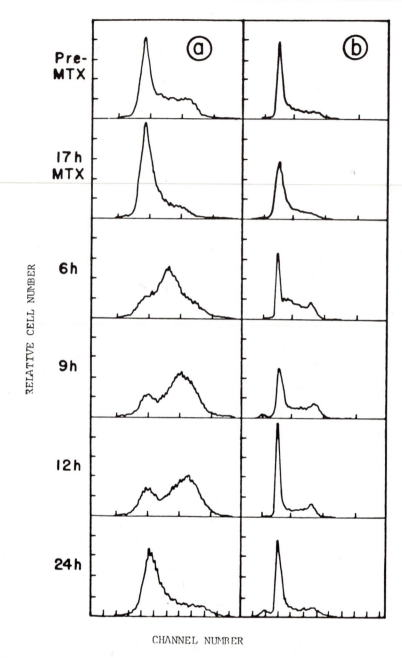

Figure 8–4. DNA histograms obtained immediately prior to and at the times indicated after exposure to 10^{-7} M methotrexate. Channel number is a measure of fluorescence due to the DNA-binding dye and is linearly proportional to DNA content. (*a*) K562 cells; (*b*) cells from the patient with ALL.

somes, and a new type of karyotype in the form of a histogram can be obtained. Up to 14 peaks (chromosomes or chromosome groups) have been identified (30).

Enzyme Analysis

Enzyme analysis by flow cytometry is possible by the use of fluorogenic substrates. These compounds, when hydrolized by enzymatic action, are rendered fluorescent and therefore detectable by flow cytometry. Table 8–2 shows a list of fluorogenic substrates commonly used in flow cytometry.

Other Applications

The reader should be aware that the list of applications of flow cytometry is greater than that presented here, but a comprehensive

Table 8–2 Fluorogenic Substrates Used in Flow Cytometry for Enzyme Analysis

Substrate	Enzyme
Flavone-3-diphosphate triammonium salt	Acid phosphatase
7-Bromo-3-hydroxy-2-naphtho-O-anisidine phosphate	Alkaline phosphatase
Fluorescein diacetate	Neutral esterase
Fluorescein dibutyrate	
Fluorescein laurate	
Benzyloxycarbonyl-alanyl-arginyl-arginyl-4-methoxy-2-naphthylamide	Acid arylaminidase
Lysyl-alanyl-4-methoxy-2-naphthylamide	Acid γ-D-glucuronidase
γ-Glutamyl-4-methoxy-2-naphthylamide	
7-Bromo-3-hydroxy-2-naphtho-O-anisidine-γ-D-glucuronide	
Nicotinamide adenine dinucleotide-sodium lactate	Lactase dehydrogenase

Adapted from Kruth (ref. 21)

review on the subject would be beyond the scope of this chapter. Among the more important applications of flow cytometry is its increasing use for the study of receptor–ligand interactions; in this regard, it is interesting to point out again that flow cytometric measurements are carried out on single cells, and subpopulations that have different concentrations of receptors can be identified. This makes flow cytometry more desirable than radiolabeled compounds for receptor–ligand interaction studies since the latter cannot discern the existence of subpopulations with different expression of the receptor. As reviewed by Kruth (21), this technology has been used to study problems such as binding of low-density proteins, cholera toxin, histamine, complement, antibody, murine leukemia virus, insulin, lectins, and antigens. With the increasing recognition of the importance of receptor–ligand interaction in cell functions, researchers should find more and more applications for flow cytometry in this area.

Physical Sorting

A remarkable characteristic of flow cytometry is its capability to separate cells according to parameters defined by the investigator. The cells are first analyzed, according to their light-scatter and/or fluorescence characteristics; the subpopulations of interest are identified, and the parameters for sorting are given to the computer. The sorters are equipped with mechanisms (usually a piezoelectric transducer) that make the cell stream vibrate at a specified rate and form a chain of single-cell-containing droplets that fall through an electric field. Droplets containing cells with the characteristics specified are charged as they travel through the electric field and are diverted to appropriate containers. With this technology the investigator can separate cells based on the presence of surface antigens, on their DNA content, or on their physiologic state. If the procedure is carried out under sterile conditions and if the substances used to treat the cells are not harmful to their viability, the sorted cells can be used for further studies, making this technology not only a powerful analytical tool but also a procedure that can be used to separate and enrich cell subpopulations with a high degree of purity suitable for further studies on more homogeneous cell populations. Instruments equipped with single-cell deposition systems allow the investigator to collect individual cells in appropriate containers (microtiter plates) for growth and cloning studies.

FLOW CYTOMETRY AND CANCER

Direct observation of cells or tissues continues to be the most reliable method for identifying malignancy. Old and new histological techniques combined with modern cytochemical techniques have greatly increased the potential for determining when a cell has undergone malignant transformation. Malignant transformation is underlined by metabolic changes that, when accompanied by the expression of new or special antigens conveniently located or exposed on the cell surface, can be used for identification or diagnostic purposes. Fluorescent microscopy, especially when performed with monoclonal antibodies, is a powerful tool for the detection of cell surface antigens (markers). Determination of the DNA distribution within a cell population provides information on the proportion of cells in each phase of the cell life cycle. Studies of the cell cycle kinetics give information on the proliferative stage of cells. This has been particularly successful with *in vitro* studies. Kinetic studies on bone marrow of leukemia patients has been proposed for monitoring response to treatment with different anti-leukemic drugs. However, analysis of this type is complicated by the fact that bone marrow aspirates usually have varying degrees of peripheral blood contamination. For this reason, use of bone marrow biopsies is the recommended procedure for collecting material for flow cytometric studies. Alterations in the genetic make-up of malignant or premalignant cells seem to be more frequent than previously thought. There is a great deal of variation in the reports on genetic alterations in malignant conditions. This is probably due in part to differences in the techniques used by different investigators, or difficulties such as the need to analyze large numbers of cells in order to document an alteration that might be present only in a small proportion of cells. As mentioned previously, this is overcome by flow cytometry since large numbers of cells can be analyzed reproducibly in a few seconds. It is generally accepted that, at the present time, flow cytometry is the most accurate, rapid, and convenient method not only for cell surface marker determination, but also for other types of studies on single cells with applications in many biological problems, as previously discussed.

Hematology and immunology have been particularly enriched with the advent of flow cytometry. The knowledge of the hematopoietic system has expanded tremendously in recent years, and its heterogeneity and complex variety of functions are now more clearly understood. The role of the different cell subpopulations in the defense mechanism has been the focus of many studies, and the understanding of the effects of diseases that alter the immune system and the distribution and function of the different cell subsets is becoming clearer. Lymphocytes are commonly characterized by a variety of tests, including determination on immunoglobuline, presence of receptors for sheep erythrocytes, and presence of surface membrane antigens. They are primarily divided into bone-marrow-derived (B) lymphocytes identified by the presence on their surface of surface membrane immunoglobuline and thymus-dependent (T) lymphocytes. Major subsets within the T lymphocytes are helper/inducer and suppressor/cytotoxic. Other groups, such as the NK (natural killer) cells, can also be identified. The characterization of lymphocytes into more precisely defined subsets is continuing, and it is foreseeable that new subsets will be defined, especially with the use of analytical techniques such as multiparameter analysis. The study of leukemia has been approached from different angles. The FAB classification, proposed by Gralnick et al. in 1977 (16) is based on cytomorphological characteristics. Correlation of disease categories proposed in this classification and results of flow-cytometric studies have not been satisfactory in all cases. Attempts in this direction have been made, but more work is necessary to find common grounds in most cases.

Flow-cytometric studies of leukemia are based on nucleic acid analysis, determination of cell surface markers, and enzyme determinations. As reviewed by Andreff and Darzynkiewics (1), acute lymphocytic leukemia (ALL) cells are characterized by low RNA content as compared to acute nonlymphoblastic leukemia (ANLL). Some proliferation is evident, as indicated by the presence of some cells in S and G2M phases. When compared to the FAB classification, a difference was seen in the proliferative state and ploidy level between the L1 and L2 ALL. In a study of 111 cases of childhood ALL, aneuploidy was reported in 34% of L1 cases and 71% in L2 cases. The proportion of cells in S phase was found to be higher (9.8%) in aneuploid than in diploid (4.3%) cases. The L3 subgroup of ALL was reported as showing high RNA content and having aneuploidy in all cases. Aneuploidy reported in cases of ALL is mostly of the hyperdiploid or tetraploid type, although hypodiploid cases have also been reported. Acute lymphoblastic leukemia can also be classified using cell markers such as the presence of surface antigens, presence of immunoglobuline, or the presence or absence of certain enzymes. According to Foon et al. (10) several major groups are recognized: unclassified acute lymphoblastic leukemia (un-ALL), common acute lymphoblastic leukemia (cALL), pre B-ALL, and T-ALL.

Acute nonlymphoblastic leukemia has also been studied by flow cytometry. High RNA content and aneuploidy levels of 30–40% have been reported (1). Correlation with cell surface markers has, however, not been very successful. Among the unclassified acute leukemias, two subgroups have been defined by flow cytometry. One group of cases is TdT (terminal deoxynucleotidyl transferase) positive and shows low RNA content. The other group, with high RNA content, is TdT negative. Aneuploidy as high as 85% was found in cases of myeloma, and the cells showed high RNA content. In cases of non-Hodgkin's lymphoma, attempts to correlate degree of malignancy with nucleic acid analysis show a probable association of low-grade malignancy with low RNA content and low incidence of aneuploidy. High-grade malignancy seems to correlate with higher RNA content and higher frequency of aneuploidy.

Information from cytometric studies can serve prognostic purposes. A study of DNA content of bone marrow cells from patients with myelodysplastic syndromes (25) showed that patients with stable conditions had more cells in S and G2M phases than patients who developed leukemia or died. Solid tumors can also be studied by flow cytometry. However, a problem of primary importance is apparent. Even though appropriate material for such studies can be obtained from normal cavities such as by bladder washing (and possibly urine) or from pleural effusion in response to invasion from cancer ailments in the vicinity, in most instances cells for cytometric studies must be obtained from biopsy material. It is therefore necessary to subject such samples to enzyme treatment in order to obtain single-cell suspensions. This is not always easy, since enzyme treatment may alter the cells, and cell clumps of different sizes usually remain. Provisions must be taken to eliminate as many clumps as possible by screening the cell suspensions before running them through the instrument or eliminating the clumps from analysis by electronic gating. The association of alterations in the DNA content and malignant transformation of cells has been the subject of many studies. It now seems evident that these two conditions often appear together and that DNA alterations depart more from the normal level as the tumor shows higher anaplastic grades. Olszewski et al. (27) in a study of 92 cases of human breast cancer found 92% of aneuploidy in the form of hyperdiploidy. Based on the DNA content they defined two groups: one group with diploid or near diploid DNA distribution, the other conforming cases with triploid, tetraploid, or higher DNA content. When compared with their histologic characteristics, more differentiated-type tumors with positive estrogen-binding characteristics showed ploidy levels closer to normal; less-differentiated estrogen-binding negative tumors showed higher DNA ploidy. Cell cycle analysis of similar cases (28) showed that malignant breast tumors had a greater proportion of cells in S and

G2M phases than benign tumors. Great variation was found among the breast cancers, but medullary carcinoma showed the highest proportion of cells in S and G2M phases, while papillary, tubular, colloid, and well-differentiated duct carcinomas showed the lowest. Estrogen receptor-negative tumors from premenopausal patients showed more cells in S and G2M, while estrogen receptor-positive tumors from postmenopausal women had fewer cells in the same phases of the cell cycle.

Diagnosis of bladder tumors is traditionally accomplished by histopathological examination of biopsy material. With the advent of flow cytometry, new avenues of study are available not only for analysis of material obtained by biopsy but also for the utilization of cells exfoliated from the tumors that can be collected through bladder washings or voided urine. One problem that complicates the use of bladder washings or urine for diagnosis of bladder cancer is the presence of inflammatory cells. This has been addressed in several ways. In 1978 Pedersen et al. (29) reported on the DNA analysis of bladder washings. They introduced a correction for the presence of leukocytes bases on a differential count performed on the material under analysis. They found a good correlation between the degree of anaplasia and invasiveness of the tumor and the presence of aneu-ploidy. Similar findings were reported by Jacobsen et al. (16), who found good correlation between the grade of atypia and ploidy level. Collste et al. (4), using acridine orange to stain the DNA and RNA to distinguish normal epithelial cells and leukocytes, also found similar results in comparing bladder washings with suspensions prepared from tumor biopsies. In some cases, bladder washings detected the presence of malignant cells when the biopsies gave negative results. They concluded that these differences were probably due to problems in sampling, supporting the concept of the multifocal nature of bladder tumors and showing that flow cytometry might be more sensitive for detecting such tumors. Carcinoma *in situ* seems to be readily detectable by flow cytometry, with percentage positive as high as 98% in cases with flat carcinoma *in situ* and 88% in cases of papillary carcinoma and carcinoma *in situ*, with an overall false-negative rate of 6% (17). In a recent review, Frankfurt and Huben (11) summarized the current work on DNA analysis in bladder cancer and discussed possible applications of flow cytometry to the diagnosis and manage-ment of the disease.

Primary bone tumors have also been studied by flow cytometry. Kreicbergs et al. (19) recently reported a study of 15 benign tumors, which included giant cell tumors, aneurysmal bone cyst, eosinophilic granuloma, non-ossifying fibroma, chondroblastoma, enchondroma, and osteochondroma, and 34 malignant primary bone tumors including osteoblastic osteosarcoma, chondroblastic osteosarcoma, fibroblastic osteosarcoma, paraosteal osteosarcoma, chondrosarcoma, adamantinoma, and Ewing sarcoma. They found that all benign tumors except one of questionable histologic type exhibited normal DNA content. Among the 34 malignant tumors, 23 showed some degree of aneuploidy, and those with diploid DNA content corresponded to low-grade malignancy. The proliferative activity of aneuploid tumors was illustrated by a higher proportion of cells in S and G2M phases, but no difference in this respect was observed between diploid-benign and diploid-malignant tumors.

So far we have mentioned some examples of cancers that have been studied by flow cytometry. More studies have been published, some with not very clear or definite results. However, refinement of the techniques continues, and it is expected that the successful application of flow cytometry to the study of cancer will show a steady increase in the near future.

CONCLUSION AND FUTURE PERSPECTIVES

Flow cytometry as a technology has evolved as a result of the interaction of many disciplines working together toward the solution of a problem. The ingenuity of dedicated scientists from fields ranging from biology to engineering, from biophysics to computer sciences, interacting much beyond the boundaries of their individual disciplines, has created a new discipline whose impact is evident in practically all fields of biology. Cell components can now be studied at the molecular level in intact cells. Physiologic processes can be monitored with great accuracy. Cell populations that might seem homogeneous when analyzed with conventional techniques are found to be different or to react differently when seen with the electronic eyes of the cell sorter. Cells with special characteristics can be singled out and separated. The rapid analysis of all this information by computers and by sophisticated analytical techniques has led to remarkable progress in just over a decade of endeavor. The benefits of flow cytometry have been more useful so far in the solution of research problems; however, applications to the solution of clinical or diagnostic problems are rapidly emerging, and one can state without doubt that, with wider use of the technology, instruments accessible to most clinical laboratories will be developed and that the technique will soon become a routine diagnostic procedure as well as continuing to be an invaluable research tool.

REFERENCES

1. Andreeff, M., and Darzynkiewicz, Z. Multiparameter flow cytometry. Part II: Application in hematology. Clin. Bull. *11*: 120–130, 1981.

2. Bass, D. A., Parce, J. W., Dechatelet, L. R., Szejda, P., Seeds, M. C., and Thomas, M. Flow cytometric studies of oxidative product formation by neutrophils: A graded response to membrane stimulation. J. Immunol. *130*: 1910–1917, 1983.

3. Calvin, M. New sources for fuel and materials. Science, *219*: 24–26, 1983.

4. Collste, L. G., Devonec, M., Darzynkiewicz, Z., Triaganos, F., Sharpless, T. K., Whitmore, W. F. Jr., and Melamed, M. R. Bladder cancer diagnosis by flow cytometry. Correlation between cell samples from biopsy and bladder irrigation fluid. Cancer *45*: 2389–2394, 1980.

5. Crissman, H. A., Egmond, J. V., Holdrinet, R. S., Pennings, A., and Haanen, C. Simplified method for DNA and protein staining of human hematopoietic cell samples. Cytometry *2*: 59–62, 1981.

6. Cupp, J. E., Leary, J. F., Cernichiari, I, Wood, J. C. S., and Doherty, R. A. Rare event analysis methods for detection of fetal red blood cells in material blood. Cytometry *5*: 138–144, 1984.

7. Darzynkiewicz, Z., and Andreeff, M. Multiparameter flow cytometry. Part I: Application in analysis of the cell cycle. Clin. Bull. *11*: 47–57, 1981.

8. Deitch, A. D., Law, H., and White, R. D. A stable propidium iodide staining procedure for flow cytometry. J. Histochem. Cytochem. *30*: 967–972, 1982.

9. Dolbeare, F., Gratzner, H., Pallavicini, M. G., and Gray, J. W. Flow cytometric measurement of total DNA content and incorporated bromodeoxyuridine. Proc. Natl. Acad. Sci. USA *80*: 5573–5577, 1983.

10. Foon, K. A., Schroff, R. W., and Gale, R. P. Surface markers on leukemia and lymphoma cells: Recent advances. Blood *60*: 1–19, 1982.

11. Frankfurt, O. S., and Huben, R. P. Clinical applications of DNA flow cytometry for bladder tumors: A review. Urology (in press)

12. Fulwyler, M. J. Flow cytometry and cell sorting. Blood Cells *6*: 173–184, 1980.

13. Gallo, J. H., Ordonez, J. V., Brown, G. E., and Testa, J. R. Synchronization of human leukemic cells: Relevance for high resolution chromosome banding. Human Genetics (in press).

14. Gallop, P. M., Paz, M. A., and Henson, E. Boradeption: A new procedure for transferring water-insoluble agents across cell membranes. Science *217*: 166–169, 1982.

15. Gerson, D.F. Determination of intracellular pH changes in lymphocytes with 4-methylumbelliferone by flow microfluorometry. In: *Intracellular pH: Its Measurement, Regulation and Utilization in Cellular Functions,* edited by R. Nuccitelli and D. W. Deamer, pp. 125–133. New York: Alan R. Liss, Inc., 1982.

16. Gralnick, H. R., Galton, D. A. G., Catovsky, D., Sultan, C., and Bennett, J. M. Classification of acute leukemia. Ann. Intern. Med. *87*: 740–753, 1977.

17. Jacobsen, A., Mommsen, S. and Olsen, S. Characterization of ploidy level in

bladder tumors and selected site specimens by flow cytometry. Cytometry *4*: 170–173, 1983.

18. Klein, F. A., Herr, H. W., Whitmore, W. F. Jr., Sogani, P. C., and Melamed, M. R. An evaluation of automated flow cytometry (FCM) in detection of carcinoma in situ of the urinary bladder. Cancer *50*: 1003–1008, 1982.

19. Kreicbergs, A., Silversward, C., and Tribukait, B. Flow DNA analysis of primary bone tumors. Relationship between cellular DNA content and histopathologic classification. Cancer *53*: 129–136, 1984.

20. Krisham, A. Rapid flow cytofluorometric analysis of mammalian cell cycle by propidium iodide staining. J. Cell. Biol. *66*: 188–193, 1975.

21. Kruth, H. S. Flow cytometry: Rapid biochemical analysis of single cells. Anal. Biochem. *125*: 225–242, 1982.

22. Loken, M. R., and Houck, D. W. Light scattered at two wavelengths can discriminate viable lymphoid cell populations on a fluorescence-activated cell sorter. J. Histochem. Cytochem. *29*: 609–615, 1981.

23. Loken, M. R., and Stall, A. M. Flow cytometry as an analytical and preparative tool in immunology. J. Immunol. Methods. *50*: R85–R112, 1982.

24. Melamed, M. R., Mullaney, P. F., and Mendelsohn, M. L., eds. *Flow Cytometry and Sorting*, New York: John Wiley, 1979.

25. Montecucco, C., Riccardi, A., Traversi, E., Danova, M., Ucci, G., Mazzini, G., and Giordono, P. Flow cytometric DNA content in myelodysplactic syndromes. Cytometry *4*: 238–243, 1983.

26. Oi, V. T., Glazer, A. N., and Stryer, L. Fluorescent phycobiliprotein conjugates for analyses of cells and molecules. J. Cell. Biol. *93*: 981–986, 1982.

27. Olszewski, W., Darzynkiewicz, Z., Rosen, P. P., Schwartz, M. K., and Melamed, M. R. Flow cytometry of breast carcinoma. I: Relation of DNA ploidy level to histology and estrogen receptor. Cancer *48*: 980–984, 1981.

28. Olszewski, W., Darzynkiewicz, Z., Rosen, P. P., Schwartz, M. K., and Melamed, M. R. Flow cytometry of breast carcinoma. II: Relation of tumor cell cycle distribution to histology and estrogen receptor. Cancer *48*: 985–988, 1981.

29. Pedersen, T., Larsen, J. K., and Krarup, T. Characterization of bladder tumours by flow cytometry on bladder washings. Eur. Urol. *4*: 351–355, 1978.

30. Shapiro, H. M., Natale, P. J., and Kamentsky, L. A. Estimation of membrane potentials of individual lymphocytes by flow cytometry. Proc. Natl. Acad. Sci. USA *76*: 5728–5730, 1979.

31. Sillar, R., and Young, B. D. A new method for the preparation of metaphase chromosomes for flow analysis. J. Histochem. Cytochem. *29*: 74–78, 1981.

32. Steinkamp, J. A., Wilson, J. S., Saunders, G. C., and Stewart, C. C. Phagocytosis: Flow cytometric quantitation with fluorescent microspheres. Science *215*: 64–66, 1982.

33. Whaun, J. M., Rittershaus, C., and Ip, S. H. C. Rapid identification and detection of parasitized human red cells by automated flow cytometry. Cytometry *4*: 117–122, 1983.

34. White, R. A theory for the estimation of DNA synthesis rates by flow cytometry. J. Theor. Biol. *85*: 53–73, 1980.

9

Chromosomal Markers in Cancer

Avery A. Sandberg

The distribution of nuclear DNA within an individual's somatic cells is maintained rigorously among the 46 chromosomes, i.e. 46,XY in the male and 46,XX in the female (Fig. 9–1) (1). Slight inter-individual variations, particularly of heterochromatin and the size of the Y, may exist between individuals, but almost invariably the maintenance of normality and cellular integrity and function is related to the stability of the 46 chromosomes within somatic cells. Even minor deviations from the normal karyotype, particularly if they occur *in utero*, lead to a number of anatomic anomalies, only a small portion of which are compatible with survival. Even then, those individuals who do survive usually have a short life span. In addition, some of the disorders with constitutional chromosome anomalies also predispose to malignancy (2), including such conditions as Wilms' tumor with 11p−, retinoblastoma with 13q−, and various lymphomas and leukemias in Bloom syndrome and ataxia telangiectasia. Thus, in these conditions in which all the somatic cells of the body are involved by chromosomal anomalies, the latter appear to predispose to the development of malignancy in a particular organ or tissue. However, the major attention of this chapter will be given to those chromosomal (cytogenetic, karyotypic) changes that are present only in the affected neoplastic cells and that are almost always accompanied by normal karyotypes in the remaining somatic cells of the patients (1). Thus, to establish karyotypic changes in malignancy, it is necessary that the affected tissue or cells be examined, since examination of such cells as circulating lymphocytes or fibroblasts will usually reveal the normal

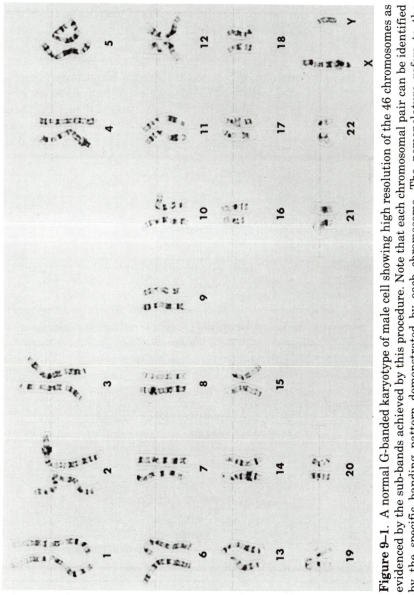

Figure 9–1. A normal G-banded karyotype of male cell showing high resolution of the 46 chromosomes as evidenced by the sub-bands achieved by this procedure. Note that each chromosomal pair can be identified by the specific banding pattern demonstrated by each chromosome. The nomenclature refers to the chromosomal arm above the centromere as p and that below the centromere as q. Each arm is then divided into regions and each region into bands and sub-bands.

karyotype of the affected individuals. In the case of leukemias it is generally necessary to obtain bone marrow material in order to establish the chromosomal changes, both at a quantitative and qualitative level. In the case of cancer, the cells of various parts of the tumor have to be examined to establish the karyotypic changes, whether they be primary or metastatic lesions. Thus, with the exception of a few situations, the karyotypic changes in cancer, lymphoma, and leukemia can only be established through a cytogenetic analysis of the affected cells or tissues per se. When a karyotypic change is suspected as possibly being of constitutional origin, then examination of circulating lymphocytes stimulated with phytohemagglutinin (PHA) is the usual approach to utilize to rule in or rule out such a possibility (1).

CHROMOSOMAL CHANGES IN LEUKEMIA

The generally recognized and established chromosomal changes associated with various leukemias are shown in Tables 9–1 to 9–3.

Table 9–1 Nonrandom Translocations Characterizing Leukemias

t(1;7)(p11;p11)	Dysmyelopoietic disorder (induced?)
t(1;19)(q21;q13)	ALL (L1)
t(1;19)(q23;p13.3)	Pre-B-cell ALL
t(2:8)(p11-13;q24)	ALL (L3)
t(2;11)(p21;q23)	Dysmyelopoietic preleukemia
t(4;11)(q21;q23)	Acute leukemia
t(6;9)(p23:q34)	ANLL (M2), myeloproliferative diseases
t(6;12)(q15;p13)	Prolymphocytic leukemia
t(8;14)(q24;q32)	ALL (L3)
t(8;22)(q24;q11)	ALL (L3)
t(9;11)(p21;q23)	AMol (M5)
t(9;22)(q34;q11)	CML, acute leukemias
t(11;14)(q13;q32)	ALL, CLL, lymphoma
t(11;21)(q22;q21)	ANNLL, myeloproliferative disorders
t(15;17)(q22;q12)	APL (M3)

Note: ALL: acute lymphoblastic leukemia; ANLL: acute nonlymphocytic leukemia; AMol: acute monoblastic leukemia; CML: chronic myelocytic leukemia; CLL: chronic lymphocytic leukemia; APL: acute promyelocytic leukemia. Designations in parentheses refer to the FAB classification of the leukemias.

Table 9–2   Nonrandom Morphologic Chromosome Changes in Leukemia

3p−, 3q−	Secondary acute leukemia
5q−	Refractory anemia, secondary acute leukemia
6q−	ALL
7q− (q33q36)	Secondary acute leukemia
9p−	T-cell ALL
11q− (q23)	ANLL (M2, M4, and M5)
12p− (p12)	ALL
12q−	ANLL
inv(14) (q11q32)	T-cell CLL
14q+ (q32)	ALL, CLL, adult T-cell acute leukemia
inv(16) (p13q22) or 16q− (q22)	ANLL with eosinophilia
i(17q)	Blastic phase of CML
20q−	Polycytemia vera
21q	Preleukemia, ANLL

Those in Table 9–1 represent translocations, usually balanced and reciprocal, associated with specific leukemic entities (Figs. 9–2 to 9–5). In almost all these conditions a translocation is often the only karyotypic change observed at the initial cytogenetic examination, pointing to the role this change may play in the genesis of the leukemia (3–5). In fact, it is now generally accepted that the specific (primary) karyotypic change is related to the genesis of the neoplasia and may be a necessary genomic alteration for malignant transformation to take place in the cell involved by the translocation. Thus, in the leukemias when translocations are present they possibly point to a specific cause capable of inducing the chromosomal change in a specific cell and ultimately resulting in the appearance of leukemia whose morphologic, laboratory, and clinical aspects reflect unique features

Table 9–3   Nonrandom Numerical Chromosome Changes in Leukemia

−5	Secondary leukemia
−7	Secondary leukemia
+8	ANLL, blastic phase of CML
+12	CLL
+21	ALL

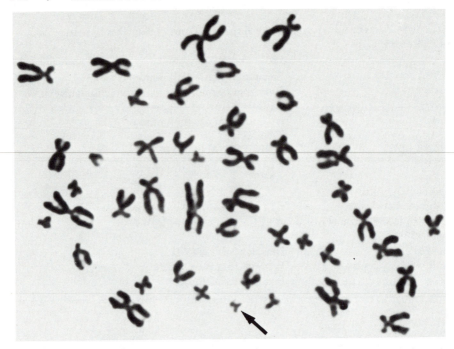

Figure 9–2. A metaphase (unbanded) showing the morphologic appearance of the Ph-chromosome (arrow) characteristic of chronic myelocytic leukemia. The telomeric segments of chromosome #9 are translocated to the Ph[1] (not shown in this schema).

associated with the chromosomal change. When additional chromosomal changes appear, besides the specific translocation, these secondary karyotypic changes are usually associated with biologic and clinical progression of the disease (6), particularly in leukemias with t(8;21) and t(9;22). Thus, one can look upon the primary chromosomal change as being related to the primary cause of the leukemia and necessary for the leukemic transformation to occur. Although some of the secondary changes may also be nonrandom and may be related to the original basic cause of the leukemia and/or the specific translocation, subsequent secondary changes tend to have an apparent randomness about them; on occasion, such changes are difficult to characterize but, nevertheless, may play a crucial role in the biology of the disease (6).

In Table 9–2 are shown those leukemias that are associated with morphologic changes of particular chromosomes, these changes being due either to deletions of one or another arm of the chromosome or the insertion or presence of extra material (Fig. 9–4). Those chromosomes that have lost or gained material are indicated by a minus or plus sign next to the arm, respectively; e.g. 11q− means that part of the long arm of chromosome #11 has been lost and 14q+ that extra material is present on the long arm of chromosome #14. Although a careful search has been made in these conditions to ascertain whether the extra or missing material is due to one type of translocation or another, generally these searches have not revealed such an event and we may assume then that the missing or extra material is the sole karyotypic change existing as the primary one in such cells. In Table 9–3 are shown a small number of leukemias in which the primary chromosome change appears to be due either to an extra chromosome or to a missing chromosome; in some of these conditions the loss of the chromosome may be preceded by partial loss of an arm and ultimately by total loss of the chromosome. An example is that of secondary leukemia, in

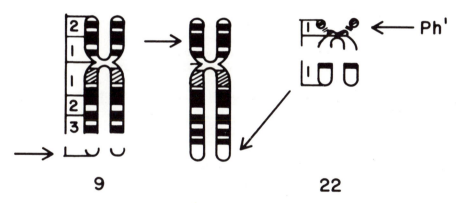

Figure 9–3. Schematic presentation of the chromosomal events leading to the genesis of the Ph[1] chromosome and the molecular events accompanying this translocation. The break in chromosome 9 affects the location of an oncogene called *abl* whereas that in chromosome 22 does not affect the oncogene *sis*. In each case the oncogene is reciprocally translocated but only activation of the *abl* gene appears to take place, whereas that of *sis* apparently is not activated since it is not involved in the breakpoints of this translocation. The Philadelphia chromosome always consists of a chromosome 22 with a break at band q11 and then followed by a reciprocal translocation of material with that of chromosome 9, though other chromosomes may be involved in this translocation. These variant Ph[1] translocations can be either simple when they involve a chromosome other than #9 or complex in which 3 or more chromosomes are involved.

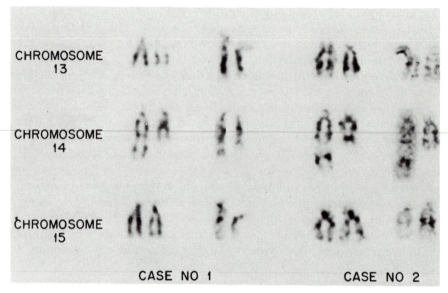

Figure 9–4. A 14q+ anomaly, resulting from extra material having been added to the long arm of chromosome #14, seen in chronic lymphocytic leukemia (CLL), lymphomas, and occasionally other diseases. Partial karyotypes from 2 CLL cases show chromosomes #13–15, with the 14q+ in each case being shown to the left of the normal chromosome #14. In CLL the nature of the extra material has been difficult to identify, although in Burkitt lymphoma it is often due to a reciprocal translocation with the long arm of chromosome #8.

which part of the long arm of chromosome #5 and/or chromosome #7 is lost and is often followed by total loss of the chromosome (7–9).

An examination of Tables 9–1 to 9–3 will reveal that the number of leukemias that have been characterized cytogenetically exceeds that based on such classifications as that of the FAB system (10) and points to the usefulness of cytogenetic analysis in establishing subentitites with the FAB system, each of which is characterized not only by a specific chromosomal change, but also by a number of clinical, laboratory, and prognostic parameters unique to the leukemia with such karyotypic changes. For example, acute myeloblastic leukemia (AML) with t(8;21) is almost invariably of the M2 variety and associated with Auer bodies in the leukemic cells and, generally, with a relatively good prognosis (1,7,11). On the other hand, AML with t(6;9) tends to have a poorer prognosis, with the patients usually not achieving lengthy complete remissions (12–14).

In chronic myelocytic leukemia (CML) the appearance of cells with chromosomal changes in addition to the Ph[1]—particularly an extra Ph[1], +8, or an isochromosome of the long arm of chromosome #17—is usually associated with or heralds the blastic phase (1). These changes may precede laboratory and clinical evidence of such a phase by months or weeks and could be used as an important criterion for the development of the blastic phase when the latter is not clinically evident.

Up to now only qualitative changes in the karyotype of leukemic cells have been discussed, but there is a quantitative aspect to these changes that is worthy of mention. It has been generally established that when the marrow, particularly in acute nonlymphocytic leukemia (ANLL), contains (for all practical purposes) no cytogenetically normal cells, the prognosis is usually much worse than that observed in those

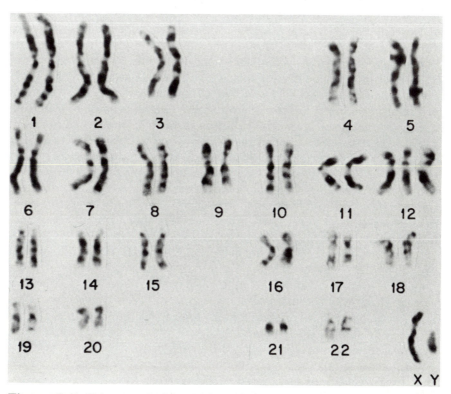

Figure 9–5. Trisomy of chromosome #12 (+12), a rather characteristic karyotypic finding in chronic lymphocytic leukemia and affecting nearly half of the cases studied to-date.

Table 9–4 Median Survival of ANLL Patients According to Karyotypic Status

No. of patients	Karyotypic classification	Median survival (months)
136	NN	7.9
79	AN	5.9
51	AA	2.4

patients whose marrow contains some or totally cytogenetically normal cells (11,15). Table 9–4 shows the general experience in dealing with this parameter of acute leukemia. A similar situation, although less clear-cut, appears also to apply to acute lymphoblastic leukemia (ALL) (16); thus, in acute leukemia the presence or absence of normal cells in the marrow could serve as a useful guide in determining not only the course of the disease but also the appropriate therapy, bone marrow transplantation, and other treatments.

Chronic lymphocytic leukemia (CLL) is a disease that has only recently been successfully studied cytogenetically (17–19). This is primarily because a number of mitogenic agents capable of stimulating the leukemic cells in this leukemia have been introduced in recent years, and these have yielded results reflected in Tables 9–1 to 9–3. In contrast to the acute leukemias and CML, these changes can be readily established on circulating blood cells when these mitogens are used (Fig. 9–5). Generally, the information obtained with bone marrow cells tends to be of a similar nature and, thus, for a number of reasons, blood cells should be preferentially examined. In this leukemia also, the appearance of secondary chromosome changes in addition to the primary one has recently been correlated with a definitely poor prognosis (20); these changes indicate, again, that in general the leukemic process tends to be at its lowest aggressiveness when the cells contain only the primary karyotypic change, with the secondary changes usually resulting in a more aggressive biologic and clinical picture and shortened survival. Often, the latter is due to failure of the cells to respond to previously used therapy or new chemotherapy.

In acute lymphoblastic leukemia, the general experience has been that those conditions associated with translocations appear to have a poorer prognosis (16), primarily due to less-than-optimal response to therapy, than that of ALL which is associated with high chromosome numbers or morphologic changes other than translocations. As indicated above, if it can be assumed that the etiology of these leukemias is reflected in the primary karyotypic changes (3–5), which differ from one condition to another, it would appear that ALL associated with translocations tends to be of a more aggressive nature than ALL associated with other karyotypic anomalies.

CHROMOSOME CHANGES
IN LYMPHOMA

The introduction of a more simplified classification of the lymphomas (21) and of improvements in techniques (22) has already yielded definite correlations between certain types of lymphoma and their specific chromosome changes. The most extensively studied lymphoma has been that of the Burkitt type in which a translocation between chromosomes #8 and #14 (Table 9–5) is commonly observed (Fig. 9–6), although variant translocations involving chromosome #8 with either chromosome #2 or #22 have also been described (Fig. 9–7) (23). In each case the involvement of chromosome #8 at band q24 is present and points to the important role played by this karyotypic event in Burkitt lymphoma. An interesting feature of these translocations is the fact that when chromosome #2 is involved only light chains of the kappa variety are expressed, whereas lambda types are expressed solely when chromosome #22 is involved in the translocation. A translocation identical to that seen in Burkitt lymphoma, i.e. t(8;14), has also been observed in other types of diffuse small and large cell lymphomas (22), although characterization of these lymphomas in relation to the karyotypic changes is still to be accomplished. A common specific translocation is t(14;18), observed in a large number of lymphomas of the follicular variety (22). Whether this change

Table 9–5   Nonrandom Translocations in Lymphoma

t(2;8)(p11–13;q24)	Burkitt lymphoma
t(8;14)(q24;q32)	Burkitt lymphoma
t(8;22)(q24;q11)	Burkitt lymphoma
t(11;14)(q13;q32)	Lymphoma (small cell)
t(12;14)(q13;q32)	Diffuse mixed T-cell lymphoma
t(14;18)(q32; q21)	Lymphoma (follicular)

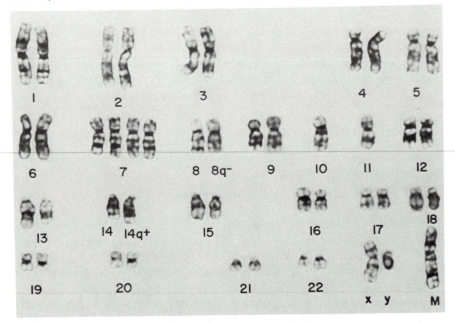

Figure 9–6. A translocation between chromosomes #8 and #14, t(8;14), in Burkitt lymphoma (BL), the involved chromosomes being shown as +8q− and 14q+. This is the most common translocation observed in BL. Secondary chromosome changes were also present in this case, i.e. +7,+7,−10,−11 and a marker (M), the latter involving an X chromosome and chromosome #1. The role played by these secondary karyotypic changes in the biologic and clinical aspects of BL has yet to be established.

characterizes a specific subgroup of these lymphomas will be established once a larger number of cases has been studied. A diffuse small cell lymphoma similar in character to CLL has been found not infrequently to be associated with a t(11;14) (22). Thus, there is little doubt that as more and more cases of lymphoma are studied the disease will be subdivided, akin to the acute leukemias, on a cytogenetic basis into definitive categories, thus bringing this group of diseases into a more defined status than that afforded by immunology and histology alone.

The T-cell lymphomas and their associated leukemias have been less categorically defined cytogenetically (Table 9–6), primarily due to the rather variable karyotypic picture obtained in different laboratories and patients. It is possible that the primary chromosomal change in these conditions is of a nature that cannot be established with presently used methodologies and may have to await some sort of molecular probing which may reveal such a primary event, with the

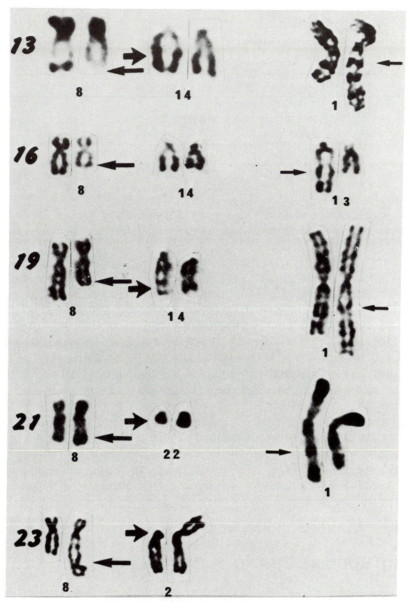

Figure 9–7. The common, t(8;14), and uncommon translocations, t(2;8) and t(8;22), which occur in Burkitt lymphoma or leukemia. Cases 13, 16 and 19 have a t(8;14), whereas case 21 has a t(2;8) and case 23 a t(8;22). In four of the cases secondary changes affecting chromosome #1 (1q+) or #13 (13q+) were seen. The nature of the translocation definitely affects the type of surface immunoglobulins produced by the cells, i.e. when chromosome #2 is involved only kappa light chains are produced, whereas with chromosome #22 involvement only lambda light chains are produced. (Courtesy of Dr. Roland Berger.)

Table 9–6 Nonrandom Morphologic and Numerical Chromosome Changes in Lymphoma

6q−	Lymphoma (diffuse, large cell, noncleaved)
9p−	T-cell lymphoma
11q−	Lymphoma (small cell, lymphocytic)
14q+ (q32)	Lymphoma (diffused?)
+12	Small cell lymphocytic lymphoma

changes described to date being more of a secondary nature. However, several recent reports have clarified to some extent the karyotypic situation in T-cell diseases. Thus, an inversion of segment q11q32 of the long arm of a chromosome #14 has been reported to characterize T-cell CLL (Table 9–2) (24–25). The variable cytogenetic findings seen in the cells of the acute leukemias associated with HTLV may potentially be explained by the incoporation of the retroviral genome into the chromosomes of the affected cells (26), with some specificity of the chromosome in which this material has been inserted recently reported in mice (27). Thus, one could look upon this event as the primary karyotypic change in this acute leukemia, with the subsequent (and observed) variable chromosome changes being secondary in nature (28).

One of the shortcomings in examining lymphomas cytogenetically is that the affected lymph nodes or lymphomatous tumors have to be examined in order to establish the chromosome changes. Often, such tissues are not readily available, and, hence, the number of cases with lymphoma which can be successfully analyzed cytogenetically is fewer than would be desirable.

CHROMOSOME CHANGES IN CANCERS

Although the number of cancers in which chromosome changes of a primary nature have been established is relatively small when compared to the leukemias, advances in recent years, particularly methodologic, are leading to more and more cancers being characterized cytogenetically. In Tables 9–7 to 9–9 are listed the specific chromosome changes observed in various cancers; the list will undoubtedly be enlarged in the near future. Thus, specific chromosome changes have recently been established in such conditions as ovarian

Table 9–7   Nonrandom Translocations Characterizing Cancers

Translocation	Condition
t(3;8)(p25;q21)	Mixed tumor of parotid
t(6;14)(q21;q24)	Serous cystadenocarcinoma of ovary
t(11;22)(q24;q12)	Ewing's sarcoma

Table 9–8   Nonrandom Morphologic Chromosome Changes in Cancer

Chromosome	Condition
1p−	Malignant melanoma
1p−(p31p36)	Neuroblastoma
1p−,i(1q)	Endometrial cancer
1q+	Breast cancer
3p−(p14p23)	Small cell cancer of lung, renal cancer
3q+(q25)	Nasopharyngeal cancer
i(5p)	Bladder cancer
5q−	Cervical cancer
6q−,i(6p)	Malignant melanoma
11p−(p13)	Wilms' tumor
11q−	Cervical cancer
i(12p)	Seminoma, teratoma
12q−(q22a24)	Large bowel cancer
13q−(q14)	Retinoblastoma
22q−	Meningioma

Table 9–9   Nonrandom Numerical Chromosome Changes in Cancer

+7	Bladder cancer, large bowel cancer
+8	Polyps of large bowel
−9	Bladder cancer
+12	Seminoma
−22	Meningioma, sarcoma

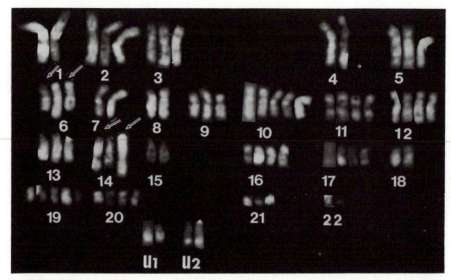

Figure 9–8. Karyotype of a cell from a serous cystadenocarcinoma of the ovary. A translocation, t(6;14), occurring in serous cystadenocarcinoma of the ovary and apparently being the specific (primary) event in this group of cancers is shown in two copies (arrows). A large number of secondary chromosomal changes is present, affecting most of the chromosomes and including two marker chromosomes (U1 and U2) whose origin could not be ascertained.

cancer (Fig. 9–8), malignant melanoma (Fig. 9–9), nasopharyngeal cancer, large bowel cancer, kidney cancer, and others (Fig. 9–10). An important advance has also recently been made in bladder cancer in which at least three separate cytogenetic entities, each constituting a primary chromosome change, appear to exist, possibly indicating etiologic differences underlying each (29). These primary changes consist of an isochromosome for the short arm of chromosome #5, trisomy of chromosome #7, and loss of chromosome #9. The loss of chromosome #9 may be preceded by deletion of the long arm of this chromosome, before it is lost from the cells.

Several reasons account for the primary karyotypic changes in cancers not having been established more readily than in leukemias (1). One important reason is the low mitotic activity of many tumors, with the result that an insufficient number of metaphases is available for analysis; when some sort of long-term tissue culture is resorted to, either the tumor cells do not grow well or they represent a subpopulation of cells with a karyotypic picture not reflecting that of the predominant cells in the primary tumor. Furthermore, cancers often have a large number of complex karyotypic changes, of both a qualitative and quantitative nature, which tend to obscure the primary change. Thus, ideally, tumors with a pseudodiploid (46 chromosomes) or hypodiploid karyotype containing only one karyotypic event are best examined for the establishment of the primary chromosomal change. Once such a change is established, it is then possible to decipher and categorize the secondary changes. Since these secondary changes probably play a crucial role in such parameters as tumor biology, metastatic spread, resistance or sensitivity to therapy, and invasiveness (Table 9–10) (6), it will be the cytogeneticists' task in the future to correlate not only the primary change, but also the secondary changes, with these parameters and attempt to decipher which chromosome or chromosomes affect each of these parameters. Since karyotypic heterogeneity in the same type of cancer has been shown to exist not only in patients with tumors of the same site and

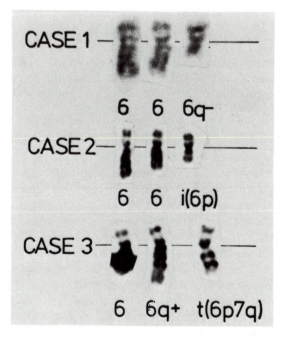

Figure 9–9. This figure shows the primary karyotypic events thought to be characteristic for malignant melanoma with 6q–, a deletion of the long arm of chromosome #6 being the most common. It appears that the primary event in malignant melanoma resides in morphologic changes of the long arm of chromosome #6.

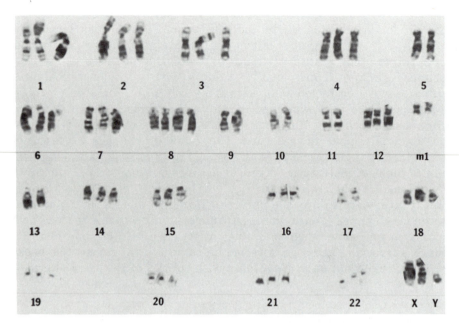

1   2   3   4   5
6   7   8   9   10   11   12   m1
13   14   15   16   17   18
19   20   21   22   X   Y

Figure 9–10. A specific change observed in testicular tumors, either teratomas or seminomas, consisting of an isochromosome of the short arm of chromosome #12, i.e. i(12p). This isochromosome (m1) has been found by us to be present in almost every tumor of the type just mentioned. In addition to the two i(12p) chromosomes, numerical changes affected most of the chromosomes, leading to a hypertetraploid number (76 chromosomes).

histology, but also within a single tumor, such chromosomal heterogeneity may affect the response of cells to various forms of therapy (30). Thus, it can easily be visualized that the preponderant number of cells within a tumor, though karyotypically different, may respond to therapy, whereas a small population of cells with a particular karyotype that endows them with resistance to such therapy may, in fact, become the predominant ones when a tumor is treated with either chemotherapy and/or radiation. Thus, deciphering the relationship of the secondary chromosome changes to the parameters mentioned above will remain an important task of cancer cytogeneticists.

The chromosome number of tumors has been utilized in correlations with such parameters as prognosis and invasiveness. Thus, several papers have appeared in which the chromosome number in bladder cancer has been correlated with these parameters and have shown that the higher the chromosome number (31–33)—and, hence, one must assume, the more complex the karyotypic picture in such a tumor—the worse the prognosis, with more likelihood of recurrence

Table 9–10 Significance of Chromosome Changes in Human Cancer

A. Primary Changes
Specific karyotypic anomalies—possibly related to etiology, location, and activation of oncogenes.

B. Secondary Changes
1. Vary from tumor to tumor (of the same site and histology) and may show considerable heterogeneity within an individual tumor.
2. May play an important role in the biology of cancer cells, e.g. invasiveness, metastatic spread, and sensitivity or resistance to therapy.
3. Probably responsible for much of the phenotypic characteristics and heterogeneity of cancer cells, e.g. biochemical aspects, inappropriate synthesis of hormones and other substances, and overproduction of normal materials.
4. The secondary karyotypic changes may be a selective proliferation of cells already existing in the earliest phases of the cancer, or they may develop *de novo*.
5. The relative heterogeneity of the secondary karyotypic changes may be a reflection of the effects of the hosts' genotypes and/or extraneous factors.

and invasiveness. Similar studies should be performed in other cancers to ascertain whether such a relationship exists.

An interesting phenomenon observed in rare tumors is the presence of either double minutes (DMS) or heterogeneously staining regions (HSR) (1). In the case of acute leukemia it has been established that the presence of DMS appears to be related to a rather poor prognosis (34). In solid tumors these changes, either DMS or HSR, appear to be associated with gene amplification for such enzymes as dihydrofolate reductase and possibly lead to resistance to chemotherapy (1). In a number of studies it has been shown that the DMS probably originate from HSR, since, depending on the experimental conditions, one appears to transform into the other (35).

ONCOGENES AND CHROMOSOME CHANGES

Recent literature has paid much attention to specific chromosome changes observed in various leukemias and cancers and their possible relationship to oncogenes (3–5). The general theory at present holds that certain viruses—which are capable of producing tumors in

Table 9–11   Tenets of Chromosomal Hypothesis of Oncogenesis

1. Each cell contains within it genetic material associated with a specific chromosomal segment and necessary for the proliferative (embryogenic?) activity of the cell, i.e. a proliferative factor (PF).
2. The proliferative factor (PF) is normally suppressed in differentiated cells by a contiguous chromosomal segment "housing" the inhibitory factor (IF). Chromosomal contiguity is required for this inhibition.
3. The chromosomal (and intrachromosomal) location of these factors is unique for each cell type.
4. Chromosomal rearrangements, such as translocations, deletions, or insertions, leading to loss of contiguity between these segments and, hence, removal of inhibition of the proliferative factor (PF) by the inhibitory factor (IF), may result in the expression of proliferative functions as *malignant transformation*. The specific chromosome change is a necessary prerequisite for malignant transformation to become *manifest* but may not be the basic cause of the neoplasia.
5. Conceptually, the proliferative factor (PF) could constitute in its dormant state an entity under the general category of a proto-oncogene, and when active, that of an oncogene.
6. In a like manner, specialized (differentiated) functions (SF) not given to a cell may be suppressed similarly by a suppressing factor (Sup F) and expressed inappropriately when inhibition is removed through chromosomal rearrangements, e.g. inappropriate (ectopic) hormone production by some cancers or leukemias.

appropriate experimental animals—have captured part of DNA present within the normal human genome. It should be stressed that these DNA sequences are present in normal cells and are probably necessary for normal function sometime during the life of the cell and do not express oncogenetic function unless abnormal conditions exist (3). It now appears that chromosome changes, particularly translocations or deletions, may activate such latent oncogenes in the cell, leading to their expression in malignant transformation. As to how such oncogenes are activated and express their oncogenetic potential is a subject that has not been settled, although a number of theories have been advanced (3–5). Whether each human malignancy is associated with an oncogene is an area of much debate, though the present author favors the hypothesis that only a chromosomal change is necessary for malignant transformation to become manifest (Table 9–11) (3); whether the chromosomal segment affected harbors material that can be characterized as an oncogene in a retrovirus may not be an essential parameter. An example of oncogene involvement is that of c-*myc* in Burkitt lymphoma, in which it has been shown that this oncogene is located at band q24 on chromosome #8, the very band that is invariably involved in the translocation associated with Burkitt lymphoma (36). Another oncogene located on the long arm of chromosome #9, c-*abl*, has recently been shown to be translocated to the Ph^1 chromosome in CML and thus has been implicated in the possible genesis of this disease (37). In fact, in those Ph^1 translocations in which chromosome #9 appears not to be involved microscopically, even with the best banding techniques, molecular probing has recently indicated that the c-*abl* is nevertheless translocated to the Ph^1 chromosome (38). If that is true, it is readily apparent that we are now entering a new era of cytogenetics in which DNA probes of one nature or another will be used to define cytogenetic events that at present cannot be visualized in the microscope. Establishing specific chromosome changes in various human cancers and leukemias has a direct bearing on oncogene research, because once the primary karyotypic

Table 9–12   Chromosomal Oncogene Locations That May Be Affected by Primary and/or Secondary Chromosome Changes in Bladder Cancer

Chromosome	Location	Oncogene
1	1p32	c-*Blym*-1
1	1p31.1–p21.1	c-N-*ras*
1	1q11–qter	c-*sk*
2	2q22–q34	c-*fos*
3	3p25	c-*raf*-1
4		c-*raf*-2
5	5q24	c-*fms*
6	6q32–q12	c-K-*ras* 1
6	6q15–qter	c-*myb*
7	7pter–q22	c-*erb* B
8	8q22	c-*mos*
8	8q24	c-*myc*
9	9q34	c-*abl*
11	11pter–15.1	c-H-*ras* 1
12	12pter–p12	c-K-*ras* 2
12	12pter–q14	c-*int*
15	15q25–q26	c-*fes*
17	17p11–q21	c-*erb* A
18		c-*erv* 1
20		c-*src*
22	22q12.3–qter	c-*sis*
X		c-H-*ras* 2

Table 9–13   Classification of Fragile Sites on Human Chromosomes That May Be Related to Translocations or Other Morphologic Karyotypic Changes

Group	Methods of induction	Chromosomal location	Population incidence
1. Folate-sensitive	Thymidylate stress: a. Folate and thymidine deficient medium b. Inhibition of dihydrofolate reductase (methotrexate, aminopterin, etc.) c. Inhibition of thymidylate synthetase (FUdR)	2q11, 2q13, 6p23, 7p11, 8q22, 9p21, 9q32, 10q23, 11q13, 11q23, 1q213, 16p12, 2p11, Xq27	Rare
2. Distamycin A inducible	a. Distamycin A b. Novobiocin c. Bromodeoxyuridine (BrdU)	16q22 17p12	Rare
3. BrdU inducible	BrdU	10q25	2–3%
4. Common or aphidicolin inducible	DNA polymerase alpha inhibition a. Aphidicolin b. Thymidylate stress	2q31, 3p14, 6q26, 7q32 1623, Xp22 Possible: 1p22, 1p32, 1p36, 1q25, 2p13, 2q33, 3p24, 3q27, 5q31, 7p31, 7q22, 8q22, 9q32, 11p13, 14q24, 22q12, Xq22	Very common

This table is based primarily on published data of Sutherland (40) and Glover et al. (41), as well as on private communications from Dr. T. W. Glover.

change is established it may serve as a guide to the molecular biologist for establishing oncogenetic events more accurately than when such changes are not known (Table 9–12). Since, undoubtedly, the secondary chromosomal changes are capable of involving a number of oncogenetic areas (39), the significance of such changes assumes further importance which to date has not been fully explored but will undoubtedly be an important area for further investigation.

Heritable fragile sites in the chromosomes can be brought out by a number of techniques (Table 9–13). There is correlation between some of the chromosomal fragile sites and their involvement in translocations or deletions seen in human neoplasia. However, much has yet to be learned about the exact relationship between the fragile sites, their expression in different cell types, and their correlation with specific karyotypic events in leukemia and cancer.

SUMMARY

Cytogenetic studies in leukemia, lymphoma, and cancer have so far revealed a picture that can be summarized as follows: each human neoplastic entity (or subentities within a disease category) is characterized by a specific chromosomal change which may be translocation, deletion, insertion, or numerical in character, as a result of a basic cause which essentially remains unknown. This primary (specific) chromosome change is necessary for malignant transformation to become manifest. Without such a karyotypic event, the cell will probably not undergo such a transformation. The primary karyotypic event may or may not be accompanied by secondary cytogenetic changes, which may or may not be nonrandom in nature. When the secondary chromosome change or changes are nonrandom they may reflect the primary karyotypic event and/or the basic cause of the disease. Most importantly, once the secondary chromosome changes appear, the leukemia, lymphoma, or cancer tends to assume a biologically more aggressive course, often characterized by karyotypic heterogeneity within a single leukemia or tumor. Such heterogeneity is particularly common in solid tumors and may be due to the fact that such tumors are observed cytogenetically at a much more advanced stage than are the leukemias. The latter are more readily diagnosed early since they produce symptoms and signs at an earlier stage of their biology than do solid tumors. Establishing the primary chromosomal change may be utilized for recognition of oncogenes and similar genetic events, and thus it is of utmost importance to ascertain such a change in as many tumors as is possible. Most importantly, as has been shown in the leukemias, cytogenetics may reveal definite subentities within each disease category characterized by clinical, laboratory, and prognostic features unique to each specific chromosomal change. Undoubtedly, a similar situation will ultimately be observed in various tumors and other cancers.

A few words should be said regarding congenital conditions associated with chromosome changes and predisposition to cancer. A case in point is the development of Wilms' tumor in individuals who are born with a constitutional disorder characterized by deletion of the short arm of chromosome #11 (11p−) or those who develop ocular retinoblastoma with the constitutional disorder of 13q−. It is possible that other constitutional disorders may be associated with development of one type of cancer or another. An interesting feature of these neoplasms that emerges from these studies is the fact that the tumor that develops contains the specific chromosome change characteristic of the leukemia or cancer, whether the individual is constitutionally affected or not. For example, Wilms' tumor has been shown to contain 11p− in individuals with normal karyotypes and 13q− in retinoblastomas under similar conditions. It is interesting to note that renal cell carcinomas often have a change in the short arm of chromosome #3 which has been observed in a family with a 3;8 translocation involving the very same band. Mention has already been made of chromosomal breakage syndromes in which no specific karyotypic event has been established and which are often associated with the development of one type of malignancy or another. In fact, neoplasia is frequent in such states as Bloom's syndrome and ataxia telangiectasia characterized by chromosomal breakage.

The cytogenetic experience in human neoplasia has revealed that in all probability each entity of leukemia/lymphoma or cancer is characterized by a primary karyotypic event, not only specific for each condition but often characterizing subgroups within each entity. This has been particularly true in the acute leukemias, and evidence is now accumulating that a similar situation may hold true for various cancers. For example, we have been able to characterize three primary karyotypic changes in bladder cancer (an isochromosome for the short arm of chromosome #5, trisomy 7, and monosomy 9), possibly indicating that cancers that appear to be homogeneous histologically, biochemically, and clinically may, in fact, consist of several subentities. The specific primary chromosomal change in each condition would indicate a different underlying causation for each of these subentities. Thus, the chromosomal changes can serve as important and crucial criteria in the characterization and classification of various human neoplastic states. In addition, as has been shown in some forms of leukemia, the cytogenetic findings, including primary and secondary, may serve as important criteria for prognosis, since they often tend to define conditions in terms of their resistance or sensitivity to therapy and, thus, survival. The probable relationship of the specific chromosome change to the direct causation of the neoplasia has already been mentioned but remains an extremely complex and elusive area. The information on the primary chromosome changes is also useful in establishing the loci for cancer genes (oncogenes) related to each specific condition. As already mentioned, this field constitutes, at present, a very active and exciting area for clinicians and basic scientists alike.

REFERENCES

1. Sandberg, A. A. *The Chromosomes in Human Cancer and Leukemia*. New York: Elsevier/North-Holland, 1980.

2. German, J. Patterns of neoplasia associated with the chromosome breakage syndromes. In *Chromosome Mutation and Neoplasia*, edited by J. German, pp. 97–134. New York: Alan R. Liss, 1983.

3. Sandberg, A. A. A chromosomal hypothesis of oncogenesis. Cancer Genet. Cytogenet. *8*: 227–285 (1983).

4. Yunis, J. J. The chromosomal basis of human neoplasia. Science *221*: 227–236 (1983).

5. Rowley, J. D. Human oncogene locations and chromosome aberrations. Nature *301*: 290–291 (1983).

6. Sandberg, A. A. Secondary chromosome changes in cancer: Their nature and significance. Science (submitted).

7. The Fourth International Workshop on Chromosomes in Leukemia. A prospective study of acute nonlymphocytic leukemia. Cancer Genet. Cytogenet. *11*: 249–360 (1984).

8. Sandberg, A. A., Abe, S., Kowalczyk, J. R., Zedginidze, A., Takeuchi, J., and Kakati, S. Chromosomes and causation of human cancer and leukemia. L. Cytogenetics of leukemias complicating other diseases. Cancer Genet. Cytogenet. 7: 95–136 (1982).

9. Rowley, J. D., Golomb, H. M., and Vardiman, J. W. Nonrandom chromosome abnormalities in acute leukemia and dysmyelopoietic syndromes in patients with previously treated malignant disease. Blood *58*: 759–767 (1981).

10. Bennett, J. M., Catovsky, D., Daniel, M.-T., Flandrin, G., Galton, D. A. G., Gralnick, H. R., and Sultan, C. Proposals for the classification of the acute leukemias. Br. J. Haematol. *33*: 451–458 (1976).

11. The Second International Workshop on Chromosomes in Leukemia. Cancer Genet. Cytogenet. *2*: 89–113 (1980).

12. Vermaelen, K., Michaux, J.-L., Louwagie, A., and Van Den Berghe, H. Reciprocal translocation t(6;9)(p21;q33): New characteristic chromosome anomaly in myeloid leukemias. Cancer Genet. Cytogenet. *10*: 125–131 (1983).

13. Schwartz, S., Jiji, R., Kerman, S., Meekins, J., and Cohen, M. M. Translocation (6;9)(p23;q34) in acute nonlymphocytic leukemia. Cancer Genet. Cytogenet. *10*: 133–142 (1983).

14. Sandberg, A. A., Morgan, R., McCallister, J. A., Kaiser-McCaw, B., and Hecht,

F. Acute myeloblastic leukemia (AML) with t(6;9)(p23;q34): A specific subgroup of AML? Cancer Genet. Cytogenet. *10*: 139–142 (1983).

15. Sakurai, M., and Sandberg, A. A. Prognosis in acute myeloblastic leukemia: Chromosomal correlation. Blood *41*: 93–104 (1973).

16. Third International Workshop on Chromosomes in Leukemia. Cancer Genet. Cytogenet. *4*: 95–142 (1981).

17. Morita, M., Minowada, J., and Sandberg, A. A. Chromosomes and causation of human cancer and leukemia. XLV. Chromosome patterns in stimulated lymphocytes of chronic lymphocytic leukemia. Cancer Genet. Cytogenet. *3*: 293–306 (1981).

18. Gahrton, G., and Robert, K.-H. Chromosomal aberrations in chronic B-cell lymphocytic leukemia. Cancer Genet. Cytogenet. *6*: 171–181 (1982).

19. Sadamori, N., Han, T., Minowada, J., and Sandberg, A. A. Clinical significance of cytogenetic findings in untreated patients with B-cell chronic lymphocytic leukemia. Cancer Genet. Cytogenet. *11*: 45–51 (1984).

20. Han, T., Ozer, H., Sadamori, N., Emrich, L., Gomez, G. A., Henderson, E. S., Bloom, M. L., and Sandberg, A. A. Prognostic importance of cytogenetic abnormalities in patients with chronic lymphocytic leukemia. N. Engl. J. Med. *310*: 288–292 (1984).

21. The non-Hodgkin's Lymphoma Pathologic Classification Project. National Cancer Institute sponsored study of classifications of non-Hodgkin's lymphomas: Summary and description of a working formulation for clinical usage. Cancer *49*: 2112–2135 (1982).

22. Yunis, J. J., Oken, M. M., Kaplan, M. E., Ensrud, K. M., Howe, R. R., and Theologides, A. Distinctive chromosomal abnormalities in histologic subtypes of non-Hodgkin's lymphoma. N. Engl. J. Med. *307*: 1231–1236 (1982).

23. Sandberg, A. A. Chromosomes in Human Neoplasia. In *Current Problems in Cancer*, Vol. 8, No. 2, pp. 1–52. Chicago: Year Book Medical, 1983.

24. Zech, L., Gahrton, G., Hammarström, L., Juliusson, G., Mellstedt, H., Robert, K. H., and Smith, C. I. E. Inversion of chromosome 14 marks human T-cell chronic lymphocytic leukaemia. Nature *308*: 858–860 (1984).

25. Ueshima, Y., Rowley, J. D., Variakojis, D., Winter, J., and Gordon, L. Cytogenetic studies on patients with chronic T cell leukemia/lymphoma. Blood *63*: 1028–1038 (1984).

26. Corcoran, L. M., Adams, J. M., Dunn, A. R., and Cory, S. Murine T lymphomas in which the cellular *myc* oncogene has been activated by retroviral insertion. Cell *37*: 113–122 (1984).

27. Cuypers, H. Theo, Selten, G., Quint, W., Zijlstra, M., Maandag, E. R., Boelens, W., van Wezenbeek, P., Melief, C., and Berns, A. Murine leukemia virus-induced T-cell lymphomagenesis: Integration of proviruses in a distinct chromosomal region. Cell *37*: 141–150 (1984).

28. Sandberg, A. A. Chromosomal changes and cancer causation: Chromatin's re-awakening. In *Accomplishments in Cancer Research*, edited by J. G. Fortner and J. E. Rhoads, pp. 157–169. Philadelphia: J. B. Lippincott, 1984.

29. Gibas, Z., Prout, G. R., Jr., Connolly, J. G., Pontes, J. E., and Sandberg, A. A. Non-random chromosomal changes in transitional cell carcinoma of the bladder. Cancer Res. *44*: 1257–1264 (1984).

30. Sandberg, A. A. Chromosomal changes in human cancer: Specificity and heterogeneity. In *Tumor Cell Heterogeneity: Origins and Implications*, edited by A. H. Owens, Jr., D. S. Coffey and S. B. Baylin, Vol. 4, pp. 367–397. New York: Academic Press, 1982.

31. Granberg-Ohman, I., Tribukait, B., and Wijkstrom, H. Cytogenetic analysis of 62 transitional cell bladder carcinomas. Cancer Genet. Cytogenet. *11*: 68–85 (1984).

32. Summers, J. L., Coon, J. S., Ward, R. M., Falor, W. H., Miller, A., III, and Weinstein, R. S. Prognosis in carcinoma of the urinary bladder based upon tissue ABH and T antigen status and karyotype of the initial tumor. Cancer Res. *43*: 934–939 (1983).

33. Sandberg, A. A. Chromosomes in bladder cancer. In *AUA Monographs*, edited by W. W. Bonney and G. R. Prout, Jr., Vol. 1, pp. 81–94. Baltimore: Williams and Wilkins, 1982.

34. Marinello, M. J., Bloom, M. L., Doeblin, T. D., and Sandberg, A. A. Double minute chromosomes in human leukemia. N. Engl. J. Med. *303*: 704 (1980).

35. Barker, P. E. Double minutes in human tumor cells. Cancer Genet. Cytogenet. *5*: 81–94 (1982).

36. Croce, C. M., Thierfelder, W., Erikson, J., Nishikura, K., Finan, J., Lenoir, G. M., and Nowell, P. C. Transcriptional activation of an unrearranged and untranslocated c-*myc* oncogene by translocation of a Cλ locus in Burkitt lymphoma cells. Proc. Natl. Acad. Sci., USA, *80*: 6922–6926 (1983).

37. de Klein, A., van Kessel, A. G., Grosveld, G., Bartram, C. R., Hagemeijer, A., Bootsma, D., Spurr, N. K., Heisterkamp, N., Groffen, J., and Stephenson, J. R. A cellular oncogene is translocated to the Philadelphia chromosome in chronic myelocytic leukaemia. Nature *300*: 765–767 (1982).

38. Hagemeijer, A., Bartram, C. R., Smit, E. M. E., van Agthoven, A. J., Bootsma, D. Is the chromosomal region 9q34 always involved in variants of the Ph[1] translocation? Cancer Genet. Cytogenet. 5(2): 95–107 (1985).

39. Slamon, D. J., deKernion, J. B., Verma, I. M., and Cline, M. J. Expression of cellular oncogenes in human malignancies. Science *224*: 256–262 (1984).

40. Sutherland, G. R. Heritable fragile sites on human chromosomes. II. Distribution, phenotypic effects and cytogenetics. Am. J. Human Genet. *31*: 136–148 (1979).

41. Glover, T. W., Bergen, C., Coyle, A., and Echo, B.: DNA polymerase α inhibition of an aphidicolin induces gaps and breaks at common fragile sites in human chromosomes. Hum. Genet. (in press).

10

Radioimmunodetection of Cancer and Potential for Therapy

Frank H. DeLand, M.D.,
& David M. Goldenberg, D.Sc., M.D.

Ninety years ago the first attempt to use antibodies raised against malignant tissue was reported by Hericourt and Richet (16). In animals, they prepared antisera against human osteogenic sarcoma and reported that these sera were effective in ameliorating two different carcinomata, a fibrosarcoma and a gastric cancer. In a subsequent publication they reported that in 50 cases treated similarly excellent results were obtained, whereas the results from the administration of normal serum were negative (17). A number of subsequent investigators were unable to demonstrate positive results consistently, possibly for the following reasons: (a) the sera did not contain antibodies that would react with the tumor tissue; (b) the sera contained nonspecific antibodies that were completely bound by other tissues; (c) because of the histological architecture of the tumor, the antibodies were unable to interface with the tumor antigens; and (d) the antibodies did not demonstrate an observable affect even though they may have localized within the tumor. As a result of these hypotheses, a number of investigations were performed to elucidate and evaluate the problems and to develop methodologies to overcome the observed inconsistencies. By labeling antibodies with a radionuclide, Korngold and Pressman demonstrated that antibodies prepared in laboratory animals against specific animal tumors did contain the antibodies that were sequestered in tumors (19). In 1958 Pressman and colleagues showed that antibodies labeled with radioactive iodine could be used in animals on a diagnostic basis, and that the localization of the antibodies in tumor could be defined by means of radionuclide scanning (29). Later, Bale and others demonstrated that tumor-localizing antibodies could be used as a therapeutic measure for treating experimental neoplasms by radioactivity (2).

Pressman and Korngold demonstrated that globulins obtained from normal sera were sequestered in different organs when components to these organs were used as specific absorbents (28). In more recent studies it has been shown that certain immunoglobulins will react with tumor-associated products such as carcinoembryonic antigen (CEA) and prostatic acid phosphotase (PAP), if these globulins have been isolated from normal human serum (26,31). Earlier, Goldenberg et al. initiated localization studies for human colorectal cancer (GW-39 tumor) in an animal model (12,13). Antibodies to CEA were prepared by hyperimmunization of goats and dually labeled to determine tumor-specific accretion as described by the paired-label method of Pressman et al. (29). In hamsters, highly specific tumor localization of antibodies to CEA was achieved, and it was observed that the concentration of the radiolabeled antibody in the tumor compared with that in the nontumor areas increased with time following injection (33). Subsequently, it was demonstrated that CEA-containing tumors could be detected and imaged by scintigraphic techniques following the administration of the radiolabeled antibody to CEA (14). To overcome some of the deficiencies as noted by Pressman (32), affinity purification of antibodies was used, and this procedure resulted in a three- to fourfold improvement in tumor localization (34). Although the purification of antibodies to CEA by affinity columns did demonstrate improved tumor localization in laboratory animals, the role of circulating antigen was at this point unknown since it was possible that the plasma CEA antigen would bind the administered antibody in humans (in contrast to tumor-bearing laboratory animals, where there are very low levels of circulating CEA). This problem of neutralization of administered radiolabeled antibodies was of paramount importance, particularly in view of the disappointing studies reported by other investigators (21,37).

CLINICAL STUDIES

The first investigations undertaken by our group were with antibodies prepared against carcinoembryonic antigen. In brief, the preparation of the CEA antibody was as follows: Hyperimmune goat IgG was prepared against CEA purified from a hepatic metastasis of a colonic adenocarcinoma. The antibody was purified by successive steps of affinity chromatography and determined to have an immunoreactivity level of approximately 70% with CEA and 11% with colon carcinoma antigen-111. The final titer of the antibody as measured by radioassay was 2×10^6, and this titer did not change after radiolabeling by the chloramine-T method. The specific activity of the IgG labeled with I-131 was demonstrated to be 5–10 Ci/g of IgG protein, and this represents approximately 1 atom of I-131 per molecule of IgG. By means of Sephadex G-200 (Pharmacea Fine Chemicals, Inc., Piscataway, N.J.) column chromatography, it was ascertained that 90–95% of the radioactivity chromatographed with IgG.

For patient examinations, 2–3 mCi of I-131–labeled antibody to CEA (2–3 µg/kg body weight) was administered intravenously. Prior to administration of the labeled antibody, each patient was tested for hypersensitivity to goat IgG by means of intradermal injection of the antibody to be used. To reduce the sequestration of free I-131 by the thyroid gland, Lugol's solution was administered orally beginning 1 day prior to the administration of the labeled antibody and continued for 7 days thereafter. In later studies perchlorate was administered prior to the labeled antibody to block secretion of radioactivity in the stomach and to augment the inhibition of sequestration of radioactivity in the thyroid gland.

A standard imaging protocol was established for two purposes: (a) to ensure that all areas of the body would be imaged and prevent omissions of regions later found to be pertinent by other diagnostic methods, and (b) to prevent any suggestions of the sites under investigation to the physician responsible for interpreting the images. The standard images obtained on each patient were anterior and posterior projections of the chest, and anterior posterior and lateral projections of the abdomen and pelvis. Studies were made routinely at 24 and 48 h following administration of the radioactive antibody preparation by gamma camera imaging. Based on data accumulated in the animal studies, it was hypothesized that the concentration of radioactivity in the target compared to that of the adjacent nontarget tissues would probably be inadequate for definition, and that some type of procedure would be required to minimize nontarget radioactivity. Thus, to increase the T/NT ratio, approximately 0.5 mCi of radioactive pertechnetate and Tc-99m–labeled human serum albumin are administered intravenously just prior to imaging at 24 and 48 h. These two radiotracers are used to simulate the nontarget distribution of radioactivity in the intra- and extravascular spaces, and Tc-99m has a gamma photon that is readily separable from that of iodine-131. The images are acquired with two pulse-height analyzers, one at 364 keV

Table 10–1 CEA Radioimmunodetection in Patients

Cancer	No. of cases	Primary site	Secondary site	Total	Percent
Colorectal	51	10/12	49/53	59/65	91
Ovarian	19	10/10	11/14	21/24	88
Lung	30	18/25	5/8	23/33	70
Pan-creatic	6	3/6	1/2	4/8	50
Mammary	6	2/5	7/9	9/14	64
Cervical	15	6/8	13/13	19/21	90
Other uterine	9	5/6	9/10	14/16	88
Total	136	54/72	95/109	149/181	82

for I-131 and the other at 140 keV for Tc-99m. After acquisition of the data and storage in the computer, the counts in the two images are equalized. The area used for equalization depends on the particular images in question, but generally a background area is chosen for this purpose. In addition we have used specific tracers to enhance the T/NT ratios. For example, when evaluating the liver for abnormal foci of increased I-131 activity, 1 mCi of Tc-99m sulfur colloid is administered. After collection of the I-131 and Tc-99m images, the liver is outlined as a region of interest, extracted from the two images, and all data outside of the liver are discarded. The level of activity of the Tc-99m and I-131 is normalized and the technetium counts subtracted from the iodine counts, pixel by pixel. Based on previous work, abnormal concentration of the I-131 is then highlighted since the T/NT ratio is increased by an average of about 5 or 6 to 1 (5).

Table 10–1 summarizes the results from examination of 136 patients with known carcinoma of a type that produces carcinoembryonic antigen. The overall group sensitivity of this procedure is 82%. For the group of tumors that include colorectal, ovarian, cervical, and other uterine cancers, the percentage of accuracy is 90%. The detection rate for this group is greater because the sites are easier to differentiate from nontarget radioactivity accumulations. On the other hand, the detection for lung, breast, and pancreas ranges from 50–70%. The reasons for these lower sensitivity rates are the interfering nontarget activity of the heart and large vessels with respect to lung cancer, the relatively high nontarget background when attempting to define primary mammary cancer, and the radioactivity in the vasculature of the upper midabdomen and secretion of iodine into the stomach when attempting to define pancreatic cancer. The problem of interfering radioactivity is related to the method of imaging: namely, the two-dimensional planar type. If these images are obtained in three-dimensions—i.e. single-proton-emission computerized tomography—then the detection rate will be higher, for two reasons: first, with emission tomography, the target-to-nontarget ratio required is approximately 2 to 1, compared to planar imaging where 6–8 to 1 is needed; second, the problem of overlying nontarget radioactivity is to a great extent solved by the separation in a tomographic plane. In a recent paper Berche and his group reported an appreciable increase in detection rate with tomography (94%) as compared to the rate in the same patients by two-dimensional planar imaging (43%) (3). By means of the previously described computer manipulation of data, the role of CEA-RAID in the detection of liver metastasis has been very encouraging. In a recent study, a retrospective evaluation in 29 patients with confirmed liver metastases, 97% of the cases were detected by the antibody method, compared with 85% by the sulfur colloid nuclear-medicine-type studies, 79% by ultrasound, and 75% by computerized tomography. It must be noted, however, that there were only 8 computerized tomography studies available for this group of 29 patients. In more recent work that has not been published we found that computerized tomography had an accuracy of 50% or less in the early detection of liver metastasis.

In view of previous experience with the sequestration of nonspecific protein molecules by tumor deposits, the question of whether or not the localization of the CEA antibody labeled with a radionuclide is a specific antibody–antigen type of reaction or is a nonspecific accumulation of a large immunoglobulin becomes of prime importance. Primus et al. examined the molecular size of the eluted radioactivity from surgical tissues by immunochemical methods, and they found that the size range of the radiolabeled molecule was larger than that of normal IgG or carcinoembryonic antigen. They concluded that this was probably due to an antibody–antigen complex (35). By means of the paired-label method, Mach et al. observed a selective concentration of antibody to radiolabeled CEA, exceeding that of normal goat radiolabeled IgG, in colorectal tumors (22).

From the immunological standpoint, the use of radiolabeled antibodies for the detection of a specific tissue such as neoplasms should have a very high level of specificity. In an analysis of 116 non-neoplastic diseases in 142 patients with cancer, only two sites

Table 10–2   AFP Radioimmunodetection in Patient Studies

Cancer	No. of cases	Serum AFP range (ng/ml)	RAID results		
			True positive[a]	False-positive	False negative
Embryo-nal	6	3.7–15,000	15/15	1	1
Hepato-cellular	5	2.5–270,000	5/5	1	0
Seminoma	3		1/5	0	4
Ovary[b]	3	0–18,000	3/3	0	0
Lung	4	2.4–8.4	2/6	0	4

[a]Total known sites of cancer substantiated by other diagnostic finding.

[b]Endodermal sinus tumor (1), Sertoli-Leydig cell tumor (1), and cystadenocarcinoma (1).

demonstrated an abnormal accumulation of radioactivity. One of these sites was an empyema and the other a diverticulosis (15). Of over 350 patients studied by us with antibodies to carcinoembryonic antigen, at least 20 have been performed with affinity-purified goat polyclonal $F(ab^1)_2$ or murine monoclonal antibodies to CEA. Although the latter two studies are not large in number, no significant difference has been observed in the detection of tumors with any one of the three forms of antibodies.

Fifty patients have been studied with antibodies to alpha-fetoprotein (AFP), both goat polyclonal IgG and mouse monoclonal IgG. Table 10–2 summarizes the results in a study of 21 patients. The overall true-positive rate of detection by this method was 74%, and the false-positive rate was 6%. Elevated levels of AFP are found particularly in hepatocellular carcinoma, embryonal carcinoma and teratomas of the testis, and certain ovarian tumors. Elevations are also seen, but not as dramatic, in cancers of the pancreas, colon, lung, and stomach and in other non-neoplastic diseases such as cirrhosis and hepatitis. In this group of patients (Table 10–2), if just those patients with tumors that synthesize and secrete AFP to any appreciable extent are considered, then the true-positive rate is 96% and the false-positive rate is 8%. This group of patients would include those with embryonal carcinoma of the testis, hepatocellular carcinoma, and ovarian carcinomas. The other two tumors reported here, seminomas and pulmonary, demonstrated a very low detection rate of only 27%. At this time it is not possible to assess whether the detection of tumors not usually associated with the production of AFP were true-positive findings and that these tumors may produce AFP, or whether the antibody used was not sufficiently specific since a large number of these studies were obtained with non-affinity-purified antibody. An important point to be made is that the level of serum AFP has essentially no adverse effect on the detection of the specific tumors with antibodies to AFP. For example, in Table 10-2 the level of serum AFP ranged from 0–270,000 ng/ml in the group of patients with embryonal carcinoma, hepatocellular carcinoma, and ovarian carcinoma, yet in this group there was only one false-negative finding. The lack of influence of the circulating antigen on the ability to detect tumors with radiolabeled antibodies has been observed in the studies with CEA, AFP, hCG, and PAP. This has been a particularly important observation, and a fortunate one. It was of appreciable concern, when the antibody studies were first initiated, that increased levels of circulating antigen would be inversely related to the ability to detect tumors by the radioimmunological method of *in vivo* imaging.

We have studied 60 patients with antibody to hCG of the goat polyclonal type. Table 10–3 summarizes our results in patients with 28 known sites of tumor, and hCG antibody studies by the RAID techniques identified 23 (82%). In those testicular tumors that have demonstrated the highest rate of detection by radioimmunoassay, i.e. embryonal carcinoma, teratocarcinoma, choriocarcinoma, and mixtures, the detection rate by *in vivo* imaging was 100%. In this group, one case—the germ cell tumor of the mediastinum—presented a very interesting problem. This young man was referred for an antibody study because of a mediastinal mass that was biopsied, but a definitive diagnosis could not be made. Concentration of I-131–labeled antibodies to hCG was observed by gamma camera imaging in the mediastinal tumor at 48 h followng i.v. administration of the antibody. The final histologic diagnosis at autopsy confirmed that this was a germ cell tumor. Of the testicular cancer patients studied by this modality, four were identified by RAID when other detection methods were negative. As with CEA and AFP, the serum level of hCG had no relationship to the ability to detect the tumors *in vivo*.

During these *in vivo* studies for the detection of cancer by means of radiolabeled antibodies, a number of patients had been referred because there was a high index of suspicion of cancer presence, particularly on the basis of a rising titer of one of the markers.

Table 10–3 hCG Radioimmunodetection in Patient Studies

Cancer	No. of cases	Serum hCG ng/ml	RAID results True-positive[a]	False-positive	False-negative
Embryo-nal cell	6	0.5–140	7	0	0
Seminoma	3	0.4–400	2	0	1
Embryo-nal + teratoma	2	5.1–3,300	4	0	0
Embryo-nal + chorio-carci-noma	2	0.5–1,721	2	0	0
Hydati-form mole	3		2	0	0
Ovary[b]	4		2	0	2
Germ cell[c]	2	2	0	0	
Lung	3	NA	2	0	2

[a]Total known sites of cancer substantiated by other diagnostic findings.
[b]Mucinous cystadenocarcinoma (1), cystic teratoma (1), and hemorrhagic cyst (1).
[c]Retroperitoneum (1) and mediastinum (1).

These patients had been evaluated extensively with many modalities of diagnostic procedures, but the site of the tumor could not be ascertained. In a series of 51 patients with colorectal carcinoma, 11 had been referred because the primary, recurrent, and/or metastatic sites could not be identified by other means. In each patient the primary tumor had been previously resected. The serum CEA levels varied from 9 to 5,500 ng/ml. In these 11 patients, the tumor was identified by the CEA RAID study, and the locations varied from the region of the original primary resection to the adjacent abdomen, pelvis, and/or liver. In all instances the diagnosis of the tumors was confirmed by other procedures. The time between the identification by RAID and subsequent confirmation varied from less than 1 week to as long as 40 weeks. Occult tumors were also detected in four patients with hCG antibodies labeled with I-131, as already discussed. In these patients the serum hCG levels ranged from 5.1 to 1,721 ng/ml. Extensive evaluations by other diagnostic modalities had been negative. The time between the identification by the RAID studies and subsequent confirmation by other procedures varied from less than 1 week to over 52 weeks. In the patient that was not diagnosed by another modality for over 52 weeks, a testicular carcinoma metastatic to the base of the right lung was found. In the hCG study the tumor was readily identified, but it required 1 year before this tumor was visible by chest radiography. It has also been our experience that it has been possible to identify recurrent or metastatic tumors, particularly in the liver, that were still not visible or palpable by direct surgical observation. In two cases, when the RAID studies indicated hepatic metastasis, multiple biopsies obtained at the first laparotomy were negative. However, a subsequent laparotomy following additional RAID studies did demonstrate the metastatic lesions. In another series of 12 patients with known or suspected hepatic metastases at the time when the diagnoses of the hepatic lesions were made by a RAID study, transmission computerized tomography was positive in only 3 and eventually became positive in 6. Of these 12 patients, 8 were absolutely confirmed, and in 3 the diagnosis was of high probability. The information gained from these RAID studies of not otherwise clinically detectable carcinoma underlines the high sensitivity of the method.

One of our more recent clinical studies has involved the use of colon-specific antigen-protein (CSAp) antibodies for the detection of colorectal carcinoma. CSAp is an antigen distinct from that of CEA and other colorectal cancer markers that have been studied and has been found to be quantitatively increased in the serum of certain colorectal cancer patients (25). As with antibodies to carcinoembryonic antigen, CSAp antibodies labeled with I-131 have also demonstrated primary and metastatic colorectal carcinoma by means of external scintillation imaging. It has been possible to image the same patients with antibodies to both CEA and CSAp. The results demonstrate that in the same patient the findings corroborate and complement each other, and it appears that one antibody may reveal some tumor sites that are missed by the other. Although we have not had the opportunity to administer antibodies to CEA and CSAp simultaneously in patients, this has been done in laboratory animals. The sequestration of radioactivity in a GW-39 tumor implanted in an animal was increased with a mixture of CSAp and CEA antibody when compared to either antibody alone. This concept of cocktails of antibodies has been put forward by a number of investigators;

however, this is the first instance in our experience where the addition of a second antibody has improved the target-to-nontarget activity.

The application of radiolabeled antibodies for lymphoscintigraphy is a logical advancement following the evidence that antibodies labeled with a radiotracer will concentrate in tumors and be defined by expernal imaging. Although lymphoscintigraphy was introduced over thirty years ago with a radiotracer-labeled colloid and extensive investigations in clinical evaluations for the detection of cancer in lymph nodes have been reported by Ege, there are many unanswered questions about the sequestration and residence time of radiocolloids within lymph nodes (6–8). The basis for a colloid type of lymphoscintigraphy is the phagocytic activities of the reticuloendothelial cells, although in some patients the phagocytosis does not appear to be appreciably functional. This variation in phagocytic function suggests that cellular changes have occurred in these lymph nodes, yet the only obvious change has been the filtration of products from tumors through the nodes that are in the regional drainage area. Laboratory experiments have demonstrated that phagocytosis of colloids can be inhibited if there is a transplanted tumor within that drainage area (4). In a series of patients with carcinoma of the breast, the lymphatic drainage from the breast following subcutaneous injection of radiolabeled sulfur colloid around the areola demonstrated no sequestration of radioactivity in 13, and no nodal metastases were found in 5 of these studies. In one patient without evidence of nodal sequestration of the radiocolloid, phagocytosis was reestablished once the primary tumor had been removed (4). Similar phenomena have been observed in experimental animals (1). Extensive investigations have been reported on the reaction of lymph nodes to the presence of tumors, and the results have been quite variable, some showing sinus histiocytosis, others follicular hyperlasia, and in some instances a combination of both. The question is whether or not the regional lymph nodes that drain a site of carcinoma demonstrate any immunologic competence or response (9). Although the results of many experiments support the concept of immunologic competence in the regional lymph nodes of patients with cancer, the marked variation in patient response to cancer probably nullifies any simplistic interpretation. Instead, the immunologic interrelationship of lymph nodes and tumor is complex, and our findings with radiotracer antibody lymphoscintigraphy reinforce this impression.

Lymphoscintigraphy with radiolabeled antibodies to tumor-associated antigens is performed in a similar manner to that with the radiotracer-labeled colloids. Approximately 250 μCi of the radiolabeled antibody is injected subcutaneously or in a fascial layer, depending on the drainage of the lymph node group in question. Since the radiolabeled antibodies are channeled into the lymphatics and subsequently into the regional draining lymph nodes, the concentration of the antibody is much higher than in the blood after intravenous injection. The high concentration of antibody plus the much slower mobility through the lymphatic system provides an environment for an optimal interaction between antibodies and antigens. Since the sequestration of the labeled antibody by the cellular components of the lymph nodes occurs before absorption into the general circulation, subtraction techniques are not usually required.

In a series of 50 patients with carcinomata of various types, 42 examinations were performed with I-131–labeled antibody to CEA and 8 with I-131–labeled normal IgG (goat). These included patients with cancer of the rectosigmoid (11), cancer of the breast (12), genitourinary cancer (14), other gastrointestinal cancers (5), pulmonary cancer (5), and vulvar cancer (3). After injection of radiolabeled antibody between the webs of the fingers and toes, images were obtained over the inguinal and axillary areas at 24 and 28 h. In every instance where there was metastatic carcinoma in the lymph nodes, sequestration of the radiolabeled antibody was demonstrated by imaging. However, in the case of tumors of the breast, gastrointestinal tract, genitourinary tract, and vulva, sequestration of antibody was also observed in nodes without evidence of metastatic carcinoma. In the case of the GI and GU tumors, the presence of radiolabeled tracers in the regional lymph nodes was closely related to the site of the tumor or resected tumor. Subsequent information was obtained in 2 of these patients; a recurrence in the area of the primary resection was demonstrated, and the lymph nodes were in the drainage pathway of the recurrence. In the carcinomas of the vulva, however, there was sequestration of radiolabeled antibody, on both the ipsilateral and the contralateral sides of the tumor, in many lymph nodes without evidence of metastatic tumor. Analysis of these lymph nodes, however, did demonstrate elevated levels of tumor antigen within the nodes, and it must be assumed that there was an antibody–antigen reaction within these nodes accounting for the detection of the radiolabeled antibody. In 2 patients with carcinoma of the cervix, both stage I, injection of radiolabeled antibody to CEA into the cuff of the cervix demonstrated indentifiable uptake of radiolabeled antibody by imaging in one patient and none in the other. Analysis of the pelvic lymph nodes from both patients indicated that there were appreciably increased levels of CEA in the patient that demonstrated sequestration of the labeled antibody and very low levels of CEA in the patient that did not.

These findings, along with those from the investigations of tracer-labeled colloids, present a rather complex picture. On the other hand, an understanding of the underlying mechanisms may contribute basic information that will influence the approach to diagnosis and therapy. It would appear that antigen secreted by a tumor is sequestered in the regional draining lymph nodes. This phenomenon was clearly demonstrated by Potamski et al. (27). The possible value of lymphoscintigraphy with radiolabeled antibodies was also suggested recently by Weinstein et al. (38). They felt that the potential advantages of the lymphatic route for the administration of radiolabeled antibodies to tumor antigens were: (a) the ability to detect less than 1 mg of cells as opposed to the hundreds of milligrams typically imaged by the intravenous route; (b) the quantity of labeled antibody required for visualization was appreciably less than that for the i.v. route; (c) the selective delivery to the lymphatic compartment dramatically reduced background interference and nonspecific interactions of the antibody; and (d) the probability that unwanted side effects such as deposition of immune complexes in the kidney would be minimized or eliminated.

Preliminary observations suggest that important information can be obtained by radiolabeled-antibody lymphoscintigraphy applicable to diagnosis, the design of therapy, and subsequent evaluation of patients with carcinoma. For example, Gitsch et al. have shown the advantages of colloid lymphoscintigraphy used as landmarks of axillary nodes during modified radical mastectomies for carcinoma of the breast (11). The greater sensitivity for demonstrating lymph nodes by means of radiolabeled-antibody lymphoscintigraphy would improve this procedure. Another example of the use of radiolabeled antibodies for lymphoscintigraphy would be an evaluation of the internal mammary lymph node chain in patients with carcinoma of the breast. From studies obtained about two months following surgery for carcinoma of the breast it should be possible to determine whether lymph node sequestration of antibodies prior to surgery was still present. If this were the case then the probability of the sequestration being due to metastasis rather than just antigen sequestration is increased. There are many other similar types of situations where presurgery and postsurgery antibody lymphoscintigraphy should contribute to diagnosis and therapy.

The development of monoclonal antibodies by Köhlar and Milstein added a new dimension in radioimmunodetection of tumor by means of tumor-associated antigens or products (18). Monoclonal antibodies offer certain advantages over those antibodies produced by conventional methods in animals, but they are also accompanied by disadvantages. Certainly the mode of producing the antibodies from a specific antigen leads to high specificity for that antigen. The advantages of antibody production, ease of purification, and the reproducibility of the purified preparation certainly is greater than that achievable with conventional antisera. From an investigative standpoint monoclonal antibodies will certainly facilitate the identification of specific cellular antigens. These latter two characteristics should contribute to the selection of the monoclonal antibody or antibodies that will provide the highest possibility of antigen–antibody reaction *in vivo* and will also provide the opportunity of engineering mixtures of monoclonal antibodies for the highest tumor sequestration. Some of these theoretical advantages, however, have not materialized at this time. In three monoclonal antibodies to carcinoembryonic antigen (obtained from the GW-39 tumor) Primus found that the individual monoclonal antibodies or the combination of the three monoclonal antibodies did not demonstrate a greater tumor-to-nontumor sequestration than the conventional antibody to CEA produced in goats (36). From the qualitative imaging standpoint, Strauss noted that there seemed to be no difference in the identification of myocardial necrosis with antibodies to myocin, whether they were monoclonal or of the conventional type (personal communication). A major advantage of monoclonal antibody production over that of conventional antibody production is the lack of extensive purification required to obtain a high specificity of the particular antibody. Also, the laboratory mechanics of producing monoclonal antibodies is certainly more desirable than having to use small laboratory animals or larger animals such as goats for immunization. An important theoretical disadvantage of a monoclonal antibody is that the localizing efficiency may be limited if there is a difference in the epitope expression between the primary and the metastatic tumor, which would not be as likely with the conventionally produced antibodies. A disadvantage that we have experienced with monoclonal antibodies has been the increased number of patients demonstrating sensitivity to the antibody and the more rapid development of antibodies to the IgG following administration of the monoclonal antibodies. In repeated doses of the same conventionally produced CEA antibody administered three to four times, no reaction has been observed. In several patients large doses of I-131–labeled antibody (25–70 mCi, 2.5–7.0 mg protein) have been administered repeatedly two or three times without evidence of hypersensitivity or anaphylactic type reaction, except in one instance.

The role of monoclonal antibodies for the detection of tumors *in vivo* by means of external scintillation imaging is still to be defined. Many of the parameters involved in the antigen–antibody reactions of monoclonal sources require further investigation. One characteristic of the radiolabeled monoclonal antibody reported by Ghose et al. and by other authors is the more rapid rate of clearance from the circulation compared to the polyclonal antibody (10). This clearance does enhance tumor images since it should improve the target-to-nontarget ratios. In another study, however, Mach et al. found that the images and tumor uptake obtained with monoclonal antibodies and polyclonal antibodies against CEA were essentially similar (23).

The use of radiolabeled antibodies to cancer-associated antigens for cancer detection poses the question of their application to therapy. The concept is very attractive. The problems associated with the therapeutic approach to cancer with specific immunoglobulins labeled with radioactive elements have been alluded to, namely the target-to-nontarget concentration of the agent. Order et al. have pioneered in the application of I-131–labeled antibodies to ferretin and CEA for tumor therapy (24). In 7 patients with melanoma, Larson et al. (20) administered 12 therapeutic doses of antimelanoma (monoclonal) fragments labeled with I-131 (34–197 mCi). Side effects to the radiation appeared to be mild; however, after multiple administrations, isotype-specific immunity was observed in 3 patients. By their dosimetry estimates, a tumor dose of 1,040 rads per 100 mCi of I-131 administered was obtained. At the time of this report, 6 of the 7 patients had died.

We have treated 12 patients with I-131–labeled specific antibodies to the type of tumor. One patient has received five therapeutic doses, three from the same batch of polyclonal antibodies produced in goats, without evidence of adverse reaction. Although we have not obtained a total obliteration of the tumors, arrest in the growth of the lesions has been observed in two patients. At this time it is not possible to define the role of radiolabeled antibodies in the therapy of cancer since advances in the types of antibodies and the radioactive labels used will be forthcoming.

The application of tumor-associated antibodies labeled with radionuclides for cancer detection and therapy is still at a very early stage. Improvements in the type of antibodies can be expected; however, it is still too early to conclude whether polyclonal or monoclonal antibodies will be the most advantageous from the standpoint of localization. For example, the higher specificity of monoclonal antibodies may be appreciably less efficient than that of polyclonal antibodies. It may require mixtures of monoclonal antibodies to obtain the most advantageous target-to-nontarget ratios. Radionuclides with energies more compatible with current imaging equipment are needed. Appreciable effort has been expended on this problem, but at present this goal has not been sufficiently successful to warrant replacement of I-131 as the major label. Undoubtedly a suitable label for the antibodies will be developed that permits the use of collimation for higher resulution (e.g. In-111). A major advance in the definition of tumors by radioimmunodetection is the introduction of emission-computed tomography. Although this approach may diminish the need for subtraction techniques, the major advantage is the three-dimensional demonstration of the distribution of radioactivity, thus overcoming the problem of obscuration of information with a two-dimensional format.

The application of radionuclide-labeled antibodies to tumors has stimulated renewed interest in the immunology of cancer. Although many problems with this diagnostic and therapeutic approach need to be resolved, evidence to date indicates that the method is valid. Prospective randomized trials of radioimmunodetection must be undertaken even though the task will prove difficult. We believe that the eventual methodology will prove to be very beneficial in the care of cancer patients.

REFERENCES

1. Agwunobi TC, Boak JL. Diagnosis of malignant breast disease by axillary lymphoscintigraphy: A preliminary report. Br J Surg 65: 379–383, 1978.

2. Bale, WF, Spar IL, Goodland RL. Experimental radiation therapy of tumor with ^{131}I-carrying antibodies to fibrin. Cancer Res 20: 1488–1494, 1960.

3. Berche C, Mach J-P, Lumbroso JD, Langlois C, Aubry F, Buchegger F, Carrel S, Rougier P, Parmentier C, Tubiana M. Tomoscintigraphy for detecting gastrointestinal and medullary thyroid cancers: First clinical results using radiolabeled monoclonal antibodies against carcinoembryonic antigen. Br Med J 285: 1447–1451, 1982.

4. Boak JL, Agwunobi TC. A study of technetium labeled sulphide colloid uptake by regional lymph nodes draining a tumor-bearing area. Br J Surg 65: 374–378, 1978.

5. DeLand FH, Kim EE, Simmons G, Goldenberg DM: Imaging approach in radioimmunodetection. Cancer Res 40: 3046–3049, 1980.

6. Ege GN. Internal mammary lymphoscintigraphy. The rationale, technique, interpretation and clinical application: A review based on 848 cases. Radiology 118: 101–107, 1976.

7. Ege GN. Internal mammary lymphoscintigraphy in breast carcinoma: A study of 1,072 patients. Int J Radiat Oncol Biol Phys 2: 755–761, 1977.

8. Ege GN. Internal mammary lymphoscintigraphy: A rational adjunct to the staging and management of breast carcinoma. Clin Radiol 29: 453–456, 1978.

9. Ellis RJ, Wernick G, Zabriskie JB, Goldman LI. Immunologic competence of regional lymph nodes in patients with breast cancer. Cancer 35: 655–659, 1975.

10. Ghose T, Ferrone S, Imai K, Novell, Jr ST, Luner SJ, Martin RH, Blair AH. Imaging of human melanoma xenografts in nude mice with a radiolabeled monoclonal antibody. J Natl Cancer Inst 69: 823–826, 1982.

11. Gitsch E, Philipp K, Pateisky N. Intraoperative lymph scintigraphy during radical surgery for cervical cancer. J Nucl Med 25: 486–489, 1984.

12. Goldenberg DM, Witte S, Elster K: GW-39. A new human tumor serially transplantable in the golden hamster. Transplantation 4: 760–763, 1966.

13. Goldenberg DM, Hansen HJ. Carcinoembryonic antigen present in human colonic neoplasms serially propagated in hamsters. Science 175: 1117–1118, 1972.

14. Goldenberg DM, Preston DF, Primus FJ, Hansen HJ. Photoscan localization of GW-39 tumors in hamsters using radiolabeled anticarcinoembryonic antigen immuno-globulin G. Cancer Res 34: 1–9, 1974.

15. Goldenberg DM, Kim EE, DeLand FH, Bennett S, Primus FJ. Radioimmuno-detection of cancer with radioactive antibodies to carcinoembryonic antigen. Cancer Res 40: 2984–2992, 1980.

16. Hericourt J, Richet C. Traitment d'un cas de sarcome par la serotherapie. CR Hebd Seances Acad Sci 120: 948–950, 1895.

17. Hericourt J, Richet C. De la serotherapie dans le traitment du cancer. CR Hebd Seances Acad Sci 121: 567–569, 1895.

18. Köhler G, Milstein C. Continuous culture of fused cells secreting antibody of predefined specificity. Nature 256: 495–497, 1975.

19. Korngold L, Pressman D. The localization of antilymphosarcoma antibodies in the Murphy lymphosarcoma of the rat. Cancer Res 24: 268–279, 1964.

20. Larson SM, Carrasquilo JA, Krohn A, Brown JP, McGuffin RW, Ferens JM, Graham MM, Hill LD, Beaumier PL, Hellström KE, Hellström I. Localization of ^{131}I-labeled p97-specific Fab fragments in human melanoma as a basis for radiotherapy. J Clin Invest 72: 2101–2114, 1983.

21. Mach J-P, Carrel S, Merenda C, Heumann D, Rosenspur U. *In vivo* localization of anti-CEA antibody to colon carcinoma. Can the results obtained in nude mice be extrapolated to the patient situation? Eur J Cancer 1 (Suppl): 113–120, 1978.

22. Mach J-P, Forni M, Ritschard J, et al.: Use and limitations of radiolabeled anti-CEA antibodies and their fragments for photoscanning detection of human colorectal carcinoma. Oncodev Biol Med 1: 49–69, 1980.

23. Mach J-P, Buchegger F, Forni M, Ritschard J, Berche C, Lumbroso JD, Schreyer M, Girardct C, Accola RS, Carrel S: Use of radiolabeled monoclonal anti-CEA antibodies for the detection of human carcinoma by external photoscanning and tomoscintigraphy. Immunol Today 2: 239–249, 1981.

24. Order SE, Klein JL, Ettinger D, Alderson P, Siegleman S, Leichner P. Use of isotopic immunoglobulin in therapy. Cancer Res 40: 3001–3007, 1980.

25. Pant KD, Shochat D, Nelson MO, Goldenberg DM: Colon-specific antigen-p (CSAp). I. Initial clinical evaluation as a marker for colorectal cancer. Cancer 50: 919–926, 1982.

26. Papsidero LD, Wojcieszyn JW, Horoszewics JS, Leono SS, Murphy GP, Chu TM. Isolation of prostatic acid phosphatase-binding immunoglobulin G from human sera and its potential use as a tumor-localizing reagent. Cancer Res 40: 3032–3035, 1980.

27. Potamski J, Harlozińska A, Starzyk H, Richter R, Wózmewski A: Correlation between immunohistochemical localization of carcinoembryonic antigen (CEA) and histological estimation of carcinomas, normal mucosal, and lymph nodes of the digestive tract in humans. Arch Immunol Ther Exp 27: 177–186, 1979.

28. Pressman D, Korngold L. Experimental hypersensitivity. Science 116: 443, 1952.

29. Pressman D, Day ED, Blau M. The use of paired labeling in the determination of tumor-localizing antibodies. Cancer Res 17: 845–850, 1957.

30. Pressman D, Pressman R. Computer programs for paired and triad radioiodine labeled techniques in radioimmunochemistry. Int J Appl Radiat Isot 18: 617–622, 1965.

31. Pressman D, Chu TM, Grossberg AL. Carcinoembryonic antigen-binding immunoglobulin isolated from normal human serum by affinity chromatography. J. Natl Cancer Inst 62: 1367–1371, 1979.

32. Pressman D. The development and use of radiolabeled antitumor antibodies. Cancer Res 40: 2960–2964, 1980.

33. Primus FJ, Wang RH, Goldenberg DM, Hansen HJ. Localization of human GW-39 tumors in hamsters by radiolabeled heterospecific antibody to carcinoembryonic antigen. Cancer Res 33: 2977–2982, 1973.

34. Primus FJ, MacDonald R, Goldenberg DM, Hansen HJ: Localization of GW-39 human tumors in hamsters by affinity-purified antibody to carcinoembryonic antigen. Cancer Res 37: 1544–1547, 1977.

35. Primus FJ, Goldenberg DM. Immunological considerations in the use of goat antibodies to carcinoembryonic antigen for the radioimmunodetection of cancer. Cancer Res 40: 2979–2982, 1980.

36. Primus FJ, DeLand FH, Goldenberg DM. Monoclonal antibodies for radioimmunodetection of cancer. In *Monoclonal Antibodies in Cancer*. Wright G, ed. New York: Marcel Dekker (in press).

37. Reif AE, Curtis LE, Duffield R, Shauffer IA. Trial of radiolabeled antibody localization in metastases of a patient with tumor containing carcinoembryonic antigen (CEA). J Surg Oncol 6: 133–150, 1974.

38. Weinstein JN, Parker RJ, Keenan AM, Dower SK, Morse III HC, Sieber SM. Monoclonal antibodies in the lymphatics: Toward the diagnosis and therapy of tumor metastases. Science 218: 1334–1337, 1982.

11

Ectopic Hormones in Cancer

Nasser Javadpour, M.D.

In 1969, the term ectopic hormone was used to describe the secretion of adrenocorticotrophine hormone (ACTH) by nonendocrine tumors. It later became apparent that a number of tumors—including oat cell carcinoma of the lung, carcinoid tumors, thymic tumors, and certain tumors of the pancreas and the stomach—may produce ectopic hormones. The criteria for establishment of ectopic hormone secretion are listed in Table 11–1. Tumors of the lung are particularly known to produce a number of ectopic hormones (Table 11-2). The discovery of APUD tumors and genetic control of these hormones has shed some light on the mechanisms of production of ectopic products from various tumors. It has assumed that certain tumors contain amino precursor uptake and decarboxylation (APUD) cells that are capable of producing ectopic products when their repressed genetic materials are turned

Table 11–1   Criteria for Ectopic Hormone Secretion

Elevated serum hormone.

An arteriovenous gradient of hormones from a given tumor.

Demonstration of higher levels of hormones in the tumor than tissue.

Demonstration of *in vitro* hormone production by the tumor.

Fall in hormone levels following the removal of the tumor.

After L. H. Rees, The biosynthesis of hormones by non-endocrine tumors: A review. J. Endocrinol. 67: 143, 1975.

Table 11–2   Ectopic Hormones That May Be Produced in Cancer of the Lung

Hormones	Reference
ACTH	Proc. Natl. Acad. Sci 75: 516, 1978
Calcitonin	Br. J. Dis. Chest 72: 263, 1978
Serotonin	Semin. Oncol. 5: 253, 1978
Renin	Semin. Oncol. 5: 253, 1978
hCG (alpha and beta)	NEJM 277: 1395, 1967
FSH	Semin. Oncol. 5: 253, 1978
Estrogen	Steroid Biochem. 10: 339, 1978
TSH	Cancer 42: 1484, 1978

back by the neoplastic process. Be that as it may, the use of ectopic hormones as tumor markers may help to detect, stage, and monitor the tumors that produce these ectopic hormones. In this chapter, we briefly discuss ectopic hormones and their clinical applications.[10–15]

ACTH

ACTH is one of the classic and most studied ectopic hormones and is produced by a variety of tumors.[9] These heterogeneous tumors include

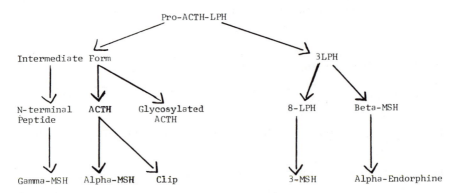

Figure 11–1. Pathway of ACTH synthesis. (From H. Imura. Ectopic hormone synthesis syndrome. Clin. Endocrinol. Metab. 9: 235, 1980.)

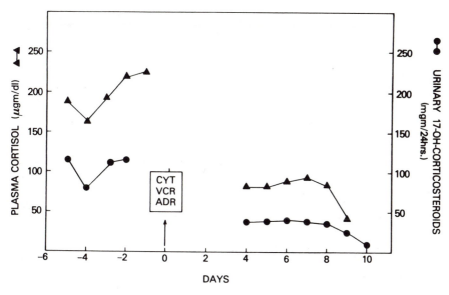

Figure 11–2. Ectopic ACTH produced by tumor of the lung. Note the fluctuation of this tumor marker with the therapy of the tumor.

tumors of the lung, pancreas, thyroid, stomach, liver, ovary, and prostate, plus a number of other tumors.

The pathway of ectopic ACTH synthesis is shown in Fig. 11-1. The treatment of ectopic production of ACTH is to remove the responsible tumor (Fig. 11–2). ACTH is used for monitoring of the tumor and of the extent of the tumor response to surgery, radiotherapy, and chemotherapy.

ANTIDIURETIC HORMONE

A number of tumors are capable of producing inappropriate antidiuretic hormones (ADH) that may be used as tumor markers in their management.[2] Although a number of non-neoplastic neoplasms may produce inappropriate ADH, 80% of all cases are related to neoplasms. The treatment of such syndromes is correction of the underlying causes.[3]

The syndrome of inappropriate ADH production includes hyponatremia, hypoosmularity, and failure of conservation of urinary sodium in the presence of hyponatremia. The total body water is increased.

Table 11–3 Mechanisms of Hypercalcemia-Associated Neoplasms

Bony metastases
Production of ectopic PTH-like material
Vitamin D and certain metabolites
Non-vitamin D steroids
Osteoblast activating factor
Prostaglandin

After L. H. Rees. The biosynthesis of hormones by nonendocrine tumors: A review. J. Endocrinol 67 : 143, 1975.

Ectopic parathyroid hormone (PTH) has been reported in a number of tumors, including renal cell carcinoma. The neoplasm may manifest as hypercalcemia, hypophosphatemia, and other metabolic changes characteristic of hyperparathyroidism. The normal PTH has a molecular weight of 9.5 kd and consists of 89 amino acids. However, the ectopic PTH has a larger molecule and can be differentiated from normal PTH by carboxyl-terminal radioimmunoassay that is designed for detecting excessive PTH produced by hyperparathyroidism. The etiology of tumor-associated hypercalcemia is shown in Table 11–3.

CALCITONIN

Calcitonin is produced by the C cell of the thyroid gland. Its serum level may increase in medullary carcinoma of the thyroid gland.[1] It decreases serum calcium and causes hypercalcuria and natriuresis with decreased bone calcium turnover. Tumors such as bronchogenic carcinoma, metastatic breast tumors, and pancreatic carcinomas are shown to produce ectopic calcitonin.[4] Calcitonin is a reliable marker in following the response of medullary carcinoma of the thyroid. Also, it may be utilized as a marker in the monitoring of other cancers producing this hormone ectopically.

A number of neoplasms may produce substances such as hCG,[6,7] LH, placental lactogens, thyroid-stimulating hormone, serotonin, and vasoactive intestinal peptide.[5] Other products such as erythropoietin, insulin, glucagon, gastrin, and renin have been reported as ectopic hormones in a number of cancers.

REFERENCES

1. Abe, K., Adachi, T., and Miyakawa, S. Production of calcitonin, adrenocorticotropic hormone and β-melanocyte stimulating hormone in tumors derived from amine precursor uptake and decarboxylation cells. Cancer Res. 37: 4190, 1977.

2. Bartter, F. C., and Schwartz, W. B. The syndrome of inappropriate secretion of antidiuretic hormone, Am. J. Med. 42: 790, 1967.

3. Beck, L. H. Hyperevicemia in the syndrome of inappropriate secretion of ADH. N. Engl. J. Med. 301: 528, 1979.

4. Bender, R. A., and Hansen, H. Hypercalcemia in bronchogenic carcinoma. A prospective study of 200 patients. Ann. Intern. Med. 80: 205, 1974.

5. Bloom, S. R., Polak, J. M., and Pearie, A. G. E. Vasoactive intestinal peptide and watery-diarrhea syndrome. Lancet 2: 14, 1973.

6. Braunstein, G. D., Vaitukaitis, J. L., Carbone, P. P., and Ross, G. J. Ectopic production of hCG by neoplasms. Ann. Intern. Med. 78: 39, 1973.

7. Braunstein, G. D., Rasor, J., and Wade, M. E. Presence in normal human testes of a chorionic gonadotropin-like substance distinct from human luteinizing hormone. New Engl. J. Med. 293: 1339, 1975.

8. Kohler, J. P., Simonowitz, D., and Polayan, D. Preoperative CEA level; A prognostic test in patients with colorectal carcinoma. Am. Surg. 46(8): 449, 1980.

9. Lipsett, M. B. Hormonal syndromes associated with neoplasia. Adv. Metab. Disord. 3: 111, 1968.

10. MacIntire, K. R., Vogel, C. L., and Primack, A. Effect of surgical and chemotherapeutic treatment of alpha-fetoprotein levels in patients with hepatocellular carcinoma. Cancer 37: 677, 1976.

11. Moertel, C. G., Schutt, A. J., and Go, V. L. W. Carcinoembryonic antigen test for recurrent colorectal carcinoma. JAMA 239: 1065, 1978.

12. Rouslahti, E., Pihko, H., and Seppala, M. Alpha-fetoprotein: Immunochemical purification and chemical properties. Expression in normal state and in malignant and non-malignant liver disease. Transplant Rev. 20: 38, 1974.

13. Silva, O. L., Becker, K. O., Primack, A., Doppman, G., and Snider, P. H. Ectopic secretion of calcitonin by oat-cell carcinoma. N. Engl. J. Med. 290: 1122, 1974.

14. Wanebo, H. J., Bhaskor, R., Pinskey, C. M., Hoffman, R. D., Stearns, M., Schwartz, M. K., and Oettgen, H. F. Preoperative carcinoembryonic antigen level as a prognostic indicator in colorectal cancer. N. Engl. J. Med. 299: 448, 1978.

15. Williams, R. R. Tumor-associated antigen levels (carcinoembryonic antigen, human chorionic gonadotropin, and alpha-fetoprotein) antedating the diagnosis of cancer in the Framingham study. J. Natl. Cancer Inst. 58: 1547, 1977.

12

The Use of
Lactate Dehydrogenase Isoenzymes
as Cancer Markers

N. M. Papadopoulos, Ph.D.

INTRODUCTION

The cytoplasmic enzyme lactate dehydrogenase (LD) is unique because it is found in all forms of life, from the unicellular organism to all human cells and fluids. LD is a component of the glycolytic cycle which is of fundamental importance in living organisms for the production of energy and sustenance of life. LD catalyzes, under aerobic and anaerobic conditions, the reversible reaction of pyruvate to lactate. This enzyme was first recognized in 1920 as an enzyme participating in metabolic reactions (26). In 1957, several studies showed that LD exists in different distinct molecular forms named isoenzymes (24). In 1959 Markert and Moller (16) reported that the various LD isoenzymes have different molecular structures, but that all perform the same catalytic function. They also demonstrated a different quantitative distribution of isoenzymes in the various tissues.

The interest in LD in relation to cancer originated from the observation by different investigators (25) that this enzyme is elevated in the sera of patients with malignant diseases. Soon thereafter it was found that total LD is elevated in the sera of patients with a variety of diseases; therefore, its value for the diagnosis of cancer is limited due to its lack of specificity. The discovery of isoenzymes has improved

I wish to thank H. M. Moutsopoulos M.D., F.A.C.P., for helpful suggestions and advice.

diagnostic discrimination and has led to their increased application in clinical practice.

ORIGIN OF
THE FIVE LD ISOENZYMES AND
METHODS FOR THEIR DETERMINATION

Two genes, a and b, provide the genetic information for the synthesis of two distinct polypeptide monomers, H and M, which have no enzymatic activity. These two monomer subunits associate with themselves to form two homogeneous tetrameric units, HHHH and MMMM, which are enzymatically active. They also associate with each other to form three hybrid tetrameric forms, HHHM, HHMM, and HMMM, which are also enzymatically active. These five LD isoenzymes are separated by electrophoresis and are numbered from 1 to 5: LD-1 is the fastest migrating toward the anode and LD-5 migrates nearest the cathode.

Several electrophoretic methods are available for the determination of LD isoenzymes. These methods utilize as support media either cellulose acetate membranes or agar, agarose, or acrylamide gels. Although the LD-isoenzyme patterns of tissues and fluids obtained by the various methods are qualitatively comparable, quantitative differences do exist. For this reason, it is important to apply the same technique for the determination of LD-isoenzyme patterns in tissues; to obtain a reference standard, in order to make meaningful comparisons; and to enhance diagnostic specificity.

Our contribution in this field has been the development of a method to determine LD isoenzymes quantitatively (18), as well as the application of this method to detect biochemical abnormalities and aid the diagnosis of disease (20). The method is divided into three parts: separation of the isoenzymes by agarose gel electrophoresis; detection of the isoenzymatic activity by tetrazolium reduction; and quantitation by densitometry, as shown in Fig. 12–1. The percentage of the individual LD isoenzymes obtained by this technique are 30, 40, 20, 6, and 4% for isoenzymes 1 to 5, respectively.

DISTRIBUTION OF LD ISOENZYMES
IN HUMAN TISSUES AND FLUIDS

The quantitative distribution of the five LD isoenzymes in various human tissues and fluids is different and characteristic for each. The release of LD isoenzymes from a tissue into the blood because of injury, inflammation, or malignancy causes a change of the normal serum pattern. The resulting pattern either resembles that of the particular tissue affected, indicating the origin of the abnormality, or is atypical, indicating an abnormal process such as malignancy. This forms the rational basis for the use of isoenzymes in diagnostic applications and as tumor markers.

LD ISOENZYMES
IN HUMAN MALIGNANCIES

Malignant transformations cause cell proliferation, alteration of the metabolism of normal cells, and excessive release of proteins and enzymes in the circulation. It has been found that serum LD-isoenzyme determinations reflect these changes. The following four types of LD-isoenzyme patterns have been associated with these changes.

Cathodic Pattern

Several investigators have confirmed that the LD-isoenzyme patterns of solid malignant tumors show a shift toward the cathodic forms LD-5, 4, and 3 when compared with the patterns of adjacent normal tissues (1,8,17,21). Since these isoenzymes are associated with anaerobic glycolysis (9), such findings are consistent with the early observations of Cori and Cori (5) who demonstrated increased anaerobic glycolytic activity in malignant tumors. It follows that the release of these LD isoenzymes in blood will cause a change in the normal serum LD-isoenzyme pattern, as shown in Fig. 12–2. The increase of LD-5 is more prominent because LD-5 has the lowest activity in normal serum. A relative increase of LD-5, 4, and 3 as a percentage of total LD could be an indicator of malignancy in the absence of other conditions that cause an increase of the same isoenzymes, such as liver and skeletal muscle abnormalities.

Intermediate Pattern

Lymphoid cell neoplasms that are manifested as lymphomas and leukemias are characterized by increased lymphocyte proliferation,

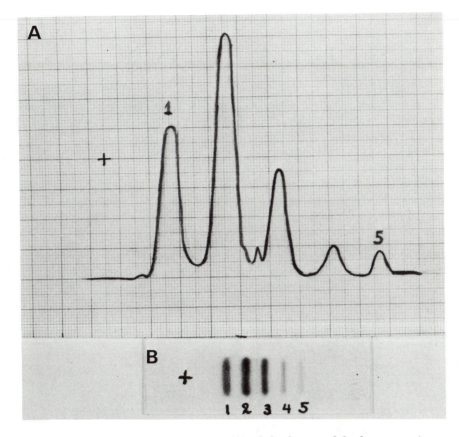

Figure 12–1. Densitometric tracing (A) of the lactate dehydrogenase isoenzyme electrophoretic pattern of a normal human serum (B).

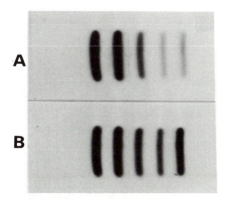

Figure 12–2. Lactate dehydrogenase isoenzyme electrophoretic patterns of: (A), a normal human serum and (B), a serum sample from a patient with colorectal carcinoma.

turnover, and release of their isoenzymes in the circulation. The serum LD-isoenzyme pattern of the patient reflects the pattern of malignant lymphocytes. This is illustrated in Fig. 12–3. The intracellular LD-isoenzyme patterns of normal human T and B lymphocytes have been determined (3,6). These patterns show a preponderance of LD-2, 3, and 4, with small differences between the T and B lymphocytes. A serum LD-isoenzyme pattern from a patient with B-cell lymphoma with a total LD activity of more than 10,000 IU/liter is included for comparison. The determination of LD-isoenzyme patterns supports the diagnosis of lymphoid neoplasms. In addition, measurements of LD isoenzymes in these patients are useful for assessing the efficacy of therapy.

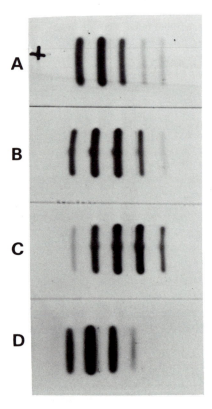

Figure 12–3. Lactate dehydrogenase isoenzyme electrophoretic patterns of: (*A*), a normal human serum; (*B*), T lymphocytes; (*C*), B lymphocytes; and (*D*), a serum sample from a patient with B-cell lymphoma.

Anodic Pattern

A specific elevation of LD-1 in the sera of patients with testicular and ovarian tumors is a unique finding among all neoplasms.

The original incidental observation of the elevation of LD-1 in the sera of patients with testicular and ovarian carcinoma (26) has recently been followed by extensive and detailed studies (12,14). In the latter studies, the original observations of serum LD-1 elevation in testicular tumors were substantiated.

A correlation was established between the stage of the disease and frequency of LD-1 increase. Furthermore, it was found that the frequency of serum LD-1 elevation was higher in advanced stages of the disease. A higher incidence of LD-1 elevation was found in the sera of patients with seminoma (12) as compared with the other nonseminomatous testicular tumors studied. In the patients with elevated LD activity, serial measurements of serum LD-1 isoenzyme reflected the response of the patient to therapy.

These data suggest that the serum LD-1 level is a useful marker for the detection of advanced stages of testicular cancer and seminoma as well as a monitor of the patient's response to treatment.

An elevation of LD-1 is also observed in patients following a myocardial infarction and in those with hemolytic disorders. For this reason, caution should be exercised in the interpretation of a laboratory finding of a serum LD-1 elevation. In a young adult, however, it is easy to differentiate clinically a suspected seminoma from myocardial infarction (Fig. 12–4).

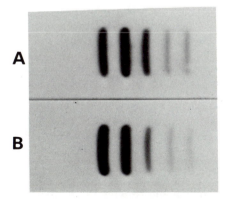

Figure 12–4. Lactate dehydrogenase isoenzyme electrophoretic patterns of: (*A*), a normal human serum and (*B*), from a patient with seminoma.

Supernumerary Pattern

A common cause of the alteration of normal human LD-isoenzyme patterns is the occurrence of additional (more than 5) LD isoenzymes in apparently normal individuals and in patients. Electrophoretic patterns with additional LD isoenzymes were also observed in neoplastic tissue extracts and in the sera of patients with malignant gliomas and carcinomas (4). Extra LD isoenzymes occurred in the electrophoretic patterns between the normal isoenzymes of the sera of patients with primary and metastatic malignancies (7). The example in Fig. 12–5 shows the serum LD-isoenzyme electrophoretic pattern from a patient with liver carcinoma.

The occurrence of supernumerary LD isoenzymes in human serum is not necessarily characteristic of neoplastic disease, because they have been reported in normal individuals (22) and in patients with various liver diseases (19,13,10). A common cause of the appearance of extra LD isoenzymes in serum electrophoretic patterns is the binding of the LD isoenzymes with serum immunoglobulins (11,15,23) or other macromolecules (2). Thus the laboratory finding of extra LD isoenzymes in the sera of normal subjects and patients should be interpreted with an appropriate clinical evaluation. If, in a normal individual, no adequate reason is found for the presence of the extra LD isoenzymes, periodic examination is indicated. The presence of extra LD isoenzymes in patients with liver disease or cancer can serve as a marker for following the course of the disease and the effect of therapy.

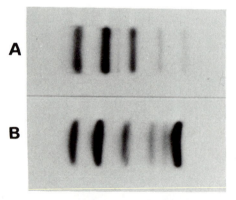

Figure 12–5. Lactate dehydrogenase isoenzyme electrophoretic patterns of: (*A*), a normal human serum and (*B*), from a patient with liver carcinoma.

CONCLUSIONS

The normal electrophoretic patterns of human serum LD isoenzymes show five equally spaced bands. They reflect the normal balance of release from cells and their catabolism.

The determination of LD isoenzymes in serum is a sensitive indicator of metabolic alterations or injury of cells, but their diagnostic discrimination for cancer is limited due to lack of specificity. From experimental evidence of numerous studies, four different types of serum LD-isoenzyme electrophoretic patterns have emerged and can be used as additional parameters to aid diagnosis and treatment of malignant neoplasms in the proper clinical setting: (a) The pattern of increased cathodic LD isoenzymes, frequently observed in solid tumors of various tissues. This change has been associated with increased anaerobic glycolysis in cancer cells of these diseases. (b) The pattern of increased intermediate LD isoenzymes, most frequently observed in malignancies involving the lymphoid cells of T- and B-cell lymphomas and leukemias. (c) The pattern of the increased anodic isoenzymes, which was found in the tissue and serum of patients with germ cell tumors of the testes. (d) The pattern with supernumerary LD isoenzymes, found in asymptomatic individuals and patients with various diseases including cancer.

REFERENCES

1. Barnett, H., and Gibson, S. Lactate dehydrogenase (LD) isoenzymes. Patterns in carcinomas of the breast. J. Clin. Path. 17: 201–202, 1964.

2. Biewenga, J., and Feltkamp, T. E. W. Lactate dehydrogenase (LD)-IgG immunoglobulin complexes in human serum. Clin. Chem. Acta. 64: 101–1116, 1975.

3. Blatt, J., Spiegel R. J., Papadopoulos, N. M., Lazarou, S. A., Magrath, I. T., and Poplack, D. G. Lactate dehydrogenase isoenzymes in normal and malignant human lymphoid cells. Blood 60: 491–494, 1982.

4. Buckell, M., and Barnes, G. K. Supernumerary fractions of lactate dehydrogenase in two malignant gliomas. Br. J. Cancer. 22: 237–243, 1968.

5. Cori, C. F., and Cori, G. T. The carbohydrate metabolism of tumors. II. Changes in the sugar, lactic acid and CO_2-combining power of blood passing through a tumor. J. Biol. Chem. 65: 397–405, 1925.

6. Csako, G., Magrath, I. T., and Elin, R. J. Serum total and isoenzymes lactate dehydrogenase activity in American Burkitt's lymphoma patients. Am. J. Clin. Pathol. 78: 712–717, 1982.

7. Fujimoto, Y., Nazarian, I., and Wilkinson, J. H. Lactate dehydrogenase polymorphism in a patient with secondary carcinoma of the liver. Enzymol Biol. Clin. 9: 214–236, 1968.

8. Goldman, R. D., Kaplan, N. O., and Hall, T. C. Lactic dehydrogenase in human neoplastic tissues. Cancer Res. 24: 389–399, 1964.

9. Goodfriend, T. L., Sokol, D. M., and Kaplan, N. O. Control of synthesis of lactic dehydrogenase. J. Mol. Biol. 15: 18–31, 1966.

10. Hoenigova, J., and Hoenin, V. Unusual band on starch gel electrophoresis of sera from patients with cirrhosis of the liver. Clin. Chim. Acta. 18: 313, 1967.

11. Lindsey, G. G., Berman, P. A. M., and Purves, L. R. An abnormal macrolactate dehydrogenase isoenzyme not due to immunoglobulin binding. Clin. Chim. Acta. 99: 153–160, 1979.

12. Lippert, M., Papadopoulos, N., and Javadpour, N. Role of lactate dehydrogenase isoenzymes in the testicular cancer. Urology 18: 53, 1981.

13. Litter, I., Jobst, K., and Barna, K. An anomalous lactate dehydrogenase isoenzyme band in acute viral hepatitis. Acta. Med. Acad. Sci. Hung. 30: 49, 1973.

14. Lie, F., Fritshe, H. A., Trujillo, J. M., and Samuels, M. L. Serum lactate dehydrogenase isoenzymes in patients with advanced testicular cancer. Am. J. Clin. Pathol 78: 178–183, 1972.

15. Lubrano, T., Ditz, A. A., and Rubinstein, H. M. Extra lactate dehydrogenase isoenzyme band in serum of patients with severe liver disease. Clin. Chem. 17: 882, 1971.

16. Markert, C. L., and Moller, F. Multiple forms of enzymes: Tissue, autogenetic and species specific patterns. Proc Natl. Acad. Sci. U.S.A. 45: 753–763, 1959.

17. Nissen, N. I., and Bohn, L. Patterns of lactic acid dehydrogenase isoenzymes in normal and malignant human tissues. Europ. J. Cancer. 1: 217–219, 1965.

18. Papadopoulos, N. M., and Kintzios J. Quantitative electrophoretic determination of lactate dehydrogenase isoenzymes. Am. J. Clin Pathol. 47: 96–99, 1967.

19. Papadopoulos, N. M. Electrophoretic demonstration of three extra lactate dehydrogenase isoenzymes in the serum of a normal individual. Clin. Chem. 20: 841–842, 1974.

20. Papadopoulos, N. M. Clinical applications of lactate dehydrogenase isoenzymes. Ann. Clin. Lab Sci. 7: 506–710, 1977.

21. Poznanska-Linde, H., Wilkinson, J. H., and Withycombe, W. A. Lactate dehydrogenase isoenzymes in malignant tissues. Nature, 209: 727–728, 1966.

22. Tanaka, F., Amino, N., and Hayahsi, C. Abnormal serum lactate dehydrogenase isoenzymes in a case of laryngeal carcinoma and thyrotoxicosis. Clin Chem. Acta. 68: 235–240, 1976.

23. Thomas, D. W., Rosen, S. W., Kahn R., Temple, R., and Papadopoulos, N. M. Macromolecular lactic acid dehydrogenase. Ann. Intern. Med. 18: 434–439, 1974.

24. Warburg, O., Wind, F., and Nejelein, E. Uber den Stoffwechsel von Tumoren im Korper. Klin. Wschr. 5: 829–832, 1926.

25. Warburg, O., and Minami, S. Versuche an Uberlebenden Carcinobgweben. Klin. Wschr. 1: 776–77, 1923.

26. Zondag, H. A., and Klein, F. Clinical applications of lactate dehydrogenase isoenzymes: Alterations in malignancy. Ann N.Y. Acad. Sci. 151: 578–586, 1968.

13

Cancers
with Clinically Useful Markers

Nasser Javadpour, M.D.

Over the past several years, it has become apparent that a number of tumor cells produce certain biologic products that can be detected in sera and localized in the cells or tumors of patients. The development of specific and sensitive radioimmunoassay and immunocytochemical techniques has made a remarkable contribution to detecting or loacalizing minute amounts of these biologic markers. These developments have helped the researchers and clinicians to utilize these markers in the detection, diagnosis, staging, and monitoring of certain cancers.[1,2]

In this chapter, we discuss the clinical utilization of markers in certain cancers. Although the criteria for a perfect marker would not allow any of the markers to be called specific for a cancer, in the context of the clinical presentation certain markers are diagnostic of cancers. For example, alpha-fetoprotein (AFP) is mainly produced by hepatoma; however, when AFP is elevated in the serum of a young patient this usually indicates the presence of testicular tumor, and differential diagnosis with other tumors that produce this marker is generally possible.[10]

The cancers that have clinically useful markers are tabulated in Tables 13–1 to 13–4 and are briefly discussed here.

TESTICULAR TUMOR MARKERS

A number of tumor markers have been found in the serum of patients with germ cell testicular cancer (Table 13–5). Among these tumor

Table 13–1 Useful Markers in Genitourinary Cancer

Cancer	Marker
1. Testicular and Ovarian Tumors	AFP, hCG, SP_1
2. Prostatic Cancer	Acid and alkaline phosphatase
3. Bladder Cancer	Cell surface antigens Chromosomal analysis
4. Adrenal Cancer	Steroids

markers, serum AFP and human chorionic gonadotropin (hCG) have been the most useful in clinical applications.[17,23,24]

At the National Cancer Institute, sensitive and specific radio-immunoassays and immunocytochemical techniques have been developed for hCG and AFP which are capable of detecting minute amounts of these markers in the sera and cancer cells of patients with testicular cancer. When these two glycoproteins are utilized together, they are the best serologic and cellular markers available in terms of diagnosis, detection of early recurrence, accurate staging, and reflecting the adequacy of treatment of testicular cancer.

Frequency of hCG and AFP in Testicular Cancer

Human chorionic gonadotropin is a glycoprotein secreted by the normal placenta. It is normally found in the serum only during pregnancy. hCG has a molecular weight of 38 kd and is composed of two dissimilar subunits, α and β. The α subunit is the basic subunit of the pituitary glycoprotein hormones: the luteinizing, follicle-stimulating, and thyrotropic hormones. The β subunit, comprising two thirds of the molecular weight, is unique to hCG and is distinct from

Table 13–2 Useful Markers in Gastrointestinal Cancer

Cancer	Marker
1. Colon and rectum	CEA
2. Liver	AFP
3. Carcinoid of intestine	5-Hydroxy tryptamin
4. Insulinoma	Insulin

Table 13–3   Useful Markers in Endocrine Cancer

Cancer	Marker
1. Thyroid	Calcitonin
2. Pituitary	Growth hormone
3. Parathyroid	Parathyroid hormone
4. Pancreas	Glycagon and insulin
5. Adrenal	Steroids and catecholamines
6. Testis	Steroids

Table 13–4   Other Cancers with Useful Markers

Cancer	Marker
1. Leukemia, lymphoma	Cell markers
2. Multiple myeloma	Bence-Jones proteins
3. Osteogenic sarcoma	Alkaline-phosphatase

Table 13–5   Testicular Tumor Markers

Specific markers
1. Alpha-fetoprotein (AFP)
2. Human chorionic gonadotropin (hCG)
3. Placental alkaline phosphatase (PLAP)
4. Gamma-glutamine transpeptidase (GGT)
5. Placental proteins number 5, 10, 15
6. Placental lactogen

Nonspecific markers
1. Lactic dehydrogenase (LPH)
2. Polyamines (putrescine, spermine, spermicline)
3. Carcinoembryonic antigen

the subunits of luteinizing, follicle-stimulating, and thyrotropic hormones, particularly in the terminal 29 amino acids. The β subunit has been isolated, purified, and used to immunize rabbits to produce an antibody specific for hCG which does not cross react with physiologic concentrations of the other glycoprotein hormones. The data from our laboratory indicate that 70% (Table 13–6) of the patients with active nonseminomatous germ cell testicular tumors had elevated serum hCG levels. Elevated levels fell to normal with effective therapy. When an elevated level persisted or normal levels rose after initial therapy, recurrent tumor was invariably found. About 7.5% (10/130) of patients with testicular seminoma had elevated serum hCG levels.

In 1963, Abelev et al. demonstrated a specific α-1-globulin in the serum of embryonic and neonatal mice which was not found in the serum of adult mice.[1] Subsequently, AFP was identified in the serum of mice bearing hepatocellular carcinoma and later in humans with hepatoma. Human AFP is a glycoprotein with a molecular weight of 70 kd and contains about 41% carbohydrate. It is produced in the liver, yolk sac, and gastrointestinal tract of the fetus. AFP is present in human fetal serum at a concentration of 3 ng/ml by the twelfth week of gestation. The concentration at birth is approximately 30 ng/ml and drops to much lower levels by 1 year of age; in normal adults it is found in concentrations of approximately 1–16 ng/ml. AFP has been clinically useful primarily as a diagnostic tool for hepatoma and certain other malignant diseases. Waldmann and McIntire, using a double-antibody RIA for AFP, found an elevated level in 72% of 130 patients with hepatoma, in 23% of 44 patients with pancreatic carcinoma, in 18% of 91 patients with gastric carcinoma, and in 5–7% of patients with colonic and bronchogenic carcinoma.[24] Of particular interest was the finding by the same authors that 75% of 101 patients with testicular germ cell tumors had elevated levels of AFP. The discovery that testicular tumors so often produce AFP is a direct result of the development of a sensitive RIA; 71% of the elevated levels were below 3,000 ng/ml, the lower limit of detectability of the previously used gel precipitation assay, and had gone undetected prior to the development of this sensitive RIA. In our series, about 70% of the patients had an elevated level of serum AFP. If an elevated level of AFP persisted after therapy, recurrent metastatic tumor was generally found.

Staging of Testicular Cancer

The effective use of surgery, chemotherapy, and radiation therapy for patients with testicular cancer requires accurate staging for therapy

Table 13–6 Frequency of Elevated hCG and AFP in Patients with Testicular Cancer

Cancer	AFP		hCG		AFP and/or hCG	
	No. of patients	Percent of patients	No. of patients	Percent of patients	No. of patients	Percent of patients
Seminoma	0/160	0	14/160	9.0	14/160	9.0
Teratoma	6/16	37.5	4/16	25.0	7/16	43.7
Embryonal carcinoma	102/145	70.3	87/145	60.0	127/145	87.5
Embryonal carcinoma with teratoma	36/56	64.2	32/56	57.0	48/56	85.7
Choriocarcinoma	0/5	0	5/5	100.0	5/5	100.0
Yolk sac tumor	3/4	75.0	1/4	25.0	3/4	75.0

and/or interpretation of end results. The conventional staging parameters, including the lymphaniogram, inferior venacavogram, and excretory urogram, often yield a considerable staging error.

With sensitive and specific radioimmunoassays of serum AFP and hCG in 118 patients with embryonal carcinoma with or without teratoma undergoing clinical and surgical staging, the staging errors have decreased to 9–14% in stage I and 5–10% in stage II cases. Various clinical observations have been made from this group of patients. The important features that tumor markers add to the clinical staging of testicular cancer are the following:

1. Clinical staging based on markers is better than clinical staging, superior to pathologic staging.
2. Persistently elevated serum markers after orchiectomy for testicular cancer invariably indicate stage II or III disease.
3. Persistently elevated serum markers after lymphadenectomy indicate stage II disease or an inadequate lymphadenectomy.
4. When lymphadenectomy is negative for tumor but post-lymphadenectomy serum markers are persistently elevated, patients invariably have stage III disease. However, surgery still remains the most accurate means of assessing retroperitoneal metastasis.
5. Perhaps the most important applications of these markers are in the monitoring of testicular tumor when serially measured.

RIA of Urinary hCG

An improved technique for detecting small amounts of hCG which is 20-fold more sensitive than the conventional RIA for detecting the β subunit of hCG has been reported. This technique utilizes concentrated 24-h urinary hCG and a highly specific RIA with an antiserum (H93) that is specifically prepared against the carboxyl terminus of urinary hCG. The urinary hCG RIA offers the potential for more sensitively monitoring the tumor burden and guiding the therapy of patients with testicular cancer.

Simultaneous serum and urinary hCG levels were measured in 12 patients with disseminated testicular cancer. Initially, these 12 patients—who had either seminoma, embryonal carcinoma, teratocarcinoma, or choriocarcinoma of the testis—had elevated levels of serum hCG. After treatment with intensive chemotherapy and/or surgery, the elevated serum hCG levels dropped to undetectable levels.

However, the 24-h urinary hCG level measured by radioimmunoassay of urine concentration was elevated in 10 of the patients, despite undetectable levels of hCG in the serum, indicating the persistence of tumor producing this marker. Indeed, there were 4 patients in whom serum hCG was undetectable, but elevated levels of urinary hCG were found; these 4 patients were proven to have persistent tumor, which by histopathological and immunoperoxidase staining contained hCG. This highly sensitive urinary hCG RIA has improved the detection of persistent tumor burden and has been rewarding in selecting the patients for whom further therapy is warranted.[10]

Monitoring the Response to Therapy

Serial measurements of serum hCG and AFP by RIAs reflect the efficacy of surgical, radiation, and/or chemotherapeutic regimens in patients with testicular tumor. When these therapies are effective, they produce an immediate decrease in serum levels of hCG and AFP which reflects the decrease in tumor size and could be as rapid as the catabolic rate for these markers. In our series, elevated markers were found often months before the patients were symptomatic or recurrence was detectable by any other clinical tests. Consequently, the markers proved to be sensitive indicators of the presence of otherwise undetectable metastases.

When following a patient with serial marker levels, an elevated level of a marker may be found before any tumor can be detected clinically. The next problem to resolve with such a patient is the location of the recurrence. The value of the α subunit of hCG is its ability to localize a tumor that is not detectable by conventional clinical tests such as IVP, inferior venacavogram, and lymphangiogram. Alpha-hCG has a short half-life (20 min) and may be used in the localization of metastases, especially metastasis in the retroperitoneal area which is not readily detectable by conventional clinical tests.

Serum AFP and hCG in Seminoma

In a prospective study at the National Cancer Institute, 130 patients with "pure seminoma" had serial quantitative measurements of hCG and AFP by specific double-antibody immunoassays originally developed at the institute. These markers were localized in different cells using the techniques of immunoperoxidase or immunofluorescence on serial sections of the tumors. Eleven of the 130 patients had elevated serum hCG. In serial sectioning of the tumor specimens, 1 of 11 patients had an element of choriocarcinoma and underwent a retroperitoneal lymph node dissection and chemotherapy; the serum hCG then dropped to normal. There were 120 patients with normal levels of AFP. However, in 1 patient the serum AFP was 152 ng/ml. In serial sectioning, an element of embryonal carcinoma was found; this patient had also been proven to have metastatic involvement. A patient with massive bulky retroperitoneal seminoma and left hydronephrosis underwent debulking and radiation.

In this study, we observed the following clinical findings: (a) The frequency of elevated hCG in the serum of patients with seminoma is about 7.5% (10/130). (b) Although the synctiotrophoblastic tumor cell occasionally found in pure seminoma is capable of secreting hCG, one must look for elements of choriocarcinoma, or embryonal carcinoma, or both. This surely changes the therapeutic approaches. (c) An elevated serum AFP in patients with seminoma indicates the presence of an element of embryonal carcinoma, which also changes the therapeutic approach. (d) The reported cases in the literature of seminoma with an elevated level of hCG are lacking either serial sections or localization of cellular hCG or both. Therefore, we must be cautious in accepting them as pure seminoma.

Multiple Markers in Seminoma

The roles of γ-glutamyl transpeptidase (GGT), placental alkaline phosphatase (PLAP), and hCG have been studied in testicular seminoma. In 89 seminoma patients with negative AFP, total serum GGT was measured and values of about 30 IU/liter were considered abnormal. Serum PLAP was measured by enzyme-linked immunoabsorbent assay, and values above 1.85 mg/ml were considered abnormal. Serum hCG and AFP were measured by double-antibody radioimmunoassays (normals <1 ng/ml and < 20 ng/ml, respectively). At the time of the study, 30 patients had detectable seminoma, 10 were histologically unconfirmed, and the remaining 49 had no evidence of tumor. Only 6 of 30 patients (20%) with active tumor had elevated levels of serum hCG. Twelve of 30 patients with active tumor (40%) had elevated serum PLAP, and 10 of the same 30 patients (33%) had elevated serum levels of GGT (Table 13–7). When these three biochemical serum markers were considered together, more than 80% of the patients with clinically active tumors had detectable serum levels of one or more of these markers. Inasmuch as the survival of

Table 13–7 False-Positive and False-Negative of PLAP, GGT, and hCG in Patients with Seminoma

	Status of 79 patients*	
	Detectable tumor	Nondetectable tumor
No. of patients	30	49
PLAP (%)	40	12
GGT (%)	33	4
hCG (%)	20	0
PLAP, GGT, and/or hCG (%)	80	14

*Ten patients who had suspected tumor, but in whom it was not confirmed histologically, were excluded from this analysis.

patients with stage III seminoma treated by radiation is only 28%, we advocate serial measurements of these serum markers along with early utilization of new chemotherapeutic regimens in such patients. However, it should be emphasized that the false-positive and false-negative rates—especially false-positive rates for GGT, due to occasional concomitant liver disease—and the biologic half-lives of these markers should be taken into consideration.

Other Markers in Seminoma

A common marker that may be useful in the management of seminoma is lactic dehydrogenase (LD). Serum lactic dehydrogenase in man is a nonspecific enzyme made up of five heterogeneous isoenzymes which can be measured electrophoretically. Cancer cells increase glycolysis, leading to an increased synthesis of lactate which may be utilized as a nonspecific tumor marker in several cancers. In seminoma, LD may be particularly useful for several reasons: (a) There is a lower frequency of serum hCG elevations in seminoma vs. nonseminoma. (b) The equipment for measuring LD is more widely available and simpler to use than that for radioimmunoassay studies. (c) The majority of patients with bulky stages II and III seminomas seen at the National Cancer Institute had elevated serum levels of LD which were useful in monitoring their therapy. The preliminary results suggest that an elevation of LD may be somewhat specific in testicular cancer compared with other neoplasms.

Limitations of Tumor Markers
in Testicular Cancer

Despite certain limitations in utilizing the markers discussed above, they appear to be the best available markers in any solid tumors. The current practices and recommendations to minimize certain problems and maximize the efficacy of RIA measurement of serum AFP and hCG from the commercial sources for testicular cancer are as follows.

1. The physician should discuss the sensitivity and specificity of a given commercial assay with the laboratory, and, perhaps, occasional inclusions of normal serum or serum with known levels of AFP and/or hCG may serve as negative and positive controls when blindly coded.

2. These markers should not replace scrotal exploration and/or retroperitoneal lymphadenectomy for histopathologic diagnosis of the primary tumor or retroperitoneal metastasis. However, elevated levels of tumor markers are indicative of the presence of tumor and the necessity for further treatment. They are also helpful in monitoring the efficacy and need for changing the therapy.

3. The problem of impurity of certain antisera against the subunit of the hCG or the possibility of high levels of luteinizing hormones (LH) in patients undergoing orchiectomy and/or chemotherapy causing a false-positive result also should be kept in mind. The false-positive results may be clarified by a testosterone suppression test, determination of serum LH, and measurement of hCG on urinary concentrate utilizing a carboxy-terminal RIA that is currently available to all urologists through the National Cancer Insitute laboratories as a courtesy.

4. In monitoring the therapy or staging in patients with testicular tumor, the physician should use frequent physical examinations, chest x-rays, and other tests as necessary, along with determination of serum AFP and hCG. In patients on chemotherapy, the normalization of these serum markers does not mean tumor-free status; in fact, on exploration of the retroperitonium and chest, it is not unusual to find cystic fibrotic material with necrosis and tumor. Therefore, normalization of serum markers should not deter the surgeon from looking for tumor. Appropriate utilization of chemotherapy, surgery, radiotherapy, and tumor markers can make a dramatic improvement in prognosis and survival of these patients.

Discordance Between Markers

The discordance between various testicular tumor markers is well known. This discordance may be explained on the basis of the findings that different cells produce these various markers. Also, during chemotherapy of a patient with elevated levels of serum hCG and AFP, one marker may return to normal although the other markers may still remain elevated. This may occur if some of the cells producing a given marker are resistant to the therapy.[11,12]

Furthermore, we have demonstrated the cellular source of various tumor markers utilizing immunocytochemical techniques.[21]

Pregnancy-Specific B₁ Glycoprotein as a Tumor Marker

In the past few years, a new placental protein—pregnancy-specific B_1 glycoprotein (SP₁)—has been purified and used as a tumor marker in our and other laboratories.[19,20] Specific RIA and immunoperoxidase (IP) techniques have been developed to identify SP₁ in the sera and tumor cells of 97 men with testicular cancer. The level of SP₁ was elevated at 11–440 ng/ml in 3 of 6 patients with choriocarcinoma, 5 of 17 patients with embryonal carcinoma and teratoma, and 5 of 50 patients with embryonal carcinoma. None of 24 sera from men with seminoma and none of five men with orchitis had elevated AFP. The highest value in a group of patients with nonmalignant disease was 9.1 ng/ml. The new biologic marker was identified in the syncytiotrophoblastic giant cell (STGC). The STGCs are seen occasionally in patients with embryonal carcinoma, teratoma, and seminoma.

It remains to be determined whether SP₁ concentrations correlate with bulk of tumor, prognosis, or result of therapy, and it also remains to be determined whether other tumor cells produce this marker.

Gonadal Stromal Tumors

It has been shown that the immunoperoxidase technique can be used to identify steroid hormones in sections of fixed embedded tissues. This advance paves the way for prospective and retrospective studies of specific sites of steroid hormone localization in a poorly understood group of gonadal neoplasms, namely, those within the sex cord–stromal category. The ability to localize specifically testosterone,

Table 13–8   Cell Origin of Steroids in Testicular Nongerm Cell Tumors

	Estrodiol	Testosterone	Progesterone
Sertoli cells	+	+	−
Leydig cells	+	+ +	±

estrogen, and progesterone has challenged many of the time-honored concepts of steroid biosynthesis by gonadal stromal tumors. In the past, specific hormone synthesis was attributed more or less to specific types of cells. These cells were thought to be responsible for estrogen synthesis, and Leydig cells for testosterone production; granulosa and Sertoli cells were regarded as inactive generally. Utilizing highly specific antibodies for testosterone, estradiol, and progesterone, it has now been shown that all these cells are functionally active and, furthermore, that most have the capacity to synthesize both estrogen and androgen. Testosterone most frequently is localized in Leydig cells, but it may also be present in Sertoli cells and occasionally in granulosa cells. Estradiol is found not only in the theca cells but also frequently in granulosa, Sertoli, and Leydig cells, whereas progesterone appears to be localized mainly in luteinized theca cells and less commonly in granulosa and Leydig cells (Table 13–8).

Other Placental Proteins

Over the past several years, we have studied a number of placental proteins—including pregnancy-specific β glycoprotein and placental proteins number 5, 10, and 15—utilizing immunoperoxidase. We have localized these markers in syncytiotrophoblastic components of the human placenta, choriocarcinoma, and syncytiotrophoblastic giant cells associated with testicular cancer (Table 13–5).

Studies of Lactic Dehydrogenase

Lactic dehydrogenase is a glycolytic enzyme found in many human tissues and fluids. The enzyme is released into serum due to tissue injury arising from inflammatory conditions, degenerative processes, toxicity, or cancer. Elevations of serum LD levels have been found to reflect growth and regression of various malignant neoplasms.[22]

Eighty patients with testicular cancer were studied with serial serum LD. Normal values were 340 ng/ml before June 1, 1978, 381 for June 1978, and 248 after July 1, 1978, due to technical improvements. Of the 80 patients, 23.8% (19) were stage I (tumor confined to the testicle), 23.8% (19) were stage II (metastatic disease in the retroperitoneal lymph nodes only), and 52.5% (42) were stage III (visceral or distant metastases). Because the NIH specifically sought patients with bulky metastatic disease during this period for protocol purposes, the bulky stage III is more heavily represented. Eight of the stage III patients had extragonadal tumors. Eleven patients had seminomas, while 69 patients had nonseminomas.

In this study, frequency of elevation of pretherapy levels of LD in patients with germ-cell testicular tumors was definitely higher in stage III patients. Only 20% (1/5) stage I patients had elevated LD levels, in comparison to 26.3% (5/19) stage II patients and 62.5% (25/40) stage III patients. However, the pretherapy frequency of elevated hCG and AFP levels was similar when comparing stages in these patients. Others have also found, in testicular tumor patients, that although LD is much more frequently elevated in advanced disease, the same findings are applicable to hCG and AFP.

Currently, no known serum marker is frequently elevated in patients with seminoma. Since seminomas do not have elevated AFP levels and seldom have elevated hCG levels, mesurement of LD provides a simple and easily available test. If the LD level is elevated, it can be utilized in the monitoring of such patients.

Although the size of the tumor found intraoperatively did not correlate with the degree of elevation in total LD in other solid tumors, an overall correlation between degree of elevation of LD and cancer burden was found in a study of 27 patients with germinal testicular tumors. However, LD was evaluated with serial serum evaluations, and tumor burden was determined by serial evaluations of calculated areas of cancer lesions measurable by physical examination, chest roentgenogram, and/or lymphangiogram. This same study also showed an overall correlation between maximum serum LD concentration and prognosis. Specifically, 4 patients with a maximum serum LD of 5,000 IU/liter had a poorer prognosis than 23 patients with a maximum serum LD of 500 IU/liter. In the study of 80 patients cited above, 43 patients who had normal pretherapy LD levels had a mean survival time (MST) of 15.1 months while the 26 patients who presented with elevated LD values had an MST of 9.2 months. However, little significant difference could be found between the 14 patients who had initial LD elevations below 900 ng/ml (9.1 months) and the 12 patients who had initial LD elevations above 900 ng/ml (9.3 months).

Therefore, whether the initial LD value was elevated or normal did play a prognostic role, whereas the actual degree of elevation did not correlate with prognosis. However, in a study of 204 nonseminomatous germinal testis tumors, initial LD levels were found to correlate with mean survival times: for initial LD values of below 225, MST was more than 8 years; for LD of 225–600, MST was 14 months; and for LD above 600, MST was 10 months. Hence, LD can be seen to play a role in pointing to poorer patient prognosis when it is elevated initially.

In conclusion, serum LD levels are elevated in a number of bulky testicular tumors and correlate well with the course of treatment. Therefore, when elevated, the LD level may be utilized as a guide for response to therapy. It is not helpful in the diagnosis, or staging, of patients with testicular tumor. However, it can be valuable in seminoma patients with no other markers. Of benefit is the fact that it is a simple and inexpensive hospital test that is easily available and provides quick results. Finally, because we have had a fair number of patients with advanced bulky testicular tumors with multiple poor prognostic features, we have been able to correlate prognosis with serum LD and it appears that elevated serum LD level is of value as a prognostic indicator. This is, perhaps, a reflection of the bulk of a tumor, since bulky disseminated tumors have a poorer prognosis. These developments have become an important part of contemporary urologic practice.

CELL MARKERS IN BLADDER CANCER

The various tumor markers available at the present time for bladder cancer are cell surface antigens and chromosomal markers.[3,7,8,14]

Cell Surface Antigens

A number of cell surface antigens that are normally expressed on the cells of most urothelium can be utilized as cell markers. Among these cell surface antigens are: ABH antigens, T antigen, and tumor-associated antigen.

The major problem in the diagnosis and management of a superficial bladder cancer has been lack of predictors to assess the potential invasiveness of such a cancer into the bladder muscle. The conventional histopathologic examination of the primary or metastatic tumor rarely predicts the potentiality of such cancer for invasion. During the past several years, it has become apparent that cellular differentiation in certain cancers is reflected in the presence or absence of certain cell surface antigens. Davidsohn and co-workers developed the specific red cell adherence test (SRCA) to determine the presence or absence of these cell surface antigens.[7] In applying the test to cancer of the cervix, they found that, as cells from the cervix undergo malignant dedifferentiation from atypia to anaplasia, a progressive loss of ABO (H) cell surface antigens appears to occur. Subsequent reports by our laboratory and by others revealed that lesions greater than stage A consistently showed absence of the ABO (H) cell surface antigen and that loss of the antigen could be correlated with advance in histologic grade. This potential ability of the SRCA test to predict which early bladder tumors might be destined to invade or metastasize prompted us to examine other conditions that might affect the observed association between ABO (H) cell surface antigen loss and cancer. However, this test has been difficult to reproduce in certain laboratories, mainly due to difficulty in preparing reactive and reliable *Ulex europaeus* extract. We believe that any given test for predicting the prognosis of cancer, including cancer of the bladder, should be most specific, sensitive, fast, inexpensive, reproducible, practical, and quantitative and easy to perform with a high accuracy rate. To our knowledge, such a test is not available for any cancer. Nevertheless, continuous effort to improve the test and accumulate accurate knowledge is essential in evaluating any given test, including the SRCA test. Currently, we are using IP and peroxidase antiperoxidase in an attempt to improve and standardize the SRCA test with appropriate quality controls. Preliminary data indicate that these techniques are superior to the conventional SRCA, especially for detection of the H blood group antigen.

T Antigen The demonstration of T-antigen expression in breast carcinoma and the loss of blood group isoantigens (A, B, or H antigen) in invasive transitional cell carcinoma prompted inquiry into the correlation between the carbohydrate precursor of the human blood group system MN and the epithelial surface blood group isoantigens. The T antigen has been identified in breast, colon, and gastric carcinomas and was felt to represent a precursor of the human blood group MN glycoproteins. Expression of these antigens was noted in 17 of 22 breast carcinomas, all of which were well differentiated. The 5 carcinomas that failed to demonstrate the antigen were poorly differentiated, possibly implying that the antigen may be further altered as the cell becomes more anaplastic. We have utilized T antigen and ABH antigens in bladder cancer.

The discovery that the T antigen was present on the surface of certain breast carcinomas, particularly those of ductal origin, lead to speculation as to its origin, its significance, and whether it was tumor-associated. Examination of other carcinomas revealed that the T antigen may be present in other epithelial-derived tumors, especially in lung, gastric, and transitional tissues.

Furthermore, it seems that in low-grade transitional cell carcinoma the T antigen is unconcealed, but, in high-grade tumors with a propensity to invade, the antigen disappears. Further studies have been under progress in our laboratory to correlate the grades and stages of bladder cancer with T antigen and with the loss of ABH cell surface antigens; while the ABH antigen loss was significantly associated with a more aggressive tumor and therefore a poorer prognosis, the presence of T antigen was not.

The avidin-biotin technique and the lectin assay have been compared in our laboratory in a double-blind study for detection of the T-antigen transitional carcinoma and to establish clinical protocols for bladder cancer. Thirty-three patients were selected with a total of 43 specimens. Tissues (a total of 43 specimens that showed no pathology) from 26 patients who had no known history of genitourinary disease were used as controls. These tissues were studied for the presence of T antigen utilizing both the avidin-biotin and the lectin techniques. The T antigen was detected in 60% of the specimens with lectin technique, as against 95% with the avidin-biotin method. In 6 patients T antigen was not detected by either method, even after treatment with neuraminidase; these patients had high-grade, high-stage tumors. The study demonstrated that the normal urothelium have concealed T antigen that can be exposed by treating the tissues with neuraminidase. However, the T antigen is unconcealed in low-grade tumor but disappears in high-grade tumor.

Simultaneous Determination of T antigen and ABO Cell Surface Antigens in Transitional Cell Carcinoma   We have studied 17 bladder tumors in an effort to assess the role of simultaneous T antigen and ABH isoantigens. A red cell adherence assay to detect T antigen on deparaffinized slides of transitional cell carcinoma of the bladder was developed. Peanut agglutinin, which has anti-T properties as well as other nonspecific binding sites, was layered over the slides, which were then washed and covered with neuraminidase-treated red cells. Red cell adherence was noted on areas of the bladder tumor that bind plant lectin. This was compared with the SRCA for ABO antigens on the same tissue samples. Of the 17 patients, 14 demonstrated loss of their cell surface ABO antigens. Of the 14, 28% demonstrated expression of the oncofetal T antigen. This would imply that T antigen may be complementary to ABH in predicting potential malignancies of bladder cancer. We are currently evaluating these antigens in bladder cancer in a prospective study utilizing immunoperoxidase.

CELL MARKERS IN PROSTATIC CANCER

The human prostatic acid phosphatase (PAP) is synthesized by the prostatic epithelial cells. It is a specific phosphatase isoenzyme, one of a large molecular family of phosphatases.[4,5,6,16] Significant concentrations of nonprostatic acid phosphatase are normally present in red blood cells, leukocytes, and the bladder. But PAP has been demonstrated to be antigenic. Therefore, specific antibody can be raised against PAP and quantitated by RIA. Currently, the false-positive rate of RIA for PAP prohibits its utilization as a screening test. The reason for these false-positive results is the synthesis of PAP by benign and normal prostatic tissue as shown by IP utilizing monoclonal antibodies to PAP (Table 13–9).

Localization of Acid Phosphatase

Immunohistochemical methods to identify acid phosphatase in prostate cancer tissue have been of increasing use. An indirect immunoperoxidase method can be used to help prove the prostatic origin of primary and metastatic carcinoma. In addition, routine hospital tissue fixation techniques do not alter the PAP. Therefore, the immunoperoxidase staining of acid phosphatase may be performed on routine hospital paraffin tissue blocks. This method can also be used to differentiate invasive bladder tumors, even those that are poorly differentiated, from prostatic carcinoma since transitional cell carcinoma does not stain on IP for PAP. The PAP appears to be more concentrated in nonmalignant prostate tissue. Therefore, immunohistochemical staining of PAP seems to be useful only to identify undifferentiated metastatic adenocarcinoma as prostatic cancer

Table 13–9   Immunocytochemical Localization in Differential Diagnosis of Various Prostatic Diseases

Prostate	Epithelial	Stroma
Normal	+	−
Benign	+	−
Malignant	+	−
Prostatitis	+	−

tumor. Also, we have found that use of the immunohistochemical technique is essential in the differentiation of intraductal transitional cell (ITCC) and adenocarcinoma of the prostate. In a double-blind study of 45 patients with a diagnosis of ITCC of the prostate, we found an 82% histologic error that could be corrected when IP was used (Table 13–10). Based on this we advocate using the immunohistochemical technique before making a diagnosis of ITCC of the prostate, because transitional cell carcinoma is negative and undifferentiated prostatic cancer is generally positive for PAP.

Although acid phosphatase was discovered over 40 years ago, there are still a number of unsolved clinical and basic problems related to its use that require rigorously controlled studies. These problems include: Does acid phosphatase correlate with the bulk of the tumor? Does elevation of this marker mean that there is a spread of the disease of a localized tumor producing this marker, and by removal of the localized disease the marker will disappear? Currently, it is known that this marker may be utilized in monitoring the disease. Also, it may be utilized to make a histopathologic diagnosis of undifferentiated metastatic tumor to be of prostatic origin on IP. There are a number of techniques utilizing various substrates. These substrates include: β glyserophosphate, phenylphosphate, p-nitrophenyl phosphate, phenylphosphate with formaldehyde or L. tartacite or phosphate. There are also a number of immunologic techniques—including various radioimmunoassays, gel precipitation, and counterimmunoelectrophoresis (CIEP)—that are available for detection of PAP.[16]

Although it appears that RIAs are more sensitive than enzymatic techniques, they may have a higher false-positive; therefore, some caution should be exercised in interpretation of the results. The measurement of bone marrow and phosphatase (BMAP) by calimetric assays has no value in the staging of prostatic cancer.

Table 13–10 Immunocytochemical Localization of Acid Phosphatase in Adenocarcinoma and Ductal TCC of Prostate

Total TCC	Positive (PAP)	Negative (PAP)
45	37*	8

*82% histologic errors.

Prostatic-Specific Antigen

Prostatic-specific antigen (PSA), which has a molecular weight of 36 kd, was isolated and characterized in 1979 from prostatic tissue. Antibodies against PSA have been raised by conventional immunologic and monoclonal techniques.[4] This marker can be detected in serum and prostatic cells of patients with prostatic cancer. The major problem, however, has been that this marker is also produced by benign prostatic tissue, rendering it nonspecific for cancer. A number of other markers—including alkaline phosphatase, creatinine kinase, lactic dehydrogenase, carcinoembryonic antigen, and ribonuclease— have been reported. These markers are nonspecific and may occasionally be useful in monitoring therapy when utilized along with other parameters.

In conclusion, elevated serum PAP, PSA, and other markers may be used for monitoring progression or response to therapy in prostatic cancer. Since these markers are not specific, they cannot be used as screening for the diagnosis of this cancer.[6] Furthermore, the elevation of these markers may alert the clinician to search for metastases. The immunocytochemical techniques may help to distinguish cancer of a prostatic origin in an undifferentiated metastatic tumor.

CANCER OF THE COLON

Carcinoembryonic antigen (CEA), a glycoprotein with a molecular weight of 200 kd, was first isolated and characterized in 1965. This tumor marker may be produced in cancers of the colon, pancreas, stomach, and lungs and in certain genitourinary cancers. It may also be elevated in a number of infections and other non-neoplastic diseases. CEA may be helpful in the monitoring and diagnosis of recurrent tumors. Due to false-positive results, it cannot be used as a screening test for colonic cancer.[18]

OTHER CANCERS

Pancreatic oncofetal antigens for the pancreas, placental alkaline phosphatase, ribonuclease, and the acute phase of proteins have been used in a certain number of cancers. These markers are nonspecific and may be helpful when elevated in serum prior to therapy and may also reflect the response to therapy.

REFERENCES

1. Abelev, G. I., Perova, S. D., Khramkova, N. I., Postnikova, Z. A., and Irlin, S. Production of embryonal alpha-globulin by transplantable mouse hepatoma. Transplantation 1: 174, 1964.

2. Abelev, G. I. Alpha-protein in oncogenesis and its association with malignant tumors. Adv. Cancer Res. 14: 295–358, 1971.

3. Bergman, S., and Javadpour, N. The cell surface antigen A, B or O (H) as an indicator of malignant potential in stage A bladder carcinoma: Preliminary report. J. Urol 119: 49, 1978.

4. Chu, T. M. Immunochemical detection of serum prostatic acid phosphatase: Methodology and clinical investigation. Invest. Urol. 15: 319, 1978.

5. Choe, B. K., Pontes, E. J., Morrison, M. D., and Rose, N. R. Human prostatic acid phosphatase: II. A double antibody radioimmunoassay. Arch. Androl. 1: 227, 1978.

6. Cooper, J. F., and Foti, G. A radioimmunoassay for prostatic acid phosphatase. J. Natl. Cancer Inst. 49: 235, 1978.

7. Davidsohn, I. Early immunologic diagnosis and prognosis of carcinoma. Am. J. Clin. Pathol. 57: 715, 1972.

8. DeCenzo, J. M., Howard, P., and Irish, C. E. Antigenic deletion and prognosis of patients with stage A transitional cell bladder carcinoma. J. Urol 114: 874, 1975.

9. Javadpour, N., Brennan, M. F., and Woltering, E. A. Recent advances in adrenal neoplasm. Curr. Probl. Surg. 17: 1, 1980.

10. Javadpour, N. The role of biologic markers in testicular cancer. Cancer 45: 1755, 1980.

11. Javadpour, N. The value of biologic markers in diagnosis and treatment of testicular cancer. Semin. Oncol. 6: 37, 1979.

12. Javadpour, N., McIntire, K. R., Waldmann, T. A., Scardino, P. T., Bergman, S., and Anderson,T. The role of radioimmunoassay of serum alpha-fetoprotein and human chorionic gonadotropin in the intensive chemotherapy and surgery of metastatic testicular tumor. J. Urol 119: 759, 1978.

13. Kurman, R. J., Scardino, P. T., McIntire, K. R., Waldmann, T. A., and Javadpour, N. Cellular localization of alpha-fetoprotein and human chorionic gonadotropin in germ cell tumors of the testis using an indirect immunoperoxidase technique. A new approach to classification utilizing tumor markers. Cancer 40: 2136, 1977.

14. Lange, P. H., Limas, C., and Fraley, E. E. Tissue blood group antigens and prognosis in low-stage transitional cell carcinoma of the bladder. J. Urol. 119: 52, 1978.

15. Millstein, C., Adetugbo, K., and Cowan, N. J. Somatic cell genetics of antibody-secreting cells: Studies of clonal diversified and analysis by cell fusion. Cold Spring Harbor Symp. Quant. Biol. 41: 793, 1977.

16. Pontes, J. E. Biological markers in prostate cancer. J. Urol. 130: 1037, 1983.

17. Perlin, E., Engeler, J. E., Jr., Edson, M., Karp, D., McIntire, K. R., and Waldmann, T. A. The value of serial measurement of both human chorionic gonadotropin and alpha-fetoprotein for monitoring germinal cell tumors. Cancer 37: 215, 1976.

18. Primus, F. J., and Goldenberg, D. M. Functional histopathology of cancer: A review of immunoenzyme histochemistry. In *Methods in Cancer Research*, H. Busch and L. C. Yeoman (editors), Vol. 20, p. 139, 1982.

19. Rosen, W. S., Javadpour, N., Calvert, I., and Kaminska, J. Pregnancy specific beta$_1$, glycoprotein (SP$_1$) is increased in certain non-seminomatous germ cell tumors. J. Natl. Cancer Inst. 62: 1439, 1979.

20. Searle, F., Leake, B. A., Bagshawe, K. D., and Dent, J. Serum-SP$_1$ pregnancy-specific-3 glycoprotein in choriocarcinoma and other neoplastic disease. Lancet 1: 579, 1978.

21. Taylor, C.R., Kurman, R. J., and Warner, N.E. The potential value of immunohistologic technique in classification of ovarian and testicular tumors. Hum. Pathol. 9: 417, 1978.

22. Von Eyben, F. E. Biochemical markers in advanced testicular tumors. Cancer 41: 648, 1978.

23. Vaitukaitis, J. L., Braunstein, G. D., and Ross, G. T. A radioimmunoassay which specifically measures human chorionic gonadotropin in the presence of human luteinizing hormone. Am. J. Obstet. Gynecol. 113: 751, 1972.

24. Waldmann, T. A., and McIntire, K.R. The use of a radioimmunoassay for alpha-fetoprotein in the diagnosis of malignancy. Cancer 34: 1510, 1974.

14

The Current Status
of Studies on Human Tumor
Nucleolar Antigens

Harris Busch

INTRODUCTION

A very fortunate series of technological advances has provided the opportunity for rapid developments in our understanding of nucleolar antigens. In part, utilization of isolated nucleoli, their fractions, and highly purified macromolecular elements has produced immunological opportunities for development of both rabbit polyclonal and mouse hybridoma monoclonal antibodies. These antibodies have been useful for more specific assessment of similarities and differences of antigens in various nuclear and nucleolar extracts as well as for comparisons of samples from different tissues. In addition, the utilization of polyclonal antibodies derived from patients, particularly with scleroderma, has provided identification of individual antigens in human tissues which had not been found earlier. With the aid of more satisfactory two-dimensional protein-separation methods as well as improvements in both silver-staining and immunoblotting, the magnitude of the

These studies were supported by the Cancer Research Center Grant CA-10893, P1, awarded by the National Cancer Institute, Department of Health and Human Services Public Health Service; the Human Tumor Nucleolar Antigen Grant, CA-27534; the Michael E. DeBakey Medical Foundation; the Davidson Fund; the Pauline Sterne Wolff Memorial Foundation; the H. Leland Kaplan Cancer Research Endowment; the Linda and Ronnie Finger Cancer Research Endowment Fund; the William S. Farish Fund; and the Sally Laird Hitchcock Fund.

number of nucleolar antigens is only now becoming apparent (Fig. 14–1).

Advances in the methods for purification of enzymes, particularly RNA polymerase I and topoisomerases, have permitted detailed analysis of their subunits, the importance of site-specific phosphorylation reactions, and the role of special nuclear kinases in activation of

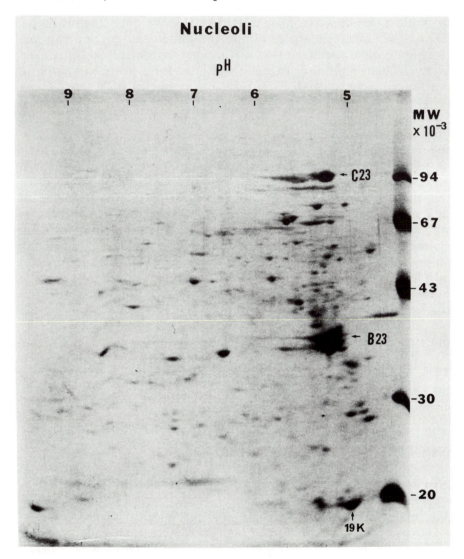

Figure 14–1. Two-dimensional gels of nucleolar proteins showing large numbers of proteins and exceptional densities of proteins C23 (110/5.3) and B23 (37/5.2) (courtesy of Dr. Y. Ahn).

particular enzyme subunits and holo enzymes. The isolation of DNA clones of rDNA gene segments, including the initiation sites, upstream promotors, and "enhancer" regions, offers the opportunity for assessment of transcription initiation factors, site-specific control elements, and upstream activators of rDNA readouts. Along with these developments, the use of antibodies in the light- and electronmicroscopic immunochemical localization of specific antigens has assisted greatly in specification of potential synthetic, packaging, and structural roles for special macromolecules. Improved immunoelectronmicroscopic techniques have sorted out the localization of special proteins involved in nucleolus organizing region (NOR) binding, the silver-staining reactions, and the spatial segregation of nucleolar events. These developments have set the stage for expansion of our information base for development of more cogent concepts of the structures and functions of macromolecular complexes such as the nucleolonemas in the nucleolus.

As information in these fields continues to increase, answers will be forthcoming as to the biological roles of specific macromolecules in the very complex but highly ordered function of the nucleolus in production, maturation, and transport of preribosomal particles as well as the mechanisms for articulation of these functions with the synthetic biological events in the cells which cannot proceed in the absence of new ribosome synthesis. Investigations into such crucial cellular processes as control of the rDNA machinery, the role of cyclic nucleotides and other messengers in activation of this apparatus, and the mechanisms for integration of nucleolar rRNA biosynthesis with biosynthesis of preribosomal and ribosomal proteins are in an early but clearly exciting stage.

Elements of the synthetic reactions of the nucleolus are listed in Table 14–1, and the nucleolar antigens that are of current interest are listed in Table 14–2.

NUCLEOLAR PHOSPHOPROTEINS

Nucleolar Phosphoproteins B23 and C23

Two major nucleolar phosphoproteins, B23 and C23, were found by older methods for two-dimensional chromatography of nucleolar proteins (Orrick et al., 1973; Kang et al., 1974; Olson et al., 1974). With either *in vivo* or *in vitro* labeling of the nucleolar proteins with ^{32}P, these two major proteins were very highly phosphorylated. Recent studies with improved two-dimensional gel methods have confirmed

Table 14–1 Synthetic Elements of the Nucleolus

1. The rDNA template
2. The enzyme RNA polymerase I
3. A variety of systems that make available nucleoside triphosphates, which are necessary as precursors of the RNA
4. Processing enzymes that produce many modifications of the RNA
5. Cleavage enzymes that split the newly synthesized RNA into precursors of the 28 and 18S rRNA
6. Trimming enzymes involved in preparation of the final product
7. Specific proteins involved in structural interaction with the rRNA precursors to produce the final conformationally correct state of the RNA

Table 14–2 Nucleolar Antigens

A. Enzymes
    1. RNA polymerase I subunits
    2. Topoisomerase
    3. Nuclear Kinases
        a. "glycogen synthase" kinase
        b. NKI
        c. NKII

B. S-Phase Antigens
    1. PCNA
    2. Protein 86/7.1, a DNA binding S-phase antigen
    3. SSB (La)

C. Nucleolar Phosphoproteins
    1. Protein 110/5.2 (C23), a silver-staining, DNA-binding protein
    2. Protein 37/5.2 (B23), a RNP particle protein, high mobility

D. Human Tumor Nucleolar Antigens
    1. Protein 68/6.3, a "decision point" antigen? U1 RNP protein
    2. Antigen 52/5.3, a "mutated protein"?
    3. Holo C23? Holo topoisomerase I

E. Human Liver Nucleolar Antigens
    1. Protein 55/7.2
    2. 70-kd topoisomerase I
    3. 76-kd protein C23

F. Other Antigens of Interest
    1. Protein P19
    2. 145-kd antigenic phosphoprotein

these earlier results (M. Son, R. K. Busch, W. S. Spohn, and H. Busch, unpublished). With commonly employed fractionation techniques, it was possible to isolate these proteins in highly purified, partially denatured forms, by HCl extraction of nucleoli, various precipitation steps, and separation on DEAE cellulose in the presence of 6 M urea. Recently, improved separations have been done under more native but still unsatisfactory conditions, such as treatment of the samples with 3 M LiCl/4 M urea.

The availability of such highly purified proteins permitted the analysis of their amino acid composition and termini and preliminary sequence studies on their peptides (Table 14–3, Fig. 14–2). Some regions of these phosphoproteins were found to be very acidic; one peptide of protein 110/5.2 (mol wt × 10^{-3}/pI) (C23) had a large number of glutamic and aspartic acid residues and three phosphoserines (Fig. 14–2). Similar highly acidic peptides were found in digests of protein 37/5.2 (B23). Protein 110/5.2 (C23) was found to have 1.3 mol% N^G,N^G-dimethylarginine (Lischwe et al., 1982).

Each of these proteins was utilized for development of polyclonal rabbit antibodies and monoclonal mouse antibodies. These antibodies,

Table 14–3 Amino Acid Compositions of Nucleolar Phosphoproteins

Amino acid	Protein 110/5.2 (C23) (mol %)	Protein 37/5.2 (B23) (mol%)
Asx	12.0	15.0
Thr	5.6	3.8
Ser	5.4	6.8
Glx	18.5	15.2
Pro	5.3	5.8
Gly	10.0	7.4
Ala	10.3	5.7
1/2-Cys	0.0	—
Val	6.0	7.2
Met	1.2	2.6
Ile	2.5	3.2
Leu	5.6	7.1
Tyr	0.8	1.3
Phe	3.5	2.6
Lys	11.8	11.1
His	0.5	2.4
Trp	0.0	—
Arg	2.9	3.1

```
                5                    10
Ala-Ala-Pro-Ala-Ala-Pro-Ala-Ser-Glu-Asp-Glu-
                15                   20
Asp-Glu-Glu-Asp-Asp-Asp-Asp-Glu-Asp-Asp-Asp-Asp-
        25                   30
    Asp-Ser-Gln-Glu-Ser-Glu-Glu-Glu-Asp-Glu-Glu-
            35                   40
        Val-Met-Glu-Ile-Thr-Pro-Ala-Lys (1)
```

Figure 14–2. Amino acid sequence of a highly acidic peptide (C23–1) of protein 110/5.2 (C23).

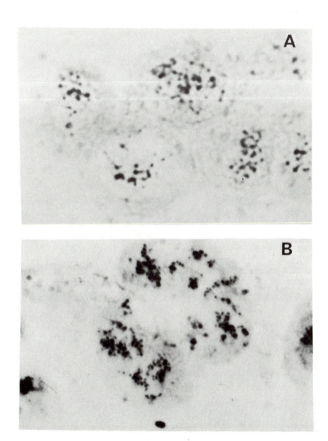

Figure 14–3. Similarities of silver staining of Novikoff hepatoma nuclei (*B*) and immunoperoxidase staining (*A*) of Novikoff hepatoma ascites cells with antibodies to protein C23.

which were very specific as shown by Ouchterlony gels and immuno-blotting procedures, were almost totally localized to nucleoli (Fig. 14–3). Their nucleolar localization differed in that protein C23 was found in the nucleolonemas where its localization corresponded precisely to that of the nucleolar "silver-staining" proteins (Lischwe et al., 1979). Indeed, pretreatment of the nucleoli with anti-C23 antibodies blocked the silver-staining reaction, but pretreatment of the nucleoli with anti-B23 antibodies did not inhibit silver staining at all. In studies on ring-shaped nucleoli of human lymphocytes, silver staining was found in the central fibrillar region of the nucleolus, as was the immuno-staining for protein C23. On the other hand, immunostaining for protein B23 was in the surrounding region at the nucleolar periphery (Smetana et al., 1984). Accordingly, protein C23 is the major nucleolar silver-staining protein.

Studies on the localization of these proteins in mitosis (Ochs et al., 1983) showed that, in prophase, protein B23 was "mobile," it distributed through the nucleoplasm, while protein 110/5.3 (C23) stayed with the nucleolus as it decreased in size. Earlier studies with silver staining of chromosomes with "secondary constrictions" showed that as the nucleolus decreased its functional activity, the silver-staining proteins tended to localize to the NOR regions of the chromosomes where they were highly specifically localized. Indeed, these proteins are the only proteins that are known to remain with the condensing mitotic chromosomes in the specific localization in which they are destined to function (Goodpasture and Bloom, 1975; Howell, 1977).

In the process of reformation of the nucleolus in telophase, protein C23 was found to accumulate in "prenucleolar bodies" which then coalesced to form the nucleolus (Busch and Smetana, 1970). Protein B23 reentered the nucleoli in late telophase (Ochs et al., 1983). These results agreed with earlier studies which indicated that protein C23 is the silver-staining nucleolar organizer region protein (Lischwe et al., 1979).

NOR Silver-staining Proteins

The development of the silver-staining procedure by Goodpasture and Bloom (1975), and its use for visualization of the NORs of chromosomes, led to development of a great deal of information on the numbers and types of NORs of various species and selected cell lines. Initially, little concern was directed to the question of what was being stained by the selective procedure of Goodpasture and Bloom (1975).

However, Howell (1977) demonstrated that the silver-staining product was neither DNA, RNA, nor histones. Treatment of various samples with DNase or RNase did not eliminate the silver-staining reactions. Removal of histones ("dehistonization") was followed by little change in the silver-staining reaction.

Howell (1977) concluded that the silver-staining reaction resulted from specific NOR proteins that were "nonhistone nuclear proteins" or possibly "acidic nuclear proteins" that are distinguished from the histones, which are basic and occur in large amounts throughout the nucleosome arrays.

In studies from our laboratory (Lischwe et al., 1979), as part of the analysis of nucleolar proteins separated on two-dimensional polyacrylamide gels, two major proteins were found that exhibited the same type of silver-staining observed with the histological procedure of Goodpasture and Bloom (1975). As correctly predicted by Howell (1977), both were acidic nonhistone proteins; the larger protein was protein C23, the smaller one was protein B23. As noted above, both were highly acidic and contained very acidic peptide chains, which were particularly rich in glutamic acid and aspartic acid. In addition, some of these regions were punctuated with phosphoserine residues (Mamrack et al., 1979).

In a particularly definitive study (Satoh and Busch, 1983), it was demonstrated that the silver-staining reaction utilized by Goodpasture and Bloom (1975) as modified by Howell (1977) and later improved by Smetana et al. (1979) had a high order of specificity for phosphoserine and phosphothreonine residues. The former are particularly common in these proteins. Accordingly, it should be apparent that the silver-staining procedure which so beautifully demonstrates the NOR regions of the chromosomes derives its "specificity" from the high concentrations of phosphoserine and phosphothreonine in these proteins and from the high concentrations of these proteins in special locations.

Initially, most of the studies done with these silver-staining methods related to the extremely important task of localizing and defining the NOR-containing chromosomes in metaphase. We reasoned that, in interphase, there should be evidence for these proteins particularly in cells with highly active NOR regions. When the same methods were applied to the interphase cells, very remarkable differences were found both for the appearance of the silver stains for cells of different tissues and, in addition, during various states of mitosis (Figs. 14–4 to 14–6).

The widest differences were noted between peripheral lymphocytes (Busch et al., 1979; Smetana et al., 1979) in which there was

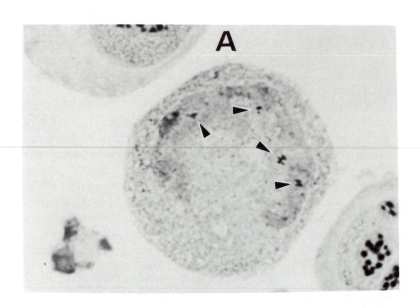

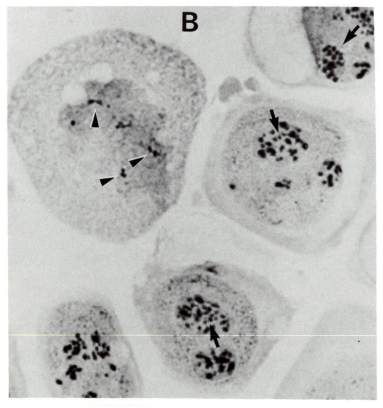

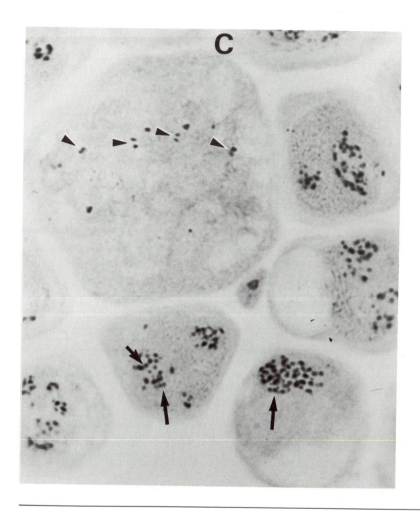

Figure14–4. (*A*): Novikoff hepatoma cell in metaphase containing four pairs of dense granules (arrowheads). (*B*): A similar cell in metaphase showing the presence of three pairs of sense granules (arrowheads) and three cells with rows of nucleolar dense granules (arrows). (*C*): Large Novikoff hepatoma cell in metaphase containing several doublets of dense granules in metaphase cells (×1,400).

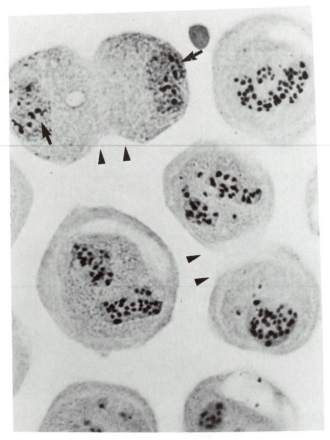

Figure 14–5. Novikoff hepatoma cells in telophase (double arrowheads) showing multiple granules (arrows) in nuclei of the daughter cells. The numbers of granules in these cells range from 28 to 67. In adjacent interphase cells, rows of granules are noted. In a pair of cells apparently in very late telophase, similar rows of granules are visible (×1,400).

frequently either one or occasionally no silver-stained granules and tumor cells which had as many as 50–60 granules per nucleolus (Figs. 14–4, 14–5). Also, notable differences were found between the appearance of the granules; i.e. in some instances they appeared to be individual units well separated from adjacent granules, and in other instances they appeared to be part of a reticulum (Figs. 14–6). With the increasing evidence that the silver-staining protein is in fact phosphoprotein C23 (Ochs et al., 1983; Spector, Ochs, and Busch, 1984), the role of this protein becomes of particularly great interest. Another protein, topoisomerase I (110/8.4), has a similar molecular weight but a different isoelectric point. The question arises as to whether these proteins may be related and whether a protein C23 has topoisomerase activity which could maintain the rDNA in extended configuration. This question is currently under study. Some interesting cross-bearing immunoreactivity has been demonstrated between these two proteins.

ANTINUCLEOLAR ANTIBODIES

Experimental Production of Polyclonal Rabbit Antinucleolar Antibodies

To determine whether nucleoli or their subfractions could induce immunological responses in rabbits, nucleoli were prepared by standard procedures developed in earlier studies in this laboratory (Busch and Smetana, 1970) and injected into rabbits in Freund's adjuvant (R. K. Busch et al., 1974). The sites of injection were initially subcutaneous and intramuscular, but in later studies injection into footpads was found to be particularly useful. The initial testing for the immunological response was by the indirect immunofluorescence assays of Hilger et al. (1972). Ouchterlony gel analysis and immunoelectrophoresis were employed to determine whether precipitating antibodies were produced (R. K. Busch and Busch, 1977).

Monoclonal Antibodies

In Vivo Immunization Balb/c mice were immunized with RNP particles and the DE–0.25 M fraction of the Tris extract of Namalwa cells. The mice were injected subcutaneously six times over a period of 3 months, each time with 0.3–0.5 mg antigen mixed with FCA. The last injections were given intraperitoneally daily for 4 days before the spleen was used for hybridization.

In Vitro Immunization For *in vitro* immunization (Towbin et al., 1979), single-cell suspensions were made from mouse spleens; the red cells were lysed with 0.17 M NH$_4$Cl. Spleen cells were incubated for 5 days in 10 ml DMEM (Gibco #380–2430) containing 1 mM sodium

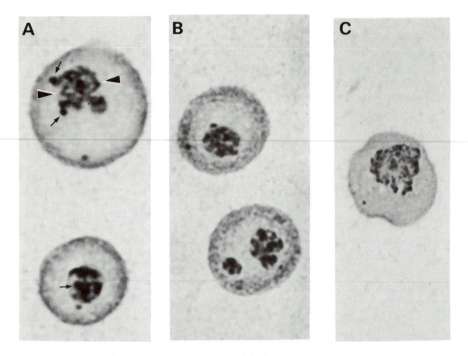

Figure 14–6. (*A*): Silver stain of spread liver cell nuclei showing a silver-stained reticulum (arrowheads) connecting a few silver-stained granules (arrows) (×1,250). (*B*): Two liver nuclei, one with a single granule; in the other, the denser silver-stained granules are associated with a less dense reticulum (×1,000). (*C*): Six-hour regenerating liver showing increased silver-staining reticulum of the enlarged nucleolus (×1,000). (*D*): Eighteen-hour regenerating liver; markedly enlarged nucleoli are noted in these cells, which contain larger numbers of granules (arrows) associated with the nucleolar silver-stained reticulum (pointers) (×1,250).

pyruvate, and 5 μg/ml streptomycin with 2% rabbit serum (Kappa Scientific, Escondido, CA) to which 10 ml mixed thymocyte culture medium and 100 g of protein B23 were added. After a 5-day incubation period, the cells were used for hybridization.

Myeloma Cell Lines Two mouse myeloma cell lines were used in these experiments; both are variants of P3 × 63 Ag cell lines. P3-X-63-Ag8.653, which is a nonsecretor line, was a generous gift from Dr. C. Reading at M. D. Anderson Hospital and Tumor Institute, Houston, TX. NS, which secretes K light chain was obtained from The Salk Institute, Cell Distribution Center, San Diego, CA. The cells were

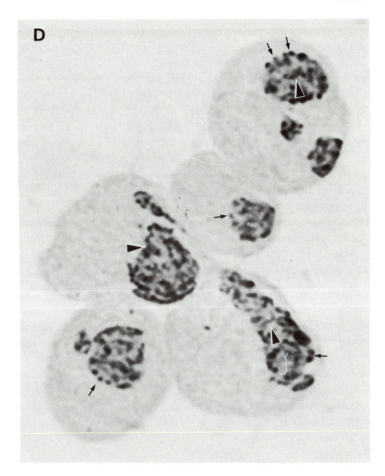

grown in supplemented DMEM medium containing 15% FCS and 20 μg/ml 8-azaguanine (Sigma Chem. Co., St. Louis, MO).

Hybridization   Approximately 50×10^6 spleen cells from a mouse immunized with Namalwa DE–0.25 M fraction were fused with 2×10^7 myeloma 653 cells with 30% PEG (mol wt 1.54 kd; J. T. Baker, Phillipsburg, NJ). After fusion, the cells were diluted in supplemented RPMI 1640 medium (Gibco #320–1875) containing 15% FCS, 10^{-4} M hypoxanthine (Sigma), 1.6×10^{-5} M thymidine (Sigma), 4×10^{-7} M aminopterin (ICN Pharmaceuticals, Inc., Cleveland, OH) (HAT), and normal spleen cells obtained from an unimmunized Balb/c mouse (1 ×

10^6 cells/ml). The cell suspension was divided into two 24-well cluster plates. Half the medium was replaced with fresh medium on days 1 and 2 and then every three days for 2 weeks.

In other experiments, about 50×10^6 spleen cells from a mouse immunized with nucleolar antigens from Novikoff hepatoma were fused with 1×10^7 NS_1 cells with 30% PEG. After fusion the cells were suspended in supplemented DMEM–HAT medium containing 15% FCS and divided into four 96-well cluster plates. Half the culture medium was replaced by fresh medium as described above.

Alternatively the spleen cells which were stimulated *in vitro* for 5 days were fused with about 10×10^6 myeloma 653 cells with 50% PEG. After fusion, the cells were suspended in supplemented DMEM–HAT medium containing 2% rabbit serum and normal spleen cells from a mouse (previously treated with 0.5 ml pristane at a concentration of 1 $\times 10^6$ cells/ml) and divided into four 96-well microtiter plates. The medium was not changed for 2 weeks, at which time the cultures were ready for testing.

Cloning of Hybridoma Cultures, Production and Purification of Monoclonal Antibodies   Those hybridoma cultures that reacted positively were subcloned by the limiting dilution method. The clones were grown either as *in vitro* cultures or as ascites tumors in Balb/c mice previously injected with 0.5 ml of 1,4-tetramethyl pentadecane (pristane) (Aldrich Chemical Co., Milwaukee, Wi). The antibodies from the culture medium or the ascites fluid were purified by precipitation with 50% ammonium sulfate.

Protein B23   The mouse monoclonal antibody against protein B23 was prepared by *in vitro* immunization. A single-cell suspension from the spleen of a CD-1 mouse was incubated in a 150-cm^3 flask containing 20 ml DMEM (Gibco), 10 ml of a 2-day supernatant from a mixed lymphocyte reaction culture, 2% rabbit serum (Quadroma, Inc.), and 400 μg of protein B23 isolated from nucleoli by DEAE cellulose column chromatography (Lischwe et al., 1981). Cells were allowed to incubate for 5 days, at which time they were harvested and fused to the parental myeloma cell line, P3-X63-Ag8.653 (Kearney et al., 1979). All hybrids were assayed for specific antibody production by the enzyme-linked immunosorbent assay (ELISA) (Engvall, 1980) and the positive hybrids were cloned twice by limiting dilution. Monoclonal anti-protein B23 antibody was obtained from the supernatant fluid of hybrid cells grown in spinner culture by precipitation with 50% ammonium sulfate. The resulting monoclonal antibody was determined to be IgG_1-Kappa utilizing a Zymed kit for typing (Zymed Laboratories).

Tissues Employed and Immunofluorescence Microscopy

In the initial studies, nucleoli from the Novikoff hepatoma cells and normal rat liver cells were employed as the immunogens. In both cases, the rabbits produced remarkably specific antisera which specifically reacted with the nucleoli and exhibited only comparatively minor extranucleolar reactions (R. K. Busch et al., 1974). When these antisera were not absorbed with other tissues, cross reactions were found so that the anti-liver nucleolar antisera produced indirect immunofluorescence in the Novikoff hepatoma cells, and the anti-hepatoma nucleolar antisera also produced immunofluorescence in the liver cells (Fig. 14–7). In addition to these cross reactions, these antisera also produced positive immunofluorescence in the normal kidney and in Walker tumor cells (Fig. 14–8).

Tumor Specificity

Ouchterlony gel analysis was used to evaluate the similarity and difference in the immunoprecipitin bands formed between the tumor and liver nucleolar antigens and their corresponding antibodies (R. K. Busch and Busch, 1977). This study was initially designed to determine whether there were antigenic differences in proteins of various fractions extracted from the nucleoli of these cells with different extractants. However, a striking finding was that there were nucleolar antigens in the Novikoff tumor (Fig. 14–9) that were not present in the liver, and vice versa. When the liver nucleolar antigens were reacted with the anti-liver antibodies, three immunoprecipitin bands were formed. When the anti-tumor nucleolar antibodies were reacted with the tumor nucleolar antigens, a single dense immunoprecipitin band was formed. Both findings were surprising. No evidence was obtained from cross reactivity of these tumor and liver antigens.

It seemed likely that if the immunizations were continued for a longer period, more antibodies would be formed. Immunoelectrophoresis (Fig. 14–10) showed that up to 14 antigens were detectable in nucleoli of Novikoff hepatoma ascites cells (Davis et al., 1978). The antisera to normal liver nucleoli detected 10 of the 14 antigens detected by the anti-Novikoff hepatoma nucleolar antiserum. Analysis

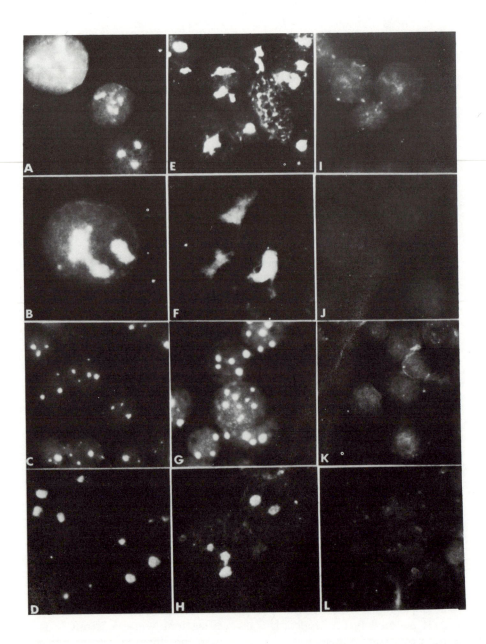

Figure 14–7. Photomicrographs of nuclei analyzed with antisera or normal sera by the indirect immunofluorescent technique. Tumor antinucleolar antisera were incubated with Novikoff hepatoma nuclei (A, ×1,800; B, ×4,500) and liver nuclei (C, ×1,800; D, ×4,500). Liver antinucleolar antisera were incubated with Novikoff hepatoma nuclei (E, ×1,800; F, ×4,500) and liver

of fetal tissues, particularly fetal liver, showed that there were antigens common to the tumor and fetal liver that were not present in the adult liver. Earlier results (Yeoman et al., 1976) showed that there are fetal nuclear antigens in tumors that are not present in normal adult rat tissues. A variety of "oncofetal" and "oncoembryonic" antigens have been studied in great detail in other systems (Fishman and Busch, 1979).

Absorption of the Antibodies

After absorption of the rabbit antisera with extracts of nucleoli and nuclei (Fig. 14–11), bright nucleolar fluorescence was still observed in the Novikoff hepatoma cells after absorption of the antiserum to Novikoff hepatoma nucleoli with normal liver nuclear products. However, the absorbed antiserum did not produce nucleolar fluorescence in the normal liver nucleoli. When the antisera to normal liver nucleoli had been absorbed with Novikoff hepatoma nuclear products to the point that no nucleolar fluorescence was evident, they still produced bright immunofluorescence in the normal liver nucleoli (Davis et al., 1978).

These studies with antinucleolar antisera—whether by immunoprecipitin band analysis, analysis of immunoelectrophoresis patterns, or evaluation of the results of absorption by immunofluorescence—indicated that antigens in the nucleoli of Novikoff hepatomas differed from those of normal liver nucleoli, and vice versa.

What Are These Tumor Nucleolar Antigens?

To advance the studies on these antigens, it was essential to purify one or more of the antigens to homogeneity. Initially the nucleoli were

---

nuclei (*G*, ×1,800; *H*, ×4,500). Normal rabbit sera were incubated with Novikoff hepatoma nuclei (*I*, ×1,800) and liver nuclei (*J*, ×1,800). Tumor antinucleolar antiserum absorbed with Novikoff tumor nucleoli was incubated with Novikoff nuclei (*K*, ×1,800), and liver antinucleolar antiserum absorbed with liver nucleoli was incubated with liver nuclei (*L*, ×1,800). (From Busch, R. K., Daskal, I., Spohn, W. H., Kellermayer, M., and Busch, H., Cancer Res., 34, 2362, 1974.)

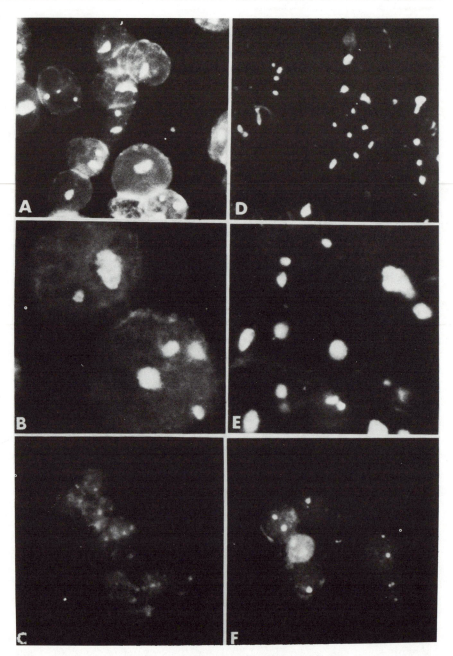

Figure 14–8. Photomicrographs of nuclei analyzed with antisera by the indirect immunofluorescent technique. Novikoff hepatoma antinucleolar antisera were incubated with Walker tumor nuclei (A, ×1,800; B, ×4,500) and kidney nuclei (C, ×1,800). Liver nucleolar antisera were incubated with Walker nuclei (D, ×1,800; E, ×4,500) and kidney nuclei (F, ×1,800). (From Busch, R. K., Daskal, I., Spohn, W. H., Kellermayer, M., and Busch, H., Cancer Res. 34, 2362, 1974.)

isolated from the Novikoff hepatoma and subjected to a series of extractions generally employed for chromatin (Rothblum et al., 1977). In the first of these steps, the nucleoli were extracted with an approximately isotonic extractant (0.075 M NaCl/0.025 M EDTA/pH 8) designed to remove divalent ions important to maintenance of the nucleolar ultrastructure. This step is one that has some advantages but is now known to produce alterations of complex structures and some enzymes. The nucleoli were then exposed to buffers of very low ionic strength (0.01 M Tris HCl, pH 7.8) designed to permit the chromatin to swell and to release nuclear particules entrapped in the chromatin. A number of nucleolar components such as RNA polymerases and kinases are very soluble in this low ionic strength buffer. Subsequent extraction procedures used a variety of salt solutions of higher ionic strengths, e.g. 0.35, 0.6, 1.0 M NaCl as well as 3 M NaCl/7 M urea. Even this last solution did not completely solubilize all the nucleolar elements, but the residue was very small (Rothblum et al., 1977; Marashi et al., 1979).

Studies on the major antigens of the Novikoff rat hepatoma nucleoli showed that more than 50% of the antigens were not extracted with either the isotonic buffer or the low ionic strength buffers employed, but they were with the 0.6 M NaCl extract which followed these initial extraction steps (Marashi et al., 1979). With affinity columns for binding the antigens, further purification of the antigen was accomplished; elution was done with putrescine at pH 11. Hydroxylapatite chromatography was used for final purification. A Coomassie® blue stained gel (Fig. 14–12A) showed that a single protein was present; it had a molecular weight of approximately 60 kd and an isoelectric point of approximately 5.0 (Marashi et al., 1979).

This was the first purification of a specific nucleolar antigen from a tumor. When the antigen in this spot was subjected to "rocket" electrophoresis, a distinctive "rocket" (Fig. 14–12B) was produced (Marashi et al., 1979). It will be of interest to determine what similarities exist between the 60-kd antigen of the Novikoff hepatoma cells and antigens of the human tumors (Chan et al., 1980).

Liver Nucleolar Antigens

There are antigens in normal liver nucleoli that differ from those of tumor nucleoli. Abelev et al. (1979) reported that liver-specific antigens exist. A 20-kd protein was reported to be rat liver specific. Studies of R. K. Busch and Busch (1977) on rat liver nuclear antigens showed that two nucleolar antigens in rat liver were not present in the Novikoff hepatoma (Fig. 14–13).

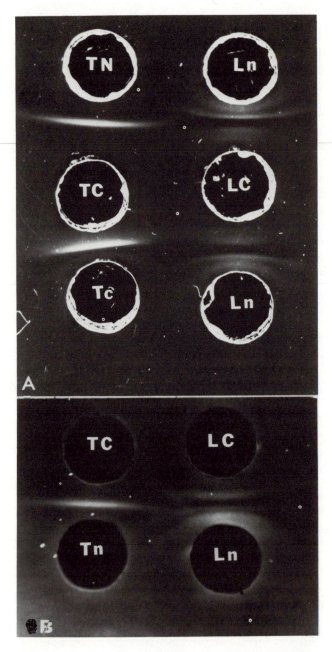

Figure 14–9. (*A*): Immunodiffusion plate which contains a 0.6 *M* NaCl extract of tumor nuclear chromatin TC in the left center well and liver chromatin LC in the right center well (300–40 μg) as antigens. The TC formed precipitin

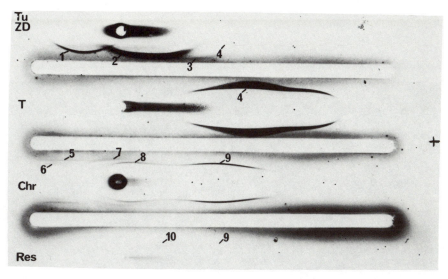

Figure 14–10. Immunoelectrophoretic profile of tumor nucleolar antigens. The Zubay-Doty (ZD), low-ionic strength Tris (T), 0.6 *M* NaCl extract of chromatin (Chr) and 2 *M* NaCl/5 *M* urea extract (Res) of Novikoff hepatoma nucleoli were analyzed by immunoelectrophoresis. The immunoelectrophoresis slide was presoaked in running buffer for 2 h. ZD (20 *μ*g) and 40 *μ*g of the other antigens were placed in the antigen wells. After electrophoresis at 100 V for 30 min, 50 *μ*l of anti-tumor nucleolar immunoglobulin at 80 mg protein per ml were placed in the antiserum troughs, and the precipitin arcs that formed in 24 h were stained with Coomassie® brilliant blue. (From Davis, F. M., Busch, R. K., Yeoman, L. C., and Busch, H., Cancer Res. 38, 1906, 1978).

bands with tumor nuclear (TN) and tumor chromatin (Tc) antibodies. The LC antigen formed at least three precipitin bands with the liver nucleolar (Ln) antibodies. The antibody wells contained 33 *μ*l. (*B*): Immunodiffusion plate which contains 0.6 *M* NaCl extracts of tumor nuclear chromatin TC in the top-left well and liver nuclear chromatin LN in the top-right well (300–400 *μ*g). The tumor chromatin antigen formed a precipitin band with the tumor nucleolar antiserum (Tn). The LCAg antigen formed at least three precipitin bands with the liver nucleolar antibodies (Ln). The antibody wells contain 33 *μ*l. (From Busch, R. K. and Busch, H., Tumori, 63, 347, 1977.)

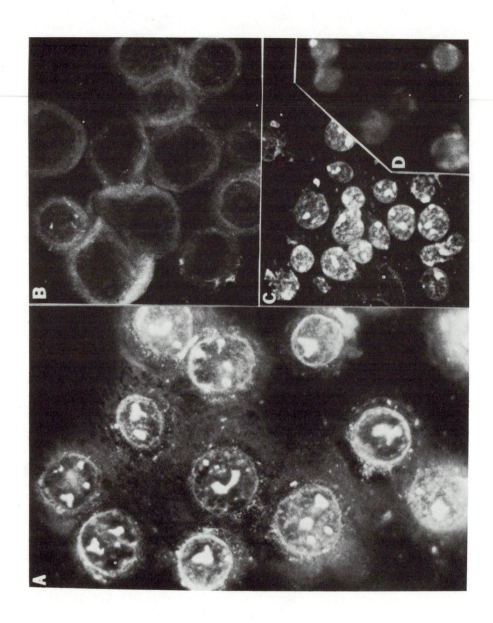

One liver antigen (Ln-1) was found in liver and kidney. Of the total antigen Ln-1, 99% was present in the cytosol and only 1% was in the nucleus. Approximately 10% was in the chromatin, from which it was extracted with 0.6 M NaCl.

When purified on affinity columns and eluted with 0.2 M Tris–HCl/0.05 M NaCl, pH 11, the antigens contained three RNA bands which were rich in guanylic and cytidylic acids. Their approximate molecular weights were 200 kd (approximately 600 nucleotides). These antigens could be snRNPs (small nuclear ribonucleoprotein particles) of undefined structure or function.

Antigen Ln-2 was found in several tissues, including spleen, Novikoff hepatoma, normal liver, and regenerating liver. Antigen Ln-3 was found in the normal and regenerating rat liver, but it was not present in the other tissues studied. Further characterization of these antigens and their associated RNA species will aid in the definition of their nucleolar and cellular functions.

mRNA for Nucleolar Antigens

To determine whether some polysomes and their mRNA for synthesis of nucleolar antigens were unique (Reiners et al., 1980), the antibodies to the Novikoff hepatoma nucleolar proteins were first absorbed with liver nucleolar proteins (Davis et al., 1978). They were then subjected to affinity chromatography on Sepharose-4B columns containing normal rat liver proteins to remove the nonspecific antibodies. The IgG which did not bind to the liver Sepharose column after 12 h of incubation at 4°C was then applied to a column containing Novikoff hepatoma nucleolar proteins. The IgG which did not bind was discarded, and the bound IgG was eluted with 1 M NaCl/3 M urea/0.2 M Tris–HCl, pH 7.5. These IgGs, which constituted 1–2% of the total IgG, were then labeled with [125]I.

Figure 14–11. Photomicrographs of cells tested with preabsorbed antinucleolar antisera by the indirect immunofluorescent technique. Preabsorbed antitumor nucleolar antiserum was incubated with Novikoff hepatoma cells (*A*) or with normal liver cells (*D*). Preabsorbed anti-liver nucleolar antiserum was incubated with Novikoff hepatoma cells (*B*) or with normal liver cells (*C*). (All photomicrographs, ×1,800.) (From Davis, F. M., Busch, R. K., Yeoman, L. C. and Busch, H., Cancer Res., 38, 1906, 1978.)

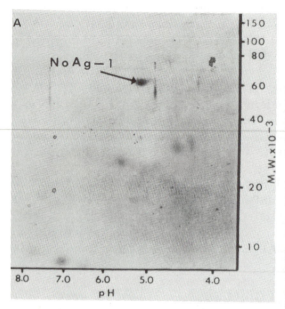

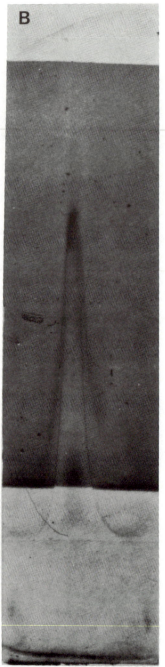

Figure 14–12. (*A*): Two-dimensional gel electrophoresis of NoAg-1, the tumor antigen. NoAg-1 (10 μg) was added to lyophilized sample buffer [9 M urea/2% ampholines (3/10 Biolyte®)/ 2 M dithiothreitol] and subjected to two-dimensional electrophoresis. (From Marashi, F., Davis, F. M., Busch, R. K., Savage, H. E., and Busch, H., Cancer Res. 39, 59, 1979.) (*B*): Rocket immunoelectrophoresis of NoAg-1 from the SDS:polyacrylamide slab gel. A 1-cm^2 area containing the single NoAg-1 spot from SDS:polyacrylamide slab gel was placed on a blank agarose gel and electrophoresed into antibody-containing agarose gel containing antinucleolar antiserum (1.0 mg/ml). A strip of agarose gel containing 1.5% Triton® X-100 was placed between the blank and antibody-containing agarose gel to trap SDS and release NoAg-1.

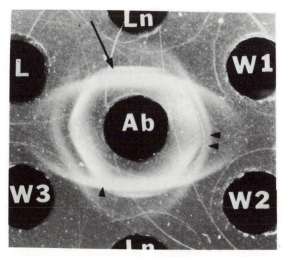

Figure 14–13. Immunodiffusion plate with Ig from antiserum to liver nucleoli in the center well. The following antigens were in the outer wells: the 0.15 *M* NaCl extract of liver nucleoli (Ln); the supernatants from the three consecutive 0.15 *M* NaCl extracts of liver pressate designated w1, w2, and w3; and the 0.15 *M* NaCl extract (1 h) of the "washed" liver pressate (L). The following immunoprecipitin bands formed between the nucleolar antibodies (Ab) and the antigens were: Ln-1 (arrow) with antigens w1, w2, w3, L, and Ln: Ln-2 (arrowhead) with antigen Ln; and Ln-3 (double arrowheads) with antigens w1, w2, w3, and L. Extraction of liver pressate with 0.15 *M* NaCl readily solubilized antigens Ln-1 and Ln-3. (From Busch, R. K., Reddy, R. C., Henning, D. H., and Busch, H., Proc. Soc. Exp. Biol. Med., 160, 185, 1979).

These antibodies bound readily with a sharply defined plateau to the polysomes of the Novikoff hepatoma cells (Fig. 14–14) but not at all to the polysomes of the normal liver cells (Reiners et al., 1980). Binding of the labeled antibodies to the regenerating liver polysomes was about one-third that of the Novikoff hepatoma. Competition studies (Fig. 14–15) showed that the tumor nucleolar and nuclear extracts effectively competed with the antibody that bound to the polysomes but the normal liver nuclear and nucleolar extracts did not compete. These studies showed a high order of specificity of the interactions of the antinucleolar antibody and IgG fractions with the tumor polysomes and the tumor products from nucleoli and nuclei (Reiners et al., 1980). In recent studies, Satoh and Busch (1983) confirmed these results and specified difference proteins by two-dimensional gel electrophoresis.

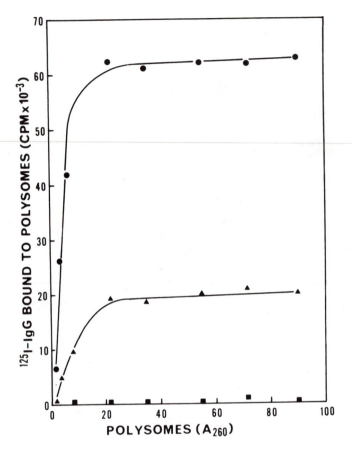

Figure 14–14. Titration of ^{125}I-labeled IgG with variable amounts of polysomes. Iodinated absorbed affinity chromatography–purified anti-tumor nucleolar IgG (2.5 .003 10^5 cpm) was incubated with tumor (●), regenerating liver (▲), and normal liver (■) polysomes. Over the range of polysomes titered, 5,800–6,600 cpm were precipitated in the absence of Mg^{2+} and were subtracted from the values for sedimented polysome–IgG complexes. (From Reiners, J. J., Jr., Davis, F. M., and Busch, H., Cancer Res. 40, 1367, 1980.)

HUMAN MALIGNANT TUMORS

Nucleolar Antigens in Human Tumors

Although the studies on the nucleolar antigens of the rodent tumors and nontumor tissues indicated that there were specific differences in these nucleolar proteins, attempts to extend these studies to human neoplasms showed that human tumor nucleoli did not exhibit bright

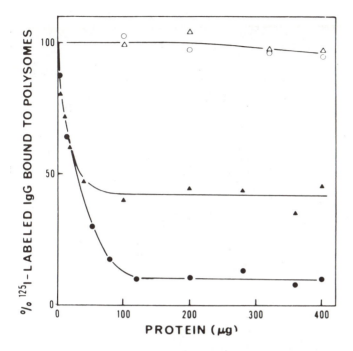

Figure 14–15. Competition by nuclear and nucleolar extracts with tumor polysomes for ^{125}I-labeled anti-tumor IgG. Competition by extracts with 20 A_{260} units of tumor polysomes for iodinated absorbed affinity chromatography–purified anti-tumor nucleolar IgG (2.5×10^5 cpm) was performed. ●, tumor nuclear extract; ▲, nucleolar 0.075 *M* NaCl/0.025 *M* EDTA extract; ○, normal rat liver nuclear extract; △, nucleolar 0.075 *M* NaCl/0.025 *M* EDTA extract. One-hundred-percent precipitation is represented by 71,000 cpm. Data are uncorrected for the 6,500 cpm (9% of maximum) sedimented in the absence of Mg^{2+}. (From Reiners, J. J., Jr., Davis, F. M., and Busch, H., Cancer Res., 40, 1367, 1980.)

fluorescence when treated with antibodies to rat tumor nucleoli. When nucleolar preparations and nuclear Tris extracts (0.01 *M* Tris–HCl, pH 8.0) of human HeLa cells were used as immunogens, the immunized rabbits developed anti–human tumor nucleolar antibodies (Davis et al., 1979; Busch et al., 1979).

Figures 14–16 and 14–17 show a bright nucleolar fluorescence (Busch et al., 1979) in a broad array of human malignant tumors following incubation of cells or sections with rabbit anti–human tumor nucleolar antibodies. These tumors include carcinomas of many types, a variety of sarcomas, and many hematological neoplasms (Table 14–4). To discriminate the nucleolar fluorescence of the tumors from

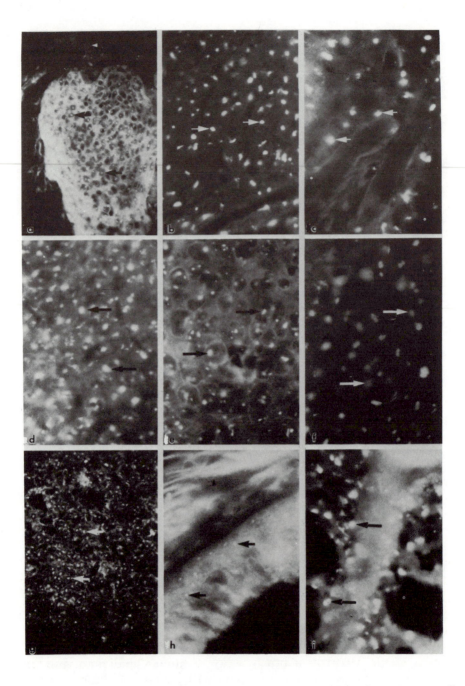

Figure 14–16 Bright nucleolar fluorescence in a series of squamous cell carcinomas and adenocarcinomas. The antibody concentration was 0.3–0.5

that of other tissues, extensive absorption of nontumor antibodies from the antisera, Ig, or IgG fractions was necessary. Because the HeLa cells initially used were grown in fetal calf serum, fetal calf serum was an essential absorbant. Since most human normal tissues were not widely available, a source of "normal" nuclei or nuclear products was necessary. Placentas are a good source of nuclei; they were a useful source of nuclear extracts for absorption (Davis et al., 1979; Busch et al., 1979). In addition, normal human serum contains some minor cross-reactive elements so that absorption was done with serum proteins or whole serum.

Antibodies to Other Tumors

For comparative purposes, two malignant tumor lines other than HeLa cells were used as sources of the antigen. The Namalwa cell line, a Burkitt tumor, was provided to us by the National Cancer Institute and the Frederick Cancer Research Center through the generosity of Drs. V. DeVita and J. Douros and Mr. Fred Klein. A human prostate carcinoma grown in tissue culture was supplied by Dr. F. Gyorkey and Mrs. P. Gyorkey. Both of these contained nucleolar antigens as demonstrated by production of antinucleolar antibodies with similar titers and specificities in rabbits.

Are the Tumor Nucleolar Antigens Present in Nontumor Tissues?

A logical question is whether antigens found in neoplastic cells represent part of a normal process of growth, cell division, or other

---

mg/ml. (*a*) Squamous cell carcinoma, skin (×160); (*b*) squamous cell carcinoma, lung (×400); (*c*) squamous cell carcinoma, metastatic to muscle (×630); (*d*) squamous cell carcinoma, esophagus (×400); (*e*) squamous cell carcinoma, metastatic to muscle (×400); (*f*) higher-power squamous cell carcinoma, lung (×630); (*g*) adenocarcinoma, prostate (×160); (*h*) adenocarcinoma, lung (×400); (*i*) adenocarcinoma, lung (high power) (×630). Arrows, positive fluorescent nucleoli; arrowheads, negative region in adjacent tissue. (From Busch, H., Gyorkey, F., Busch, R. K., Davis, F. M., and Smetana, K., Cancer Res., 36, 3024, 1979.)

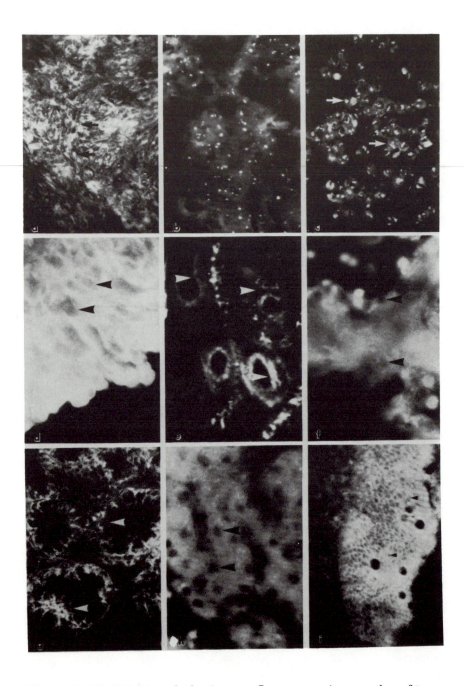

Figure 14–17. Bright nucleolar immunofluorescence in a number of tumors, and lack of nucleolar fluorescence in a number of nontumorous tissues. (a)

normal physiological events. Our theory of carcinogenesis (Busch, 1976) pointed out that cancer is probably the result of extensive misapplication of normal gene readouts as a dysplastic phenomenon involving fetal genes rather than a process involving "totally new" events, such as integration of a viral genome or other gene aberration. A search has been made for the antigens in a variety of normal, growing, and fetal tissues. Table 14–5 shows that the nucleolar antigens were not found in a broad array of nongrowing nontumor tissues.

For studies on growing nontumor tissues, bone marrow, skin Malpigian layers, and intestinal epithelium were analyzed, but the nucleolar antigens were not found in these cells. In studies on bone marrows of patients with leukemias, the neoplastic cells contained the antigens but their nontumor counterparts in the same maturation series did not contain the antigens (Smetana et al., 1979). Studies on cells of patients with acute infectious mononucleosis and lymphoid hyperplasia showed that neither exhibited bright nucleolar fluorescence.

When cultured fetal cells were studied, i.e. the IMR-90 and WI-38 diploid fetal fibroblast lines, they exhibited the same brightly positive nucleolar fluorescence (Busch et al., 1979). Such studies, along with evidence to be presented in the section on staining of gels, indicated that the nucleolar antigens in the malignant tumors could reflect activation of some fetal genes which could be important in neoplasia (Busch et al., 1979; Busch 1976). Whether such genes are equivalent to "onc genes" (Bishop, 1983; Duesberg, 1983), clearly requires further study.

Breast Cancer

The need for a "preliminary" evaluation of the possible diagnostic use of the fluorescence assay for the human tumor antigens led to efforts to

---

brain, glioblastoma ($\times$160); (*b*) adenocarcinoma of stomach, liver metastasis ($\times$400); (*c*) HeLa cells, S3 culture ($\times$400); (*d*) bronchial epithelium, newborn ($\times$400); (*e*) bronchial glands ($\times$400); (*f*) thyroid adenoma ($\times$630); (*g*) intestinal crypts ($\times$400); (*h*) adenoma, parathyroid ($\times$400); (*i*) gastric epithelium (hyperplastic) ($\times$160). Arrows, positive fluorescent nucleoli; arrowheads, negative nucleus or negative regions in cells. (From Busch, H., Gyorkey, F., Busch, R. K., Davis, F. M., and Smetana, K., Cancer Res. 36, 3024, 1979.)

Table 14–4 Bright Nucleolar Fluorescence in Human Malignant Tumor Specimens

I. Carcinomas

  1. Lung
- Adenocarcinoma (3)
- Oat cell (4)
- Squamous cell (22)

  2. Gastrointestinal
- Oral cavity (8)
- Pharynx (4)
- Esophagus, squamous cell (5)
- Stomach, adenocarcinoma (5)
  - Metastasis: liver
  - Metastasis: liver node
- Colon, adenocarcinoma (9)
  - Metastasis: liver (2)
  - Transplantable carcinoma (GW-39)
- Liver, primary carcinoma (3)
- Pancreas (4)

  3. Genitourinary
- Kidney (4)
- Prostate, adenocarcinoma (22)
- Bladder (4)

  4. CNS
- Glioblastoma (1)
- Astrocytoma (5)

  5. Endocrine
- Breast (3)
- Cervix (4)
- Parathyroid (1)
- Thyroid (5)

  6. Skin
- Basal cell (8)
- Eccrine gland (1)
- Squamous cell (7)
  - Metastasis: lymph node
- Melanoma, malignant (4)
  - Cerebral metastasis (1)
- Sweat gland (3)

II. Sarcomas

  1. Chondrosarcoma (1)
  2. Fibrosarcoma (4)
  3. Giant cell tumor (1)
  4. Granulocytic myoblastoma (2)
  5. Leimyosarcoma (4)
  6. Lymphoma (10)
  7. Meningiosarcoma (1)
  8. Myoblastoma (2)
  9. Osteogenic (6)
  10. Pulmonary blastoma (1)
  11. Reticulum cell sarcoma (1)
  12. Synovial sarcoma (1)

III. Hematological neoplasms

  1. Acute lymphocytic leukemia (2)
  2. Acute myelocytic leukemia (7)
  3. Acute monocytic leukemia (2)
  4. Chronic myelocytic leukemia (5)
  5. Hodgkin's disease (9)
  6. Leukemia: CLL (12), hairy cell (1)
  7. Mycosis fungoides
  8. Plasmacytomas (7)

Table 14–5   Negative Nucleolar Fluorescence in Human Tissues

I. Normal tissue	II. Hematologic
1. Lung	1. Bone marrow
2. Gastrointestinal	2. Lymph nodes
Stomach	Lymphocytes
Intestine	Hyperplastic lymph nodes
Small, crypts of	3. Benign growing tissues
Lieberkuhn	Thyroid, goiter
Large	Prostate, hyperplastic
Liver	
Pancreas	III. Inflammatory diseases
3. Genital urinary	1. Chronic ulcerative colitis
Kidney	2. Glomerulonephritis
Bladder	3. Granuloma and fibrosis of
Prostate	lung
4. Endocrine	4. Liver: cirrhosis, hepatitis
Thyroid	5. Lupus profundus (mammary
Breast	gland and skin)
Placenta	6. Pemphigus: bullous
5. Skin	7. Ulcer, gastric

make a "blind" evaluation. At the Michigan Cancer Foundation, a prospective study is in progress on human breast cancer. A large series of patients with breast cancer are being analyzed for relationships between the pathology of the neoplasm and the course of the disease. With the fine cooperation of Drs. P. Furmanski, R. Wiegand, W. Isenberg, and J. Russo (Busch et al., 1981), sections of normal breast tissue as well as benign and malignant tumors were analyzed for bright nucleolar fluorescence by the indirect immunofluorescence technique. These investigations were approved both by the Human Research Committee of Baylor College of Medicine and the Committee for Protection of Human Subjects of the Michigan Cancer Foundation.

Cryostat sections of the tissues were kept at $-20°C$; they were cut at 2μ and fixed for 12 min in acetone at $4°C$. The tumors were evaluated histopathologically by a panel of five pathologists who provided a consensus diagnosis and designation of tumor grade based on H&E staining. The specimens were treated with either Ig or IgG fractions from antisera absorbed with human placental nuclear extracts, fetal bovine serum, and human serum.

Before the "blind" study was initiated, known samples of breast carcinomas were examined. In 19 out of 20 of these, bright nucleolar fluorescence was found to be either distributed throughout the sections or, in a few instances, in cell masses in particular portions of the sections. The 95% positive result for nucleolar fluorescence was similar to the first result (Busch et al., 1979) in which 81 out of 84 samples (96%) were positive in the variety of malignant tumors.

Figure 14–18 presents micrographs of bright nucleolar fluorescence observed in the breast carcinomas. In some cases, the specimen consisted of cells with irregular, large, brightly fluorescent nucleoli (H. Busch et al., 1981). In others, the neoplastic cells were either in focal lesions or randomly distributed. Occasionally, cords of tumor cells were distributed throughout the specimens.

In some sections, the neoplastic cells were confined to small areas or were not visible. False-negatives resulted from failure of the antibodies to penetrate the cells as a result of sample thickness, proteolysis, or "waxy deposits." In other instances, the region containing the tumor cells was lost or was only at the periphery of the specimen. Examination of several slides from a single specimen was useful.

Normal Breast Tissue and Benign Tumors

In the normal breast tissue, the same antibodies produced no brightly fluorescent nucleoli. Some sections contained "minispots" that represented artifacts. The antinucleolar antibodies apparently were non-specifically absorbed by basement membrane elements; fluorescent boundaries were occasionally visible around the terminal ducts as either a thin or a thick limiting membrane or both (Fig. 14–19).

In the benign tumors, the results were generally similar to those for normal breast tissues. The lining membranes were larger and irregular by comparison to those observed in normal breast tissues. "Limiting membranes" were visible in most cases. Some fluorescent "spots" which appear to be artifacts were observable in the benign tumors, usually in small confined areas but occasionally in larger areas. The antibodies may be bound to some relatively nonspecific collagenous or keratinoid macromolecule which has common antigenic determinants to those of the nucleolar antigens.

In a few benign breast tumors, nucleolar fluorescence was apparent. These nucleoli were smaller and fewer in number than in the malignant tumors. Such nucleolar fluorescence was found in only a few benign tumors, but it may be related to activation of fetal genes in a few benign tumors. Tables 14–6 and 14–7 show that it is possible to distinguish between most benign and malignant tumors on the basis of overall nucleolar diameters. It is not possible to specify for any one cell whether it is malignant or not simply by observing the nucleolar size or fluorescence.

"Blind" Study

In this study, 80 breast samples were evaluated. Of these, 55 were carcinomas and 25 were either normal breast or benign tumor specimens (Busch et al., 1981).

The code for this study was kept in Detroit, and the samples were evaluated in Houston. The results were reported in four series containing 13 to 29 samples per group. In the first group (Table 14–8), the 14 samples reported as positive were correctly identified as carcinomas and the 6 reported as negative were all correct except for 1 sample, a benign tumor that contained some fluorescent nucleoli.

In the next series, 29 samples, all those reported as negative were normal or benign tumors. Of the 18 carcinomas, 1 was a false-negative. In the third series of samples (Table 14–7), which contained 15 carcinomas and 2 benign tumors, the reported results were all correct. In part, increased experience was helpful, but other criteria such as limiting membranes and limiting structures in the normal tissues and benign lesions aided in the conclusions.

The last group (13 samples) contained fewer malignant cells and two benign tumors which exhibited nucleolar fluorescence. In this series, only 77% of the specimens were correctly diagnosed. In two malignant tumors, nucleolar fluorescence was not observed. In the overall series, 52 out of 55 of the carcinomas were correctly identified; the overall percentage was 94.6% correct. This result correlated well with the initial studies. However, in the benign lesions, 2 of 27 were incorrectly diagnosed; the overall correct percentage was 92%.

Bladder Carcinoma

In recent independent studies by D. Yu, P. T. Scardino, T. Peitro, and S. Jurco (unpublished), nucleoli isolated from HeLa S3 cells were used to produce rabbit antisera capable of binding nucleoli of transitional cell carcinomas (TCCa) of the bladder. Absorption of the rabbit antiserum was done with normal serum, normal human serum, and human placental nucleoli. This antinucleolar antiserum exhibited strong reactivity in immunoperoxidase and immunofluorescence assays performed on specimens of human bladder cancer. In frozen tissue sections of 24 patients with TCCa and 8 individuals without tumor, nucleolar staining was observed in all malignant specimens but was not observed in 7 of the normal specimens. Cytologic examination of bladder-washing specimens from 47 normal individuals and from 14 patients with TCCa showed that nucleolar staining was absent in 43 of 47 (91%) normal specimens. In addition, 42 cytologic smears were

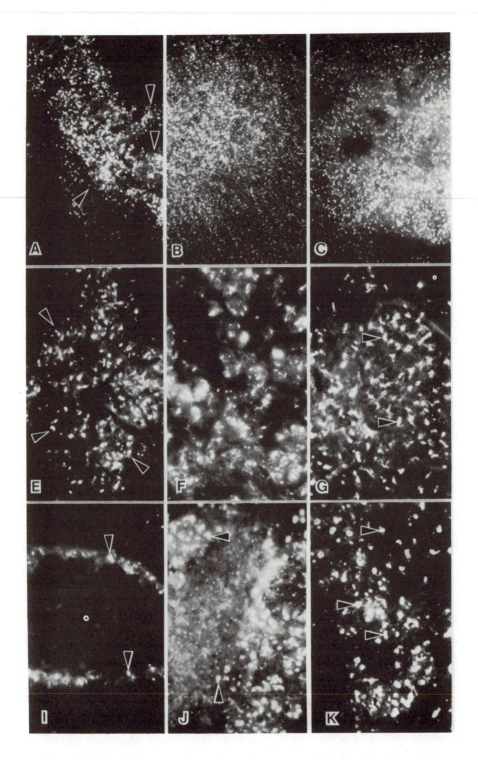

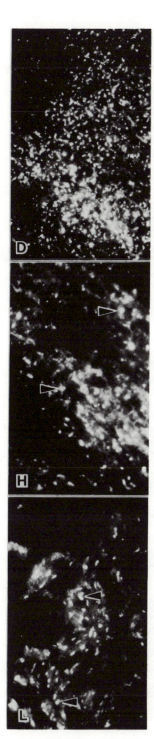

Figure 14–18. (*A–D*): Low power (×160) views of bright nucleolar fluorescence in breast carcinomas illustrating clustering of cells, extensions from masses (A-pointers), and variable densities within masses. (*E–H*): High power views of bright nucleolar fluorescence of fields within breast carcinomas showing abortive pseudolobular formations (*E,F*) and nucleolar irregularity (*G,H*) (×400). (*I–L*): Ductule in carcinoma (*I*), two sizes of brightly fluorescent nucleoli (*J*), large nucleoli (*K*), and irregular nucleoli (*L*); pointers—brightly fluorescent nucleoli (×400).

251

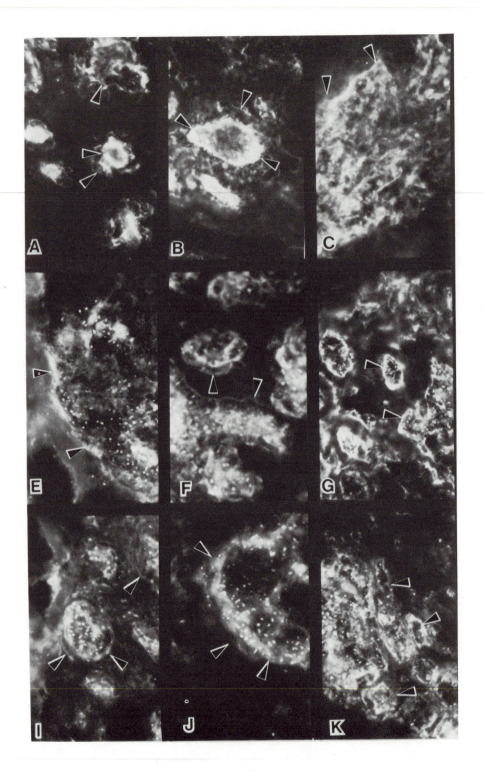

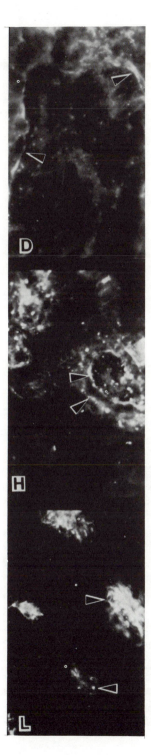

Figure14–19. Varying types of fluorescence observed in benign breast tumors and normal breast tissues. (*A,B*): Normal breast tissue; central nonfluorescent areas are surrounded by a dense fluorescent "boundary" (pointers) around which there are light fluorescent elements (pointers) (*A*, ×160; *B*, ×400). (*C*): Adenosis. Pointers show dense outer "boundary." Within the structures are "macrospherules" and semiparallel "fibrillar" elements (×160). (*D*): Fibrocystic disease. Pointers show dense boundaries surrounding inner areas containing "microspherules" (×160). (*E*): Sclerosing adenosis. Pointers show dense boundaries surrounding inner areas containing "microspherules" (×160). (*F*): Adenosis. Area containing "microspherules" surrounded by thin boundaries (pointers) (×160). (*G*): Fibrocystic disease. Dense "boundary" layer (pointers) surrounding areas containing microspherules (×160). (*H*): Normal breast tissue. Dense and less dense "boundaries" (pointers) surrounding areas containing "microspherules" (×160). (*I*): Sclerosing adenosis. Note boundary layers (pointers) surrounding areas containing microspherules. (×160). (*J*): Sclerosing adenosis. Dense and less dense "boundaries" (pointers) surrounding areas containing "microspherules" (×400). (*K*): Normal breast tissue. Large number of structures containing "microspherules" surrounded by "boundary elements" (×400). (*L*): Normal breast tissue. Fluorescent structures (pointers) seen in normal breast tissue specimens (×400).

Table 14–6   Maximum Nucleolar Diameters in a Series of Human Breast Carcinomas

Sample	(1) < 2.5 μm	(2) > 2.5 μm	(3) Ratio (2)/(1)
589–1	15	11	0.68
588	6	17	2.8
78	3	13	4.3
79	14	30	2.1
76	10	34	3.4
70	7	20	2.8
75	7	26	3.7
598	30	42	1.4
596	21	44	2.1
589–2	36	24	0.66
4	33	34	1.0
5	27	59	2.2
7	10	34	3.4
8	17	33	1.9
9	15	33	2.2
10	29	42	1.5
		Mean	2.3

stained by the Papanicolaou technique and interpreted by an experienced cytopathologist. The false-positive rate was 20.6%, and the false-negative rate 37.5%. When compared to the results of nucleolar-antigen staining in these same patients, the Papanicolaou stain was significantly ($p < 0.05$) less accurate. These results suggest that there are tumor nucleolus-associated antigens present in HeLa cells and transitional cell carcinomas which are generally absent (or in low concentration) in normal human urothelial cells, and that antisera to these antigens may be useful in the cytologic diagnosis of human transitional cell carcinoma.

The technical problems encountered in these studies included a high background fluorescence in some samples and failure to develop satisfactory fluorescence in others. Some errors in diagnosis of the malignant tumors resulted from failure of the antibodies to penetrate the samples as shown by fluorescence along the borders, excessive thickness of the samples, and necrosis of the specimen. These problems were similar to those noted in earlier studies on a broad range of malignant tumors (Busch et al., 1979).

Table 14–7 Maximum Nucleolar Diameters in a Series of Benign Breast Tumors

Sample	(1) < 2.5 μm	(2) > 2.5 μm	(3) Ratio (2)/(1)
Fibrocystic disease			
65	45	1	0.05
(2 others)	—	—	0
Cystic disease			
55	95	6	0.06
(7 others)	0	0	0
Adenosis			
49–42	65	13	0.2
63	38	2	0.05
Mazoplasia			
38	9	1	0.10
2	0	0	0
Sclerosing adenosis			
73–1	39	4	0.11
73–2	61	7	0.11
		Mean benign tumors	0.036
Normal breast tissue			
42	40	2	0.05
(9 others)	0	0	0
		Mean	0.005

Ratio 3—carcinomas/normal breast 460
Ratio 3—carcinomas/benign tumors 66.7

ISOLATION AND CHARACTERISTICS OF HUMAN MALIGNANT TUMOR ANTIGENS

What Are the Nucleolar Antigens?

Studies were designed to characterize chemically the nucleolar antigens in malignant human tumors. Although it would be highly desirable and ultimately possible to isolate and purify the antigens from fresh human tumors, it was necessary to develop purifications from a satisfactory source. The initial attempts at characterization

Table 14–8   Results of Evaluation of Bright Nucleolar Fluorescence in Unknown Specimens (Blind Study) of Benign and Malignant Breast Specimens

Specimens studied in order of difficulty	Positive	Negative	Percentage correct
I. Less difficult			
A. Generalized fluorescence or absence of fluorescence	14	6(1)	95
B. Less generalized fluorescence or unusual structures	18(1)	11	96
C. More localized fluorescence or more unusual structures	16	2	100
	48(1)	19(1)	97
II. More difficult			
Limited fluorescence or limited visualization of cells; questionable regions	7(2)	6(1)	77
Overall correct			94

with nucleolar products from HeLa cells showed that the cell mass required was expensive, and serious problems emerged.

Fortunately, the Frederick Cancer Research Laboratories were producing interferon from Namalwa cells, a Burkitt tumor line. Quantities of such cells from 100–250 g were made available. The nuclear preparations from these frozen cells were less elegant than those from fresh cells, but these cells were a source of antigens at that time (Chan et al., 1980). Because they were NDV (Newcastle Disease Virus) treated, it was not surprising that some artifacts arose, such as a 38-kd antigen which was virus-related (Deb et al., 1983).

Isoelectric Focusing of the Nucleolar Antigens

The studies on the nucleolar antigens of the Novikoff hepatoma suggested that multiple antigens might exist in the human tumor nucleoli. Isoelectric focusing of the antigens was undertaken initially (Chan et al., 1980); proteins were incorporated into the gels so that antigens would not be lost by loading on either the basic or acidic side; 8 *M* urea was added to the ampholine solution to enhance the resolution. The ampholines could modify some antigens and make them unrecognizable by the antibodies.

After electrophoresis, the gels were washed three times with isotonic saline, immersed in acetone to shrink them, and then soaked in the anti-tumor nucleolar antibodies (antiserum, Ig fraction, or IgG fraction). Excess antiserum was then removed from the gel by washing six times with buffered saline, and the fluorescein- or peroxidase-conjugated goat-antirabbit antibody was added to the preparation. Antigens were found in the gel either by the fluorescence or by the peroxidase staining methods (Fig. 14–20).

Identification of Antigen 68/6.3

The major antigen focused at pI 6.3, and a minor band focused at pI 6.1. The antigens were not detected with preimmune serum and were not found in the normal liver cells, nuclei, or nucleolar proteins focused on corresponding gels (Fig. 14–21).

In addition to these two bands, other immunostained bands were occasionally observed at pI 6.6, 5.5, 5.7, and 5.9. Some were also observed following incubation with preimmune serum.

Densitometric Scanning of the Fluorescent Antigens

Figure 14–21 shows that in the isoelectric focusing gel of the nucleolar proteins of the HeLa cells, a fluorescent peak was present at pI 6.3 when the gel was treated with immune serum but not with the preimmune serum. Corresponding analysis of the nucleolar proteins of the normal liver did not show the presence of a corresponding antigen. Staining of the same gels with Coomassie® blue staining indicated that there were 36 protein bands, which on two-dimensional gels separated into more than 60 peptides.

Studies on Namalwa nuclear 0.01 *M* Tris extracts demonstrated the presence of the same major and minor antigens (Fig. 14–22). Because of the interest in whether fetal cells contain these antigens, a similar analysis was made of IMR-90 fetal human fibroblasts. Both

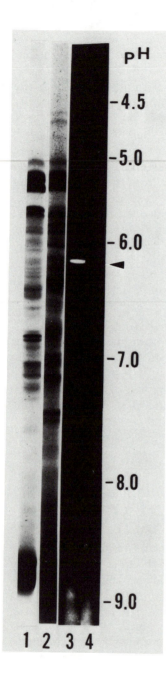

Figure 14–20. Identification of the human tumor nucleolar antigens pI 6.3 and pI 6.1 on 4% polyacrylamide IF gels. The HeLa nucleoli were treated with DNase and RNase, and the proteins were then analyzed by IF. The gels were reacted with immune or preimmune serum and then with fluorescein-conjugated goat anti-rabbit IgG. Photographs were made with a green filter under a long-wavelength UV lamp. Lane 1, Coomassie® blue-stained HeLa nucleolar proteins; lane 2, Coomassie® blue-stained human liver nucleolar proteins; lane 3, tumor proteins with immune serum; lane 4, tumor proteins with preimmune serum. (From Chan, P. K., Feyerabend, A., Busch, R. K., and Busch, H., Cancer Res., 40, 3194, 1980.)

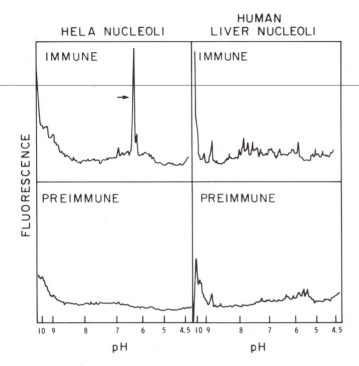

Figure 14–21. Fluorometric tracing of IF gels of nucleolar proteins of HeLa cells and human liver. The nucleolar proteins of HeLa and human liver were analyzed on IF gels and immunostained with fluorescein-conjugated goat anti-rabbit IgG. The pI 6.3 antigen band (arrow) is present in the HeLa nucleolar proteins. A corresponding fluorescent band was not found in human liver nucleolar proteins.

nucleolar antigens with pI values of 6.3 and 6.1 were demonstrable in these cells. These results provide support for the presence of oncofetal or "oncoembryonic" antigens in human malignant tumors. At what period in fetal life these antigens are normally produced is not yet known.

Purification of the Human Tumor Nucleolar Antigens

A purification procedure was developed for preservation of antigenicity and production of a homogeneous product. Initially, ammonium

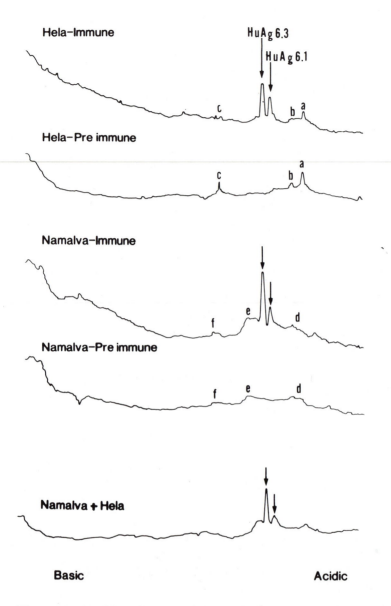

Figure 14–22. Identification of the nucleolar antigens pI 6.3 and 6.1 in the Namalwa cells. The Tris extract of the Namalwa nuclei was analyzed on IF gels. The gels were immunostained with peroxidase-conjugated goat anti-rabbit IgG and scanned with an absorption wavelength of 475 nm. It is noted that the pI 6.3 and the pI 6.1 of the HeLa sample comigrated with those of the Namalwa sample. Several weakly immunostained bands (a,b,c in the HeLa sample and d,e,f, in the Namalwa sample) and the heavily stained bands at the

sulfate fractionation was used. At a concentration of 40% ammonium sulfate, none of the antigen was precipitated. Accordingly, this sediment was discarded.

The 40–100% fraction contained the antigen. After sedimentation, it was chromatographed on a DEAE-cellulose column. A stepwise NaCl gradient was used. The antigens were eluted with 0.15 M NaCl. This fraction contained the pI 6.3 and 6.1 antigens. A Coomassie® blue-stained band which corresponds to this fraction was identified; this band was shown to be concentrated in the 0.15 M NaCl fraction but not in the other fractions.

To test whether the antigens were in the 0.15 M NaCl elutes, the antibodies were initially treated with different NaCl-eluted fractions (Fig. 14–23) and then used for the double-antibody immunostaining of the gels. The antibody fraction absorbed with the 0.15 M NaCl eluate did not stain the antigen bands, indicating that the antigens in this fraction bound antibodies (Fig. 14–23*A,B*).

Two-Dimensional Electrophoresis of the Antigens

Initially, the two antigens were detected on isoelectric focusing gels; they were subjected to two-dimensional analysis on 12% SDS (sodium dodecyl sulfate) gels. Two faint spots were visible on the two-dimensional gel in the pI 6.3 and 6.1 regions (Fig. 14–24). Their molecular weights compared to known standards were approximately 54 and 52 kd, respectively.

Affinity Gel Purification of the Antigens

Affinity gel purification was successfully employed with the Ig fraction of the tumor antibodies (Fig. 14–25). Small amounts of the antigens were in the flow-through fraction, but the fraction eluted with 3 M NaSCN contained highly purified antigens. To further improve the separation of the ^{125}I-labeled antigens from the nonspecifically binding proteins, the 0.15 M NaCl eluate was bound first to an affinity gel containing preimmune serum. The unbound fraction was then bound to the affinity gel containing the immune serum. The two major

---

basic side of the IF gel were found in both immune and preimmune gels. These bands were not consistently found in different experiments.

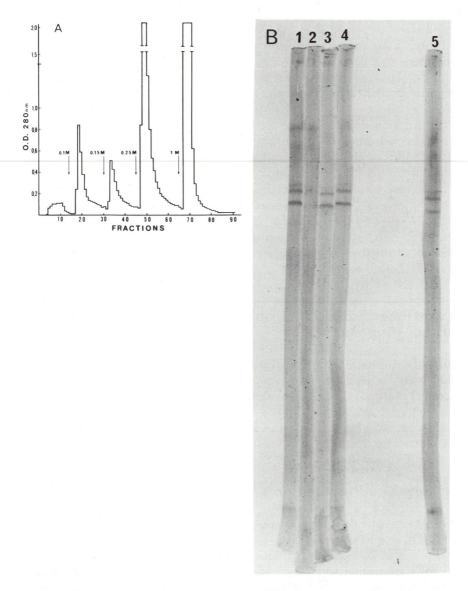

Figure 14–23. (*A*): Interrupted gradient elution of the nucleolar 0.01 *M* Tris extract proteins from DEAE cellulose. (*B*): Immunoperoxidase stain of the antigen using the antiserum preabsorbed with DE–0.15 *M* fractionated by IF gels and subsequently immunoperoxidase stained using the antisera preabsorbed with various DEAE fractions (Figure 14–23A). Lane 1, antiserum preabsorbed with DE–0.1 *M*; lane 2, antiserum preabsorbed with DE–0.15 *M*; lane 3, antiserum preabsorbed with DE–0.25 *M*; lane 4, antiserum preabsorbed with DE–1 *M*; lane 5, control antiserum.

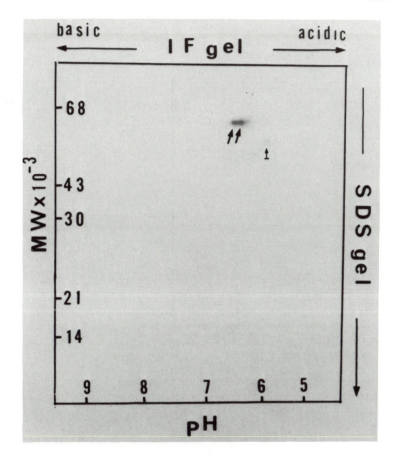

Figure 14–24. Two-dimensional gel electrophoresis of the nucleolar antigens purified from human tumors as in Fig. 14–25; note the dense doublet at pI 6.3 and the single spot at pI 6.1.

antigens detected on the two-dimensional gel of the 3 *M* NaSCN eluate were the 54/6.3 and 52/6.1 antigens (Fig. 14–24).

Separation of the Antigens into Individual Components

To further purify these antigens, preparative isoelectric focusing gels were used. With these, "single-spot" antigens were obtained (Fig. 14–26A,B).

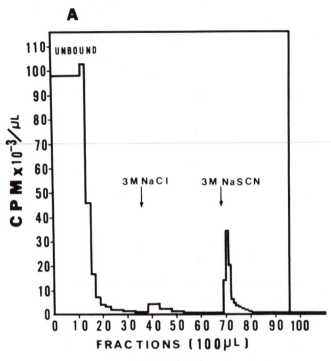

Figure 14–25. Partial purification of the human antigen on the anti-0.15 *M* NaCl extract antibody-affinity column. The human antigen was eluted with 3 *M* NaSCN after a 3 *M* NaCl wash.

Relation of the Nucleolar Antigens to the "src Gene" Product

When the nucleolar antigen was shown to have a molecular weight of approximately 60 kd and a pI of 6.3, it became of interest to compare it with other reported proteins of similar molecular weight and isoelectric points. The antigen in the Novikoff hepatoma nucleoli has a very similar molecular weight (Marashi et al., 1979). Its lower pI of 5.1 may reflect differences in amino acid content or modifications which also may account for the differences in its immunological properties.

The "src gene" (Collett at al., 1978; Collett and Erikson, 1978) has a similar molecular weight and pI, but it differs in cellular localization inasmuch as it is a membrane protein (Krueger et al., 1980), localized to the nuclear envelope and juxtanuclear reticular membrane structure in rat cells (Krueger et al., 1980). It is on the plasma membrane of

Rous sarcoma virus-transformed chicken fibroblasts. Collett and Erickson (1978) found that the "src gene" product was a protein kinase. The human tumor pI 6.3 and 6.1 nucleolar antigens were not phosphorylated and were not kinases.

To compare the structure of the nucleolar antigens with the "src gene" product, the ^{125}I-labeled antigens were subjected to partial proteolysis with staphylococcal V8 protease and chymotrypsin. The cleavage products did not parallel those of the src gene product (Collett et al., 1978; Collett and Erikson, 1978).

Purification of the Antinucleolar Antibodies

The excellent antibody response of rabbits, sheep, and goats led to the hope that purification of these antibodies would be useful. Affinity columns were developed in which RNP particles of the 0.01 M Tris extracts were employed as adsorbants. These antibodies are specific for the tumor antigens, but they did not react with 0.01 M Tris extracts of other tissues after the absorptions.

Competitive studies on antibody binding to nuclear RNP particles obtained from the 0.01 M Tris extracts was a useful inhibition assay for antibody specificity. It was found that 70–80% of the binding activity of the purified antibody was blocked by pretreatment with the pI 6.3 and 6.1 antigen preparation, which suggests that only a small amount of other antigens was recognized by that purified antibody preparation.

Complexity of Immunological Analysis for Neoplastic Cells

As noted several times above, there are always problems in immunological assays from the point of view of both false-positives and false-negatives. One such problem in this study has been a variable but reproducible nucleolar fluorescence in isolated human liver nuclei. The problem has not been resolved by any technique that also permits retention of the nucleolar fluorescence in malignant cells and loss in liver nuclei, despite the lack of the antigen in liver nucleoli, but it is under continuing study.

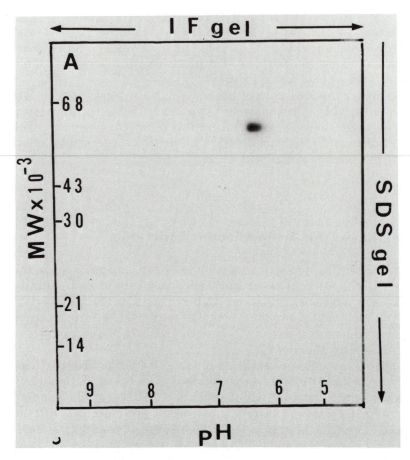

Figure 14–26. Two-dimensional gel electrophoresis showing "single-spot" purification of human tumor nucleolar antigens by preparative isoelectric

CURRENT STUDIES
OF ISOLATED HUMAN TUMOR ANTIGENS

Studies on Functions of Specific Antigens

Kinase Activity of 52- to 55-kd Phosphoproteins   Inasmuch as nucleolar kinases were identified in earlier studies (Olson et al., 1978) and we subsequently showed that some nuclear phosphoproteins have topoisomerase activity (Durban et al., 1981, 1983; Mills et al., 1982), attempts have been made to identify which nucleolar antigens exhibit protein kinase or topoisomerase activity. With combined affinity and

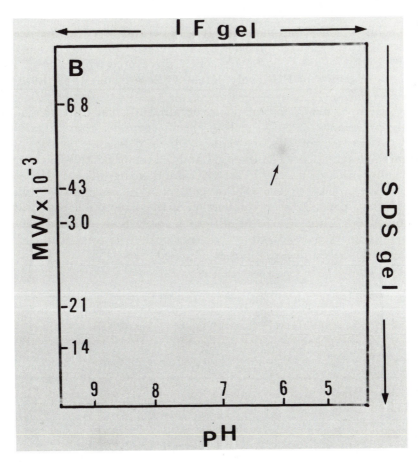

focusing gels. The dense pI 6.3 doublet is shown on the left (*A*), and the pI 6.1 antigen is shown above (*B*).

other techniques, cAMP-independent kinase 52/5.3 (Fig. 14–27) was isolated from Namalwa cells. It catalyzed the phosphorylation of rabbit muscle glycogen synthase in the amino terminal domain. Anti-nucleolar antibodies inhibited its activity 80%. The nuclei of HeLa cells contained 64% of the total cellular kinase; 11% was in the nucleoli. The specific activity of the nucleolar kinase was twice that of the nuclear supernatant and four times that of the cytoplasmic kinase.

It was notable that this kinase was optimally released from nucleolar RNP particles by nuclease digestion, which suggests that the kinase is tightly associated to the RNA. Further studies will be directed to determination of the nucleolar substrates for this kinase, particularly its possible role in catalyzing synthesis or processing of nucleolar preribosomal particles. It is important to learn whether the real substrates for this kinase are common nucleolar phosphoproteins 110/5.2 (C23), 37/5.2 (B23), a recently discovered 145/7 phosphoprotein, or subunits of RNA polymerase I (Rose et al., 1983; Rose and Jacob, 1984).

Attempts are being made to obtain sufficient amounts of the antigenic kinase 52/5.3 to define specific peptides that contain the epitope portion of the molecule and to determine whether the differences found between the liver and the tumor peptides account for the differences in antigenic activity found earlier (Takahashi et al., 1983). We propose to test whether control of the functional activity of this kinase depends upon the portion of the structure containing the epitope which appears to be different in normal human liver and human tumors. It is possible that this protein is related to the p53 antigen described by Crawford et al. (1981, 1982).

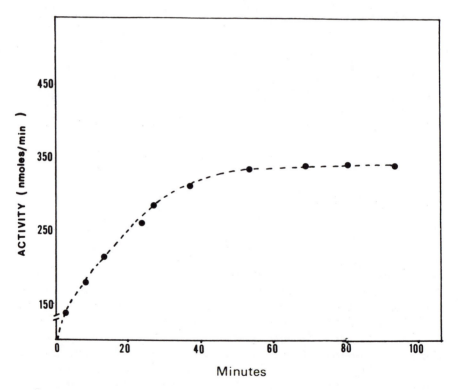

Figure 14–27. Increasing kinase activity with increasing amounts of protein 52/5.3. This glycogen synthase kinase was found to contain two bands. The location to the nuclear RNP particles suggests that it may play a role in specific phosphorylation proteins during maturation of RNP particles.

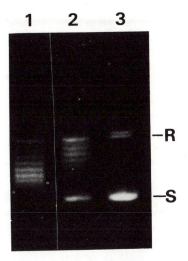

Figure 14–28. Nucleolar topoisomerase I activity. Topoisomerase I activity was purified from nucleolar 0.35 M NaCl extracts of Novikoff ascites cells by treatment with calcium phosphate gel (0.5 M phosphate buffer eluate) and phosphocellulose chromatography (0.8 M KCl eluate) according to the procedure for purification of nuclear topoisomerase I (Durban et al., 1981). Nucleolar activity eluted slightly earlier from phosphocellulose (0.8 M KCl) than nuclear topoisomerase I (1.0 M KCl). Purified topoisomerase I fractions were incubated with 100 ng of supercoiled pBR322 plasmid DNA for 20 min at 37°C and DNA forms were analyzed by agarose-gel electrophoresis (Durban et al., 1983). Lane 1, nucleolar topoisomerase I (approximately 5 ng); lane 2, nuclear topoisomerase I (approximately 1 ng); lane 3, plasmid pBR322 control. S: Position of supercoiled DNA; R: relaxed form. (Courtesy of Drs. David Roll and Egon Durban.)

Topoisomerases　An important possibility that has recently emerged is that a correlation exists between the dynamic unfolded state of the nucleoli of cancer cells and their topoisomerase activity. Morphological distinctions have long been known (Busch and Smetana, 1970) between the spherical small nucleoli characteristic of nondividing cells and the remarkably irregular, large, pleiomorphic nucleoli of malignant tumors. These differences may correlate with the increased topoisomerase activity or with the phosphorylation states of these proteins (Durban et al., 1983).

Previous studies in this laboratory demonstrated that fetal topoisomerases appear in rat and human tumors (Durban et al., 1981, 1983). Topoisomerase I (Fig. 14–28) is a phosphorylated 110/8.4 protein and is similar in molecular weight to nucleolar phosphoprotein

110/5.2, which is localized to the NORs and the fibrillar centers within the nucleolus, the suggested location of the "active" rDNA genes. The amount of the silver-stained proteins (110/5.2) (C23) correlated with the activity of the nucleolus (Busch et al., 1979).

To analyze the structure of these proteins, cleavage reactions are being carried out with both protein 110/5.2 (C23) and topoisomerase I (110/8.4). The peptides containing the epitopes are purified on SDS-gels, HPLC, and ion-exchange columns to provide peptides in sufficient amount and purity for analyses of amino acid sequences of the antibody binding sites. Attempts are in progress to develop monoclonal antibodies to these peptides for further studies on their structure and function.

Protein 110/5.2 (C23) was suggested by Bugler et al. (1982) to be a precursor of ribosomal proteins, but this suggestion awaits confirmation.

Antigens Associated with Nucleolar RNP Processing Reactions Protein 37/5.2 (B23) was previously found to be associated mainly with nucleolar RNP particles. It is readily extractable with 0.01 M Tris–HCl, pH 7.8 or salt solutions up to 0.35 M. Its nucleolar localization is distinct from that of protein 110/5.2, a phosphoprotein that is assocated with NOR regions, and newly formed RNP particles.

The availability of the epitope for interaction with monoclonal antibodies, both *in vivo* and *in vitro*, and the relative ease with which this protein can be purified suggested its use as a model for analysis of antibody–epitope interaction. For these studies, sufficient amounts of this protein were isolated for cleavage with a variety of proteolytic enzymes including trypsin, chymotrypsin, thermolysin, V8 protease, and pepsin. After immunoblots showed that partial cleavage with V8 protease permitted retention of antigenic activity, the major immunoreactive peptide of approximately 4 kd was isolated initially by DEAE chromatography and then by reverse-phase (C18) HPLC. The purified peptide was placed in a Beckman spinning-cup sequencer (890-B) using polybrene as a carrier. The PTH-amino acids from the sequencer were identified on an HPLC system using an IBM-cyano column. Its preliminary sequence is (P.K. Chan et al., unpublished):

Lys Phe Lys Lys Gln Glu Lys Thr Pro Lys Thr Pro Lys Gly
        (10)

Pro Asp Asp Val Glu His Ile Lys Ala Lys Pro Gln Ala Asp
        (20)

Ile Glu Lys Pro (Glu) (Ala) Leu Pro
        (30)

Our goal is to expand this sequence for evaluation of its relationship to the whole protein and particularly to identify the region of the peptide which reacts specifically with the antibody. For this purpose, partial cleavages are being made of this peptide with the proteases indicated above as well as stepwise trimming on the amino terminal with leucine aminopeptidase and on the C-terminal with carboxypeptidases.

For further characterization of the epitope, we are attempting to crystallize protein 37/5.2 and the antigenic peptide and to learn more about the spatial relationships of the amino acids in the antigenically active region.

Cell Cycle-Related Nucleolar Antigens

Proliferating Cell Nuclear Antigen   A proliferating cell nuclear antigen (PCNA) was identified with autoantibodies from a patient with systemic lupus erythematosus. Specific antiodies were purified by affinity chromatography in which Novikoff hepatoma nucleolar proteins were conjugated to Sepharose 4B (Chan et al., 1983). The purified anti-PCNA antibodies produced bright nucleolar fluorescence in tumor cells as shown by indirect immunofluorescence. PCNA was found in nucleoli of human cell lines, Hep-2, and Namalwa, and in a solid human renal and a prostate carcinoma. Both strong and weak nucleolar fluorescence areas were found in the renal and prostate carcinomas, indicating that there are varying degrees of proliferation among tumor cells. Two human colon carcinoma cell lines, *O* (an aggressive, fast-growing clone of human colon carcinoma cell line) and CBS (a slow-growing human colon carcinoma cell line), with different growth rates were compared. The fast-growing colon carcinoma cells, *O*, exhibited a higher percentage of nucleolar fluorescence (28.5%) than the slow-growing colon cells (13.6%). By enzyme-linked immunosorbent assays, this cell extract had a higher PCNA antigen content (2.8-fold) than the CBS cell extract which, in turn, had a higher content than that of human liver extract. PCNA was also found in a human fetal lung fibroblast cell line (IMR-90). Very weak or negative nucleolar fluorescence was observed in rat Novikoff hepatoma cells. Although normal rat livers did not exhibit PCNA fluorescence, nucleolar fluorescence was observed 18 h after partial hepatectomy.

Lymphomas (lymphocytic non-Hodgkin's malignant lymphoma) and leukemic (chronic lymphocytic, acute and chronic myeloid, myelomonocytic leukemia) cells were studied by indirect immunofluorescence to evaluate the presence of PCNA and human malignant tumor nuclear antigens (HMTNA) in their nucleoli (Smetana et al.,

1983). Most cells in lymph node smears of lymphocytic non-Hodgkin's malignant lymphoma (NHML) developed bright nucleolar fluorescence with HMTNA antibodies. PCNA was detected in nucleoli of a limited number of cells which apparently represent the proliferating cell population in these lymphomas. In bone marrow smears of patients with chronic lymphocytic leukemia, most cells exhibited nucleolar fluorescence for HMTNA. PCNA was present in nucleoli of a limited number of cells. In the bone marrow smears of patients with myeloid or myelomonocytic leukemias, most blast cells also developed a bright nucleolar fluorescence with HMTNA antibodies, and PCNA was present only in a small percentage of these cells. Leukemic cells with PCNA in their nucleoli may represent a proliferating cell population in the late G_1–early S phase.

S-phase Specific Nucleolar Antigen ("RZ2")   Monoclonal antibodies were produced by long-term immunization of mice with bovine serum albumin-conjugated HeLa nucleoli. A monoclonal antibody from recloned cells, designated RZ2 (86/6), demonstrated marked variations in the nucleolar fluorescence of Hep-2 cells on ANA slides (Zweig et al., 1984). Approximately one-third of the cells had bright nucleolar labeling, but the remaining cells had little or no nucleolar labeling. The antibody also produced a weak granular nuclear-labeling pattern in most cells. Both labeled and unlabeled nucleoli appeared similar in morphology by phase microscopy. Cell synchronization studies using either serum deprivation or double thymidine block showed that the antibody did not produce nucleolar fluorescence in the G_0 or G_1 phases, but bright nucleolar fluorescence was found during the S phase. The nucleolar fluorescence disappeared in the G_2 and M phases. The antibody also produced fluorescence in growing nontransformed WI-38 cells and in approximately 1% of the cells in normal human liver tissue sections, which suggests that it recognizes an antigen common to cycling human cells. No fluorescence was observed in Novikoff rat hepatoma cells, which suggests that the antibody may be species-specific. Immunoblot analysis of proteins isolated from both purified nucleoli and whole cells showed that the antigen has a molecular weight of approximately 86 kd.

Isolation and Functional Analysis of S-Phase Nucleolar Antigens

Isolation and Functional Analysis of PCNA   The proliferating cell nucleolar antigen is currently being identified by immunoblotting techniques. The antigen has an approximate molecular weight of 120 kd. PCNA is present in small concentrations in nucleoli, and assessment of its structure and function await purification of this protein in sufficient amounts for more satisfactory analytical studies. Because the antigen appears to be present in Novikoff hepatoma nucleoli as well as in human tumor nucleoli, attempts are being made to use the former for purification of the PCNA and its epitope. The availability of the antibody to PCNA has been limited because Dr. Eng Tan, who provided the original antiserum, has only limited supplies. Accordingly, this antibody is being used to provide affinity purification of small amounts of the antigen, which will then be used for development of monoclonal antibodies to aid in evaluation of the structure and function of this antigen.

Isolation and Functional Analysis of Protein 86/6.1   Protein 86/6.1, like PCNA, is of interest because it is present in growing and dividing cells. This antigen is characterized by the fact that it is present in nucleoli only at the S phase, where it may be important to rDNA synthesis. The monoclonal antibody to protein 86/6.1 may be a useful marker for growing and replicating cells. We are studying the presence of 86/6.1 in peripheral blood smears and bone marrow samples of leukemic patients in remission and relapse as well as under treatment. Interestingly, like kinase 52/5.3 protein, protein 86/6.1 is optimally released from the nucleolus by nuclease digestion, which suggested that it was tightly associated to either nucleolar DNA or RNA. Preliminary studies have provided evidence that it is DNA-bound since it is released by DNase but not by RNase.

Characterization of "Difference Proteins" of Nucleoli of Normal and Cancer Cells

Problems of Proteases   A key problem in dealing with human normal tissues and malignant tumors has been proteolytic degradation of many nuclear proteins and antigens. Very recently, this problem has been largely overcome by extraction with buffers containing both nonspecific and thiol protease inhibitors: 0.5 mM PMSF, 5 μg/ml leupeptin, 5 μg/ml aprotinin, 1 mM EGTA, 1 mM p-OH mercuribenzoate or 0.1 mM p-Cl-mercurisulfonic acid, 1 mM N-ethylmaleimide or 0.5 mM TLCK. To protect phosphate bonds, 10 mM α-glycerophosphate is also added. Improved one-dimensional gel patterns contained proteins of molecular weight up to 350 kd. Although the possibility exists that antigenicity could be affected by these reagents, thus far we have not experienced significant alterations in the immunoblots.

In the best preparations, HeLa extracts contained a 100-kd antigen in much greater amounts than in the liver extracts, and a 68-kd antigen was in the LeLa nucleoli that was not found in the liver nucleoli. Normal human liver nucleoli contained 75- and 55-kd antigens that were not found in the HeLa nucleolar preparations.

Further studies are in progress on these nucleolar proteins of HeLa cells and normal human liver cells. Standard methods for purification of these proteins are being used to accumulate sufficient amounts for chemical characterization and enzymatic and structural analysis. A combination of affinity procedures with polyclonal and monoclonal antibodies is being used for their purification.

In additional studies, we plan to evaluate by biochemical and immunochemical methods whether the 68-kd antigen of HeLa cells is the same as the antigen 68/6.3 purified previously (Chan et al., 1982). Proteins of this molecular weight have been suggested by Croy and Pardee (1983) to be involved in "restruction point control." In addition, some lamins, keratin-like proteins, a subunit of RNA polymerase I (Rose et al., 1983; Jacob et al., 1983), and a protein of U1-snRNP (Busch et al., 1982b) also have molecular weights of 68 kd. Other possibilities for the 100-kd antigen include topoisomerase I, α-actinin, protein 110/5.2, or previously unidentified proteins. We are attempting to purify sufficient amounts of these antigens for enzymatic and biochemical analysis.

Development of Additional Monoclonal Antibodies

We have developed several nucleolus-specific monoclonal antibodies using standard methods of fusion and subcloning (Kohler and Milstein, 1975). Satisfactory antibodies have been obtained for nucleolar phosphoproteins 110/5.2, 37/5.2, and 86/6.1 and for several other nucleolar antigens. Our goals in developing monoclonal antibodies to nucleolar proteins are to: (a) facilitate purification of nucleolar proteins by affinity chromatography; (b) improve immunocytochemical localization of the antigens; (c) identify tumor-related epitopes; and (d) make use of specific antibodies as immunochemical probes to study functions of the proteins.

One difficult problem has been the relatively low immunogenicity of nucleolar proteins, presumably because many nucleolar proteins are evolutionarily conserved. Differences between nucleolar proteins from malignant and normal tissues may reflect quantitative differences

(Busch et al., 1979) or expression of fetal proteins and other isotypes (Busch et al., 1979, 1982) which may be only weakly immunogenic.

To increase specific antibody response to weak immunogens, augmentation of immunogenicity is being done by chemical modification, addition of carrier molecules to produce hapten carriers (Green et al., 1982), and immunization *in vitro* to avoid *in vivo* suppressor activity (Reading, 1982; Goding, 1980). At present, nucleolar antigens are being chemically coupled to KLH or BSA to maximize immunogenicity for *in vivo* immunization. Studies are also to be carried out on modifications, such as acetylation, halogenation, SH blocking, and nucleophilic substitution (Kiefer, 1979). Both *in vivo* and *in vitro* immunization are being used for the development of monoclonal antibodies to nucleolar proteins.

Goding (1980) and Stahli et al. (1980) suggested that the best time for fusion is 3–4 days after boosting as an optimal time for antigen-induced proliferation. In our present protocol, mice are primed with antigen at 3-week intervals over a 3-month period and then rested for 3 weeks. The animals are then injected with high doses of antigen both i.p. and i.v. over a 4-day period. After the animals are sacrificed, the lymphocyte fraction from spleens is used for the fusion.

The amount of immunogen may be a limiting factor in producing autologous antibodies (Stahli et al., 1980). This problem has been avoided in some cases by *in vitro* immunization (Reading, 1982) where small quantities of antigen are in close contact with the reactive cells.

Investigation of Potential Nucleolar Glycoprotein Antigens

Until recently, glycoproteins had not been demonstrated in the nucleolus either directly or indirectly. As part of the analysis of immunoblots of antibody–antigen interactions, analysis of lectin-binding proteins was done as well as direct analysis for carbohydrate (periodate oxidation and reaction with ammoniacal silver). Several discrete glycoproteins were identified in the extracts. One of these corresponds in molecular weight (100 kd) to a nucleolar antigen identified by immunostaining. The demonstration of the sugar content of such proteins as well as their immunostaining offers an opportunity for purification by double-affinity procedures employing lectin-affinity columns using elution with salts and mannosides, then binding to antibody-affinity columns and elution with NaSCN, urea, or other eluents.

Studies will be done to determine the function and chemistry of these glycoprotein antigens. We are now attempting to develop specific monoclonal antibodies for immunodetection of these glycoprotein antigens in normal and tumor cells for improved purification and to evaluate the evidence for their nuclear and nucleolar localization. In addition, comparisons will be made with cell surface, cytoplasmic, and nuclear envelope glycoproteins. Analyses will be done on the activity of the purified proteins to evaluate whether they are protein kinases, RNA polymerases, DNA polymerases, topoisomerases, or similar enzymes important to nucleolar function. Comparisons will be made with nontumor tissues to evaluate growth and cancer relatedness.

Characterization of Nucleolar Antigens in Normal Human Tissues Not Found in Human Malignant Tumors

To define nucleolar antigens that are enriched in normal human tissues and that are either low in amount or absent from human tumors, antibodies were produced against normal human liver nucleoli (R. K. Busch and Busch, 1981). A 55-kd antigen recognized by these antibodies was found in high concentrations in nucleolar 0.075 M NaCl/0.025 M EDtA, 0.01 M Tris–HCl, pH 7.8, or DOC-DTT extracts of human liver nucleoli and not in HeLa or other carcinoma cells. This antigen was present in normal human kidney, spleen, and placenta. Most of the antigen was extracted from normal human liver nuclei or nucleoli with 0.075 M NaCl/0.025 M EDTA. It was purified to homogeneity by preparative slab gel electrophoresis or by affinity chromatography on antibody-Sepharose columns as shown by two-dimensional polyacrylamide gel electrophoresis. The amino acid composition had an A/B ratio of 1.6 and a proline content of 6.5%. The tryptic peptide map of isolated antigen 55/7.3 was unique; it differed markedly from the tryptic peptide map of human serum albumin.

It is possible that this protein may have a regulatory function. Studies will be done on its effects on nucleolar RNA polymerase I and on whole nucleolar RNA synthesis *in vitro* and by microinjection into tumor cells (Bennett et al., 1983).

DISCUSSION

Are There Abnormal Proteins in Cancer Cells?

The central issue in discussions of mutations in neoplastic disease is the demonstration of an abnormal protein. Ever since a single mutation was found in sickle cell anemia, corresponding searches have been made for a variety of proteins in cancers. Thus far, with the isolated instance of a tumor culture cell line change in P21 at position 12, no "abnormal" proteins have been detected in human cancer cells. Even when the proteins are "fetal," they are normal fetal proteins.

Quantitative Features of Neoplastic Disease That Offer Approaches to Therapy

From the beginning, cancer treatment has been based on a "rational empiricism." At present, more quantitative analyses of tumor markers and intracellular elements have been developed. With immunoassays, enzymatic assays, and other quantitative procedures, anti-cancer drugs may be assayed for greater selectivity and less toxicity than those currently available.

The Nucleolus and Cancer Chemotherapy

Important quantitative differences in nucleolar synthesis of preribosomal particles exist between cancer cells and other cells. In comparisons of synthesis of the nucleolar pre-RNA precursors of ribosomal RNA in rapidly growing malignant tumors and normal tissues, 15-fold greater biosynthetic rates were found in the tumors (Busch and Smetana, 1970). Similar results were obtained in analysis of the numbers of "silver-staining" granules in neoplastic tissues and normal cells (Busch, 1978a, 1978b; Busch et al., 1979).

The finding of common nucleolar antigens in a broad range of human tumors (Busch et al., 1979, 1982) provides opportunity for attack on the epitopes of these antigens (Lane and Hoeffler, 1980; Takahashi et al., 1983; Chan et al., 1982; Watt and Schimmer, 1981). As with other antigens, it is essential that their relationships to "fetal" and "onc-gene" products be defined as well as their roles as "restriction point controls" (Hammond et al., 1979; Croy and Pardee, 1983) of cancer cells.

In other studies, it has been found that the concentrations of specific nucleolar phosphoproteins such as protein B23 (37 kd/pI 5.2) and RNA polymerase I are much higher in malignant tumors than in nontumor tissues. Accordingly, the possibility exists that advantage can be taken of the quantitative differences in concentrations of nucleolar enzymes, precursor proteins, structural proteins, or phosphoproteins in the design of new anti-cancer drugs. One of the current possibilities from the "altered promoter" concept of "c-onc-genes" is that large amounts of specific proteins are produced in human cancer.

For drug design that hopefully can lead to more meaningful and specific therapeutic agents, immunochemistry may become particularly useful. The increasing development of information on the chemistry of epitopes, along with improved methods for isolation and sequence analysis of peptides containing the epitopes, offers an important new dimension for drug design.

Can Such Information Be Useful in a Quantitative Sense?

Studies noted above suggest that specific attack on particular genes could be of value whether they are normal genes functioning excessively or "onc-genes"; specific site-directed attack on DNA is only a dream as yet. Hopefully, directed attack on specific proteins or peptides can be developed with the aid of novel peptides or a variety of analogs based on peptide structure.

Such approaches will be facilitated with new technology emerging from analysis of the spatial (three-dimensional) relationships of functional portions of amino acids and drugs designed to approach such structures. If drugs can be directed against particular immunoreactive peptides such as epitopes recognized by monoclonal antibodies, their potential for success will be greater, particularly if the epitopes are functionally important. This approach has already been used for localization of nucleolar antigens (Busch et al., 1982) and transforming proteins of Rous sarcoma virus (Nigg et al., 1983; Puck et al., 1981) and leukemia virus (Versteegen et al., 1982).

Epitope Attack

Can we utilize the information derived from epitopes to develop new drugs? Inasmuch as an epitope is a small portion of a protein or other macromolecule which is recognized by a specific antibody, it has attachment sites for its antibody with high specificity for interaction. When the protein or macromolecule is properly cleaved with proteases or specific cleavage reagents, these epitopes can be preserved intact with high immunoreactivity for the antibodies. The epitope content of a given peptide can be quantitated by immunochemical assays such as ELISA (enzyme-linked immunoassay) or radioimmunoassays.

In addition, the antibodies can be utilized for "affinity" binding for the peptides containing the epitopes. Purification of the epitopes on ion-exchange columns, thin-layer chromatography, and affinity techniques can be followed with the aid of immunochemical procedures.

To gather sequence information about the epitopes, several procedures are useful. If the sequence of the protein or its DNA has been established, limited confirmatory evidence from the amino acid composition or sequence data may be sufficient. However, secondary cleavage reactions and more defined sequence information obtained from stepwise analysis of the peptide may be required to define the amino acid sequence unequivocally.

Information on the amino acid sequence of the epitope is essential for development of potential therapeutic information. The goal of such procedures is to precisely position reactive groups. The importance of such sequence information becomes apparent when one thinks of the numbers of possible di-, tri-, and tetrapeptides. Assuming that each position in a peptide sequence could be filled by 1 of 20 amino acids, there are 40 possible dipeptides, 8,000 possible tripeptides, and 160,000 possible tetrapeptides. For the chemist to produce replicas of such structures, on a hit-or-miss basis, would be impossible. Even defining the NH_2- and $-COOH$ terminals would be an advantage for such synthesis, although the more information that becomes available about conformation and sequence, the more satisfactory the chemistry that can be applied.

It is only a matter of a relatively short time before important epitopes will be identified and utilized for approaches to chemotherapy (Versteegen et al., 1982). In addition to nuclear and nucleolar antigens that are being identified and characterized (Busch et al., 1982; Wojtkowiak et al., 1982), nucleolar phosphoprotein B23 (37 kd/pI 5.2)—which is a large stained spot in two-dimensional gels of HeLa nucleolar preparations—is of special interest as a target. Protein B23 is found in nucleolar preribosomal RNP particles (Prestayko et al., 1974) and, in addition, is distributed quite homogeneously in the nucleolar mass. Recently, monoclonal antibodies have been developed to protein B23 which bind to specific peptides as shown by immunochemical analysis, as noted above. Inasmuch as the rapidly growing malignant tumors have the property of high rates of nucleolar biosynthetic reactions in which protein B23 plays an important role, it would seem that inhibition of the activity of this protein would also repress nucleolar function, inhibition of precursor particle formation, and inhibition of RNA-binding activity.

This approach, if successful, can be extended to molecules that are "cancer markers", v-*onc* and c-*onc* gene products, fetal isozymes, and other molecular species that are cancer associated. Such procedures will offer a target-directed approach to the improvement of cancer therapy.

Whether such approaches will offer a quicker path to success in cancer treatment than the "empirical" or "screening" approaches used for evolution of the current series of anti-cancer drugs (Maness et al., 1983) is at present only speculative.

REFERENCES

Abelev, G. I., Engelhardt, N. V., and Elgort, D. A. In *Methods in Cancer Research*, Vol. 18, Busch, H., Ed. New York: Academic Press, 1979.

Bennett, F. C., Busch, H., Lischwe, M. A., and Yeoman, L. C. J. Cell Biol. *97*: 1566, 1983.

Bishop, J. M. Cell *32*: 1018, 1983.

Bugler, B., Caizergues-Ferrer, M., Bouche, G., Bourbon, H., and Amalric, F. Eur. J. Biochem. *128*: 475, 1982.

Busch, H. Cancer Res. *36*: 4921, 1976.

Busch, H. Cancer Res. *36*: 4291, 1978a.

Busch, H. Life Sci. *23*: 2543, 1978b.

Busch, H., Busch, R. K., Chan, P. K., Isenberg, W., Wiegand, R., Russo, J., and Furmanski, P. Clin. Immunol. Immunopathol. *18*: 155, 1981.

Busch, H., Busch, R. K., Chan, P. K., Kelsey, D., and Takahashi, K. Methods Cancer Res. *19*: 110, 1982.

Busch, H., Daskal, Y., Gyorkey, F., and Smetana, K. Cancer Res. *39*: 857, 1979.

Busch, H., Reddy, R., Rothblum, L., and Choi, V. C. Ann. Rev. Biochem. *57*: 617, 1982.

Busch, H., and Smetana, K. *The Nucleolus*, New York: Academic Press, 1970.

Busch, R. K., and Busch, H. Proc. Soc. Exptl. Biol. Med. *168*: 125, 1981.

Busch, R. K. and Busch, H. Tumori *63*: 347, 1977.

Busch, R. K., Daskal, I., Spohn, W. H., Kellermayer, M., and Busch, H. Cancer Res. *34*: 2362, 1974.

Chan, P. K., Feyerabend, A., Busch, R. K., and Busch, H. Cancer Res. *40*: 3194, 1980.

Chan, P. K., Frakes, R. L., Busch, R. K., and Busch, H. J. Cancer Res. Clin. Oncol. *103*: 7, 1982.

Chan, P. K., Frakes, R. L., Tan, R. M., Brattain, M. G., Smetana, K., and Busch, H. Cancer Res. *43*: 3770, 1983.

Collett, M. S., Brugge, J. S., and Erikson, R. L. Cell *15*: 1363, 1978.

Collett, M. S., and Erikson, R. L. Proc. Natl. Acad. Sci. U.S.A. *75*: 2021, 1978.

Crawford, L. V., Pim, D. C., and Bulbrook, R. D. Int. J. Cancer *30*: 403, 1982.

Crawford, L. V., Pim, D. C., Gurney, E. G., Goodfellow, P., and Taylor-Papadimitriou, J. Proc. Natl. Acad. Sci. U.S.A. *78*: 41, 1981.

Croy, R. G., and Pardee, A. B. Proc. Natl. Acad. Sci. U.S.A. *80*: 4699, 1983.

Davis, F. M., Busch, R. K., Yeoman, L. C., and Busch, H. Cancer Res. *38*: 1906, 1978.

Davis, F. M., Gyorkey, F., Busch, R. K., and Busch, H. Proc. Natl. Acad. Sci. U.S.A. *76*: 892, 1979.

Deb, J. K., Chan, P. K., and Busch, H. Proc. Soc. Exptl. Biol. Med. *172*: 535, 1983.

Duesberg, P.H. Nature *304*: 219, 1983.

Durban, E., Mills, J. S., Roll, D., and Busch, H. Biochem. Biophys. Res. Comm. *3*: 897, 1983.

Durban, E., Roll, D., Beckner, G., and Busch, H. Cancer Res. *41*: 537, 1981.

Engvall, E. In *Methods in Enzymology*, Vol. 80, p. 419. New York: Academic Press, 1980.

Fishman, W. H., and Busch, H. (eds.). *Methods in Cancer Research*, Vol. 18, New York: Academic Press, 1979.

Goding, J. J. Immunol. Meth. *39*: 285, 1980.

Goodpasture, C., and Bloom, S. E. Chromosoma *53*: 37, 1975.

Green, N., Alexander, H., Olson, A., Alexander, S., Shinnick, T. M., Sutcliffe, J. G., and Lerner, R. A. Cell *28*: 477, 1982.

Hammond, G. L., Wieben, E., and Markert, C. L. Proc. Natl. Acad. Sci. U.S.A. *76*: 2455, 1979.

Hilgers, J., Nowinski, R. C., Geering, G., and Hardy, W. Cancer Res. *32*: 98, 1972.

Howell, M. W. Chromosoma *62*: 361, 1977.

Jacob, S. T., Stetler, D. A., and Rose, K. M. Isoenzymes Curr. Top Biol. Med. Res. *7*: 263, 1983.

Kang, Y.-J., Olson, M. O. J., and Busch, H. J. Biol. Chem., *249*: 5580, 1974.

Kearney, J. F., Radbruch, A., Leisegang, B., and Rajewsky, K. J. Immunol. *123*: 1548, 1979.

Kiefer, H. In *Immunological Methods*, p. 137, New York: Academic Press, 1979.

Kohler, G., and Milstein, C. Nature *256*: 495, 1975.

Krueger, J. G., Wang, E., and Goldberg, A. R. Virology *101*: 125, 1980.

Lane, D. P., and Hoeffler, W. K. Nature *288*: 167, 1980.

Lischwe, M. A., Richards, R. L., Busch, R. K., and Busch, H. Exp. Cell Res. *136*: 101, 1981.

Lischwe, M. A., Roberts, K. D., Yeoman, L. C., and Busch, H. J. Biol. Chem. *257*: 14600, 1982.

Lischwe, M. A., Smetana, K., Olson, M. O. J., and Busch, H. Life Sci. *25*: 701, 1979.

Mamrack, M. D., Olson, M. O. J., and Busch. H. Biochemistry *18*: 3381, 1979.

Maness, P. F., Perry, M. E., and Levy, B. T. J. Biol. Chem. *258*: 4055, 1983.

Marashi, F., Davis, F. M., Busch, R. K., Savage, H. E., and Busch, H. Cancer Res. *39*: 59, 1979.

Mills, J., Busch, H., and Durban, E. Biochem. Biophys. Res. Comm. *109*: 1222, 1982.

Nigg, E. A., Sefton, B. M., Hunter, T., Walter, G., and Singer, S. J. Proc. Natl. Acad. Sci. U.S.A. *79*: 5322, 1983.

Ochs, R., Lischwe, M., O'Leary, P., and Busch, H. Exptl. Cell Res. *146*: 139, 1983.

Olson, M. O. J., Hatchett, S., Allan, R., Hawkins, T. C., and Busch, H. Cancer Res. *38*: 3421, 1978.

Olson, M. O. J., Prestayko, A. W., Jones, C. E., and Busch, H. J. Mol. Biol. *90*: 161, 1974.

Orrick, L. R., Olson, M. O. J., and Busch, H. Proc. Natl. Acad. Sci. U.S.A. *70*: 1316, 1973.

Prestayko, A. W., Klomp, G. R., Schmoll, D. J., and Busch, H. Biochemistry *13*: 1945, 1974.

Puck, T. T., Erikson, R. L., Meek, W. D., and Nielson, S. E. J. Cell Phys. *107*: 399, 1981.

Reading, C. L. J. Immunol. Meth. *53*: 261, 1982.

Reiners, J. J., Jr., Davis, F. M., and Busch, H. Cancer Res. *40*: 1367, 1980.

Rose, K. M., and Jacob, S. T. In *Molecular Aspects of Cellular Regulation*, Vol. 3, p. 209, 1984.

Rose, K. M., Maguire, K. A., Wurpel, J. N. D., Stetler, D. A., and Marrquez, E. D. J. Biol. Chem. *258*: 12976, 1983.

Rose, K. M., Stetler, D. A., and Jacob, S. T. Phil. Trans. R. Soc. Lond. [Biol.] *302*: 135, 1983.

Rothblum, L. I., Mamrack, P. M., Kinkle, H. M., Olson, M. O. J., and Busch, H. Biochemistry *16*: 4716, 1977.

Satoh, K., and Busch, H. Cell Biol. Int. Rept. *5*: 857, 1981.

Satoh, K., and Busch, H. Cancer Res. *43*: 2143, 1983.

Smetana, K., Busch, R. K., Hermansky, F., and Busch, H. Life Sci. *25*: 227, 1979.

Smetana, K., Gyorkey, F., Chan, P. K., Tan, E., and Busch, H. Blut *46*: 133, 1983.

Smetana, K., Ochs, R., Lischwe, M. A., Gyorkey, F., Freireich, E., Chudomel, V., and Busch, H. Exper. Cell Res. *152*: 195, 1984.

Spector, P. L., Ochs, R., and Busch, H. Chromosoma *90*: 139, 1984.

Stahli, C., Staehelin, T., Miggiano, V., Schmidt, J., and Haring, P. J. Immunol. Methods *32*: 297, 1980.

Takahashi, K., Chan, P. K., Busch, R. K., and Busch, H. J. Cancer Res. Clin. Oncol. *105*: 67, 1983.

Tonbin, H., Staehelin, T., and Gordon, J. Proc. Natl. Acad. Sci. *76*: 4350, 1979.

Versteegen, R. J., Copeland, T. D., and Oroszlan, S. J. Biol. Chem. *257*: 3007, 1982.

Watt, V. M., and Schimmer, B. P. J. Biol. Chem. *256*: 11365, 1981.

Wojtkowiak, Z., Duhl, D. M., Briggs, R. C., Hnilica, L. S., Stein, J., and Stein, G. S. Cancer Res. *42*: 4546, 1982.

Yeoman, L. C., Jordan, J. J., Busch, R. K., Taylor, C. W., Savage, H. E., and Busch, H. Proc. Natl. Acad. Sci. U.S.A. *73*: 3258, 1976.

Zweig, S. E., Rubin, S., Yanera, M., and Busch, H. Proc. Amer. Assoc. Cancer Res. *25*: 248, 1984.

15

Future Perspectives in Laboratory and Clinical Research Searching for New Markers

Nasser Javadpour, M.D.

The quest for new tumor markers will continue in laboratory and clinical investigations. There is a need for new markers in certain cancers to help in screening, detecting, staging, and monitoring the tumor better and forecasting the prognosis more accurately. In searching for tumor markers, one may need to localize them to the cells of origin and prove with *in vitro* studies that a given marker is synthesized by its assumed cell of origin. Also, to avoid false-positive results, it is desirable to prove that the normal cell does not synthesize the marker. Furthermore, the marker should be easily obtainable from body fluid or other noncancerous secretions that will cause the increase of such a marker.

It would be ideal to have a marker that was specific for a cancer; nevertheless, even though a given marker may be synthesized by a number of different cancer cells, it can still be useful in a given clinical setting. For instance, alpha-fetoprotein (AFP) is produced by hepatoma and by certain testicular cancers; however, the distinction between these two types of cancer in a young man usually does not pose any problem.

The marker should have a relatively short half-life and be antigenic, and a radioimmunoassay would have to be developed for its measurement. The marker should undergo rigorous clinical trials with controlled patients, preferably on prospective protocols asking specific questions. The answers to these questions should have an important impact on the subsequent management of patients. The method of detection should be cost-effective and easily performed in a conventional laboratory.

There are certain leads that are important in attracting the attention of an investigator to a particular marker: examples of such leads include hCG, AFP, gamma-glutamyl transpeptidase, F9-antigen, and various placental proteins and placental enzymes. In other words, the fact that testicular cancer originates from somatic and placental parts of the embryo makes it an ideal cancer to carry the placental and embryonic markers.

A number of markers have already made important contributions to the diagnosis of certain cancers. Furthermore, with the advent of monoclonal antibodies, the detection of these markers is becoming more reliable. Finally, various techniques of conjugating radioisotopes or a particular cytotoxic agent provide the potential for radioimmuno-detection and the delivery of specific agents to cancer cells.[1]

REFERENCE

1. Javadpour, N. Immunocytochemical localization of various markers in cancer cells and tumors. Diagnostic and therapeutic strategy in urologic cancer. Urology 21: *1*: 1983.

Index